500 Single Best Answers in
MEDICINE

500 Single Best Answers in

MEDICINE

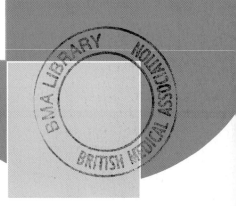

Sukhpreet Singh Dubb Final Year Medical Student, Imperial College School of Medicine, London

Kumaran Shanmugarajah FY1 AICSM, Chelsea and Westminster Hospital, London

Darren K Patten Academic Clinical Fellow and Core Surgical Trainee, London Deanery, Department of Biosurgery and Surgical Oncology, St Mary's Hospital, Imperial College Healthcare Trust, London, UK

Michael Schachter BSc MB FRCP Department of Clinical Pharmacology, National Heart and Lung Institute, Imperial College London

Cristina Koppel BSc MBBS (AICSM) Neurology Registrar, Fellow in Medical Education, Chelsea and Westminster Hospital, Imperial College School of Medicine, London

Editorial Advisor
Karim Meeran Professor of Endocrinology, Imperial College London

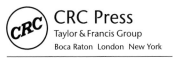 **CRC Press**
Taylor & Francis Group
Boca Raton London New York

CRC Press is an imprint of the
Taylor & Francis Group, an **informa** business

Dedication

To my parents and brother, who during the darkest nights have forever remained the brightest stars.
Sukhpreet S Dubb

To my parents – thank you for your support and encouragement
Kumaran Shanmugarajah

To my family and friends, your priceless support and inspiration made this possible.
Darren K Patten

To the memory of my parents
Michael Schachter

For Alexander and Andreas
Cristina Koppel

Contents

Foreword

A continuing pursuance of clinical excellence can be a long and difficult path to follow. Nevertheless, it is something we all aspire to in order to use our best knowledge in serving our patients. But first, one has to pass the qualifying examination!

This book helps to test your knowledge and aims to provide a question and answer format that closely follows the curriculum for Finals. It reflects the clinical scenarios that medical students will encounter when they first start as doctors and also face in Finals. It follows the single best answer format; a format of questioning that is more like real life. The authors have given comprehensive and informative answers, as well as reasons for the choice of the correct answer. It is very readable.

It is also refreshing to see that the authors have combined together to write this text from a wide range and level of knowledge – from a final year medical student to a professor. They will all remember what Finals entailed, from the sheer anxiety to the excitement of getting the knowledge of medicine into focus. I am sure this book will be useful and enjoyable. Good luck for Finals!

Professor Parveen J Kumar CBE, BSc, MD, FRCP, FRCPE
Professor of Medicine & Education
Barts & the London School of Medicine and Dentistry
Queen Mary, University of London

Preface

Medical schools have undergone a number of changes in deciding upon the ideal format for testing clinical knowledge in examinations. Multiple choice questions (MCQs) in the past were the most common modality by which medical students were examined. Although able to test a broad range of topics and being cost efficient for marking purposes, MCQs have largely been abandoned in favour of extending matching questions (EMQs) and more recently the single best answer (SBA) question format.

EMQs and SBAs overcome the ambiguity that occurs in MCQ exams, as well as being able to provide more clinical question stems reflecting real-life situations. The SBA format is highly favoured in examinations at both the undergraduate and postgraduate level since students must not only demonstrate their clinical knowledge and understanding but also make sound judgements which are more congruent with clinical practice.

500 Single Best Answers in Medicine provides a significant number of high quality SBA questions that comprehensively examines the typical undergraduate curriculum. Each question not only provides an opportunity to apply clinical knowledge and correctly identify the single best answer to a question, but also to learn why the other answers are wrong, greatly increasing the clinical acumen and learning opportunity of the reader. This book aims to provide medical students with a useful source for exam revision as well as supplementing the reader's knowledge such that they feel fully prepared for the undergraduate medical written examinations.

Sukhpreet Singh Dubb and Professor Karim Meeran

Acknowledgements

Professor Karim Meeran
Professor of Endocrinology
Department of Medicine
Imperial College London

Dr Michael Schachter
Senior Lecturer in Clinical Pharmacology
St. Mary's Hospital London
Imperial College NHS Healthcare Trust

Dr Maisse Farhan
Accident and Emergency Consultant
St. Mary's Hospital London
Imperial College NHS Healthcare Trust

Dr Frederick Tam
Consultant Nephrologist
Hammersmith Hospital
Imperial College NHS Healthcare Trust

Dr Richard Russell
Consultant Chest Physician
Heatherwood and Wexham Park Hospitals NHS Foundation Trust

Dr Jane Currie
Fellow in Medical Education
Chelsea and Westminster Hospital
Imperial College London

We would also like to thank Dr Joanna Koster, Stephen Clausard and the rest of the
Hodder Arnold team whose support and advice have made this project possible.

List of Abbreviations Used

5 ASA	5-aminosalicylic acid	CML	chronic myeloid leukaemia
AAA	abdominal aortic aneurysm	CMV	cytomegalovirus
ABG	arterial blood gas	CN	cranial nerve
ABPA	allergic bronchopulmonary aspergillosis	CNS	central nervous system
		COPD	chronic obstructive pulmonary disease
ACEI	angiotensin converting enzyme inhibitor	CRP	C-reactive protein
ACTH	adrenocorticotropic hormone	CSF	cerebrospinal fluid
		CT	computed tomography
ADH	anti-diuretic hormone	CT PA	CT pulmonary angiogram
AFP	alpha fetoprotein	DCM	dilated cardiomyopathy
AIDS	autoimmune deficiency syndrome	DIC	disseminated intravascular coagulation
AIH	autoimmune hepatitis	DIP	distal interphalangeal joint
ALL	acute lymphoblastic leukaemia	DMARD	disease-modifying antirheumatic drug
AMA	anti-mitochondrial antibody	DVT	deep vein thrombosis
AML	acute myeloid leukaemia	EBV	Epstein–Barr virus
ANA	anti-nuclear antibodies	ECG	electrocardiogram
ANCA	anti-neutrophil cytoplasmic antibodies	ERCP	endoscopic retrograde cholangiopancreatography
ARDS	acute respiratory distress syndrome	ESR	erythrocyte sedimentation rate
ASO	anti-streptolysin O	FBC	full blood count
BCC	basal cell carcinoma	FEV_1	forced expiratory volume in one second
BEP	cisplatin		
Beta-hCG	beta-human chorionic gonadotrophin	FVC	forced vital capacity
		GABA	gamma-aminobutyric acid
BMI	body mass index	GBM	glomerular basement membrane
BNF	british National Formulary		
BPPV	benign paroxysmal positional vertigo	GCS	glasgow Coma Scale
		GH	growth hormone
CCP	citrullinated peptide antibody	GMP	guanosine monophosphate
		GORD	gastro-oesophageal reflux disease
CEA	carcinoembryonic antigen		
CFTR	cystic fibrosis transmembrane conductance regulator	GTN	glyceryl trinitrate
		HbA1c	glycated haemoglobin
		HCC	hepatocellular carcinoma
CLO	campylobacter-like organism	HIV	human immunodeficiency virus

HPV	human papilloma virus
HRCT	high-resolution CT chest
HSV	herpes simplex virus
HUS	haemolytic uraemic syndrome
IBD	inflammatory bowel disease
ICP	intracranial pressure
ICS	inhaled corticosteroid
INO	intranuclear opthalmoplegia
INR	international normalized ratio
ITP	immune thrombocytopenic purpura
IV	intravenous
IVU	intravenous urography
JVP	jugular venous pressure
KUB	kidneys, ureter and bladder
LABA	long-acting beta agonist
LADA	latent autoimmune diabetes of adults
LAMA	long-acting muscarinic antagonist
LFT	liver function tests
LMN	lower motor neurone
LP	lumbar puncture
LRTI	lower respiratory tract infections
MC&S	microscopy, culture and sensitivity
MCH	mean cell haemoglobin
MCP	metacarpophalangeal joint
MCV	mean cell volume
MG	myasthenia gravis
MI	myocardial infarction
MLF	medial longitudinal fasciculus
MND	motor neurone disease
MR	magnetic resonance
MRCP	magnetic resonance cholangiopancreatography
MRI	magnetic resonance imaging
MSH	melanocyte stimulating hormone
NSAID	non-steroidal anti-inflammatory drug
NSCLC	non-small cell lung carcinomas
NSTEM	non-ST elevation myocardial infarction
OCP	oral contraceptive pill
PAN	polyarteritis nodosa
PBC	primary biliary cirrhosis
PCI	percutaneous coronary intervention
PD	Parkinson's disease
PE	pulmonary embolism
PEF	peak expiratory flow
PEFR	peak expiratory flow rate
PET	positron emission tomography
PFO	patent foramen ovale
PIP	proximal interphalangeal joint
POMC	pro-opiomelanocortin
PPI	proton pump inhibitor
PSA	prostate-specific antigen
PSC	primary sclerosing cholangitis
PTH	parathyroid hormone
PV	per vaginum
RA	rheumatoid arthritis
RAPD	relative afferent pupillary defect
RBC	red blood cell
RF	rheumatoid factor
SAH	subarachnoid haemorrhage
SAMA	short-acting muscarinic antagonist
SBP	spontaneous bacterial peritonitis
SCC	squamous cell carcinoma

SIADH	syndrome of inappropriate anti-diuretic hormone	TOE	transoesophageal echocardiography
SLA	soluble liver antigen	TSH	thyroid stimulating hormone
SLE	systemic lupus erythematosus	TTP	thrombotic thrombocytopenic purpura
SMA	smooth muscle antibody		
SSRI	selective serotonin reuptake inhibitor	U&E	urea and electrolytes
STEMI	ST elevation myocardial infarction	UC	ulcerative colitis
		UMN	upper motor neurone
T2DM	type 2 diabetes mellitus	URTI	upper respiratory tract
T3	tri-iodothyronine level	US	ultrasound scan
T4	tetraiodothyronine	UTI	urinary tract infection
TB	tuberculosis	V/Q scan	ventilation perfusion scan
TFT	thyroid function test		
TIBC	total iron-binding capacity	VZV	varicella zoster virus
TIPPS	transjugular intrahepatic portosystemic shunting	WBC	white blood cell
		WCC	white cell count
TNF	tumour necrosis factor	WHO	World Health Organization

Common Reference Intervals

Investigation/Test	Range	Units
Alanine transaminase (ALT)	0–31	IU/L
Albumin	33–47	g/L
Alkaline phosphatase (ALP)	30–130	IU/L
Amylase	70–400	U/L
APTT	22.0–29.0	secs
Aspartate transaminase (AST)	0–31	IU/L
Bicarbonate	22–29	mmol/L
Bilirubin	0–17	umol/L
Calcium	2.15–2.65	mmol/L
Chloride	95–108	mmol/L
Cholesterol	<5	mmol/L
Cholesterol HDL ratio	0–5.00	
C-reactive protein	0–10	mg/L
Creatinine	60–110	umol/L
Eosinophils	0.0–0.4	×10
Ferritin	10–120	ug/L
Free T4	9.0–26.0	pmol/L
Gamma GT	2.0–30	IU/L
Glucose fasting	3.0–6.0	mmol/L
Glucose random	3.0–8.0	mmol/L
Haemoglobin A1C	4.3–6.1	%
HDL cholesterol	1.00–2.20	mmol/L
Hgb	11.4–15.0	g/dl
Insulin	3.0–17.0	mU/L
Iron	7.0–27	umol/L
LDL cholesterol	2.0–5.0	mmol/L
Lymphocytes	1.0–3.5	×10
MCH	26.7–32.9	pg
MCV	83.0–101.0	fl
Monocytes	0.3–1.0	×10
MPV	8.0–12.0	fl
Neutrophils	2.0–7.5	×10
Osmolality serum	275–295	mOsm/kg
Osmolality urine	50–1200	mmol/kg
$PaCO_2$	4.7–6	Kpa
$PaCO_2$	35–45	mmHg
PaO_2	>10.6	Kpa
PaO_2	75–100	mmHg
pH	7.35–7.45	
Phosphate	0.80–1.40	mmol/L
Platelets	120–400	10^9/L

Investigation/Test	Range	Units
Potassium	3.8–5.5	mmol/L
Prolactin female	0–750	mU/L
Prolactin male	150–500	mU/L
Prothrombin time	9.0–12.0	secs
RBC	3.74–4.99	×10
Serum vitamin B_{12}	160–800	ng/L
Sodium	135–145	mmol/L
Total iron binding capacity	49–78	umol/L
Total protein	64–83	g/L
Transferrin Sat	20–45	%
Triglycerides	0.00–1.80	mmol/L
TSH	0.3–4.2	mU/L
Urea	2.5–7.0	mmol/L
WBC	4.0–11.0	10^9/L

SECTION 1: CARDIOVASCULAR

Questions

QUESTIONS

1. Myocardial infarction

A 65-year-old man presents with central crushing chest pain for the first time. He is transferred immediately to the closest cardiac unit to undergo a primary percutaneous coronary intervention. There is thrombosis of the left circumflex artery only. Angioplasty is carried out and a drug-eluding stent is inserted. What are the most likely changes to have occurred on ECG during admission?

    A. ST depression in leads V1–4
    B. ST elevation in leads V1–6
    C. ST depression in leads II, III and AVF
    D. ST elevation in leads V5–6
    E. ST elevation in leads II, III and AVF

2. Heart failure (1)

A 78-year-old woman is admitted with heart failure. The underlying cause is determined to be aortic stenosis. Which sign is most likely to be present?

    A. Pleural effusion on chest x-ray
    B. Raised jugular venous pressure (JVP)
    C. Bilateral pedal oedema
    D. Bibasal crepitations
    E. Atrial fibrillation

3. Valve lesion signs

A patient is admitted with pneumonia. A murmur is heard on examination. What finding points to mitral regurgitation?

    A. Murmur louder on inspiration
    B. Murmur louder with patient in left lateral position
    C. Murmur louder over the right 2nd intercostal space midclavicular line
    D. Corrigan's sign
    E. Narrow pulse pressure

4. CHAD2 score

A 79-year-old woman is admitted to the coronary care unit (CCU) with unstable angina. She is started on appropriate medication to reduce her cardiac risk. She is hypertensive, fasting glucose is normal and cholesterol is 5.2. She is found to be in atrial fibrillation. What is the most appropriate treatment?

    A. Aspirin and clopidogrel
    B. Digoxin
    C. Cardioversion
    D. Aspirin alone
    E. Warfarin

5. Chest pain (1)

A 55-year-old man has just arrived in accident and emergency complaining of 20 minutes of central crushing chest pain. Which feature is most indicative of myocardial infarction at this moment in time?

    A. Inverted T waves
    B. ST depression
    C. ST elevation
    D. Q waves
    E. Raised troponin

6. Shortness of breath (1)

A 66-year-old woman presents to accident and emergency with a 2-day history of shortness of breath. The patient notes becoming progressively short of breath as well as a sharp pain in the right side of the chest which is most painful when taking a deep breath. The patient also complains of mild pain in the right leg, though there is nothing significant on full cardiovascular and respiratory examination. Heart rate is 96 and respiratory rate is 12. The patient denies any weight loss or long haul flights but mentions undergoing a nasal polypectomy 3 weeks ago. The most likely diagnosis is:

    A. Muscular strain
    B. Heart failure
    C. Pneumothorax
    D. Angina
    E. Pulmonary embolism

7. Murmurs (1)

A 59-year-old man presents for a well person check. A cardiovascular, respiratory, gastrointestinal and neurological examination is performed. No significant findings are found, except during auscultation a mid systolic click followed by a late systolic murmur is heard at the apex. The patient denies any symptoms. The most likely diagnosis is:

    A.   Barlow syndrome
    B.   Austin Flint murmur
    C.   Patent ductus arteriosus
    D.   Graham Steell murmur
    E.   Carey Coombs murmur

8. Chest pain (2)

A 60-year-old man presents to accident and emergency with a 3-day history of increasingly severe chest pain. The patient describes the pain as a sharp, tearing pain starting in the centre of his chest and radiating straight through to his back between his shoulder blades. The patient looks in pain but there is no pallor, heart rate is 95, respiratory rate is 20, temperature 37°C and blood pressure is 155/95 mmHg. The most likely diagnosis is:

    A.   Myocardial infarction
    B.   Myocardial ischaemia
    C.   Aortic dissection
    D.   Pulmonary embolism
    E.   Pneumonia

9. Chest pain management

A 49-year-old man is rushed to accident and emergency complaining of a 20-minute history of severe, crushing chest pain. After giving the patient glyceryl trinitrate (GTN) spray, he is able to tell you he suffers from hypertension and type 2 diabetes and is allergic to aspirin. The most appropriate management is:

    A.   Aspirin
    B.   Morphine
    C.   Heparin
    D.   Clopidogrel
    E.   Warfarin

10. Ventricular tachyarrhythmia

While on call you are called by a nurse to a patient on the ward complaining of light headedness and palpitations. When you arrive the patient is not conscious but has a patent airway and is breathing with oxygen saturation at 97 per cent. You try to palpate a pulse but are unable to find the radial or carotid. The registrar arrives and after hearing your report of the patient decides to shock the patient who recovers. What is the patient most likely to have been suffering?

    A. Torsades de Pointes
    B. Ventricular fibrillation
    C. Sustained ventricular tachycardia
    D. Non-sustained ventricular tachycardia
    E. Normal heart ventricular tachycardia

11. Jugular venous pressure

A 67-year-old man presents to accident and emergency with a 3-day history of shortness of breath. On examination you palpate the radial pulse and notice that the patient has an irregular heart beat with an overall rate of 140 bpm. You request an electrocardiogram (ECG) which reveals that the patient is in atrial fibrillation. Which of the following would you expect to see when assessing the JVP?

    A. Raised JVP with normal waveform
    B. Large 'v waves'
    C. Cannon 'a waves'
    D. Absent 'a waves'
    E. Large 'a waves'

12. Heart failure (2)

A 78-year-old woman is admitted to your ward following a 3-day history of shortness of breath and a productive cough of white frothy sputum. On auscultation of the lungs, you hear bilateral basal coarse inspiratory crackles. You suspect that the patient is in congestive cardiac failure. You request a chest x-ray. Which of the following signs is not typically seen on chest x-ray in patients with congestive cardiac failure?

    A. Lower lobe diversion
    B. Cardiomegaly
    C. Pleural effusions
    D. Alveolar oedema
    E. Kerley B lines

13. First degree heart block

A 56-year-old man presents to your clinic with symptoms of exertional chest tightness which is relieved by rest. You request an ECG which reveals that the patient has first degree heart block. Which of the following ECG abnormalities is typically seen in first degree heart block?

    A. PR interval >120 ms
    B. PR interval >300 ms
    C. PR interval <200 ms
    D. PR interval >200 ms
    E. PR interval <120 ms

14. Mitral stenosis

You see a 57-year-old woman who presents with worsening shortness of breath coupled with decreased exercise tolerance. She had rheumatic fever in her adolescence and suffers from essential hypertension. On examination she has signs which point to a diagnosis of mitral stenosis. Which of the following is not a clinical sign associated with mitral stenosis?

    A. Malar flush
    B. Atrial fibrillation
    C. Pan-systolic murmur which radiates to axilla
    D. Tapping, undisplaced apex beat
    E. Right ventricular heave

15. Hypertension (1)

A 48-year-old woman has been diagnosed with essential hypertension and was commenced on treatment three months ago. She presents to you with a dry cough which has not been getting better despite taking cough linctus and antibiotics. You assess the patient's medication history. Which of the following antihypertensive medications is responsible for the patient's symptoms?

    A. Amlodipine
    B. Lisinopril
    C. Bendroflumethiazide
    D. Frusemide
    E. Atenolol

16. Palpitations

A 62-year-old male presents with palpitations, which are shown on ECG to be atrial fibrillation with a ventricular rate of approximately 130/minute. He has mild central chest discomfort but is not acutely distressed. He first noticed these about 3 hours before coming to hospital. As far as is known this is his first episode of this kind. Which of the following would you prefer as first-line therapy?

    A.   Anticoagulate with heparin and start digoxin at standard daily dose
    B.   Attempt DC cardioversion
    C.   Administer bisoprolol and verapamil, and give warfarin
    D.   Attempt cardioversion with IV flecainide
    E.   Wait to see if there is spontaneous reversion to sinus rhythm

17. Murmurs (2)

A 76-year-old male is brought to accident and emergency after collapsing at home. He has recovered within minutes and is fully alert and orientated. He says this is the first such episode that he has experienced, but describes some increasing shortness of breath in the previous six months and brief periods of central chest pain, often at the same time. On examination, blood pressure is 115/88 mmHg and there are a few rales at both bases. On ECG there are borderline criteria for left ventricular hypertrophy. Which of the following might you expect to find on auscultation?

    A.   Mid-diastolic murmur best heard at the apex
    B.   Crescendo systolic murmur best heard at the right sternal edge
    C.   Diastolic murmur best heard at the left sternal edge
    D.   Pan-systolic murmur best heard at the apex
    E.   Pan-systolic murmur best heard at the left sternal edge

18. Postmyocardial infarction (1)

A 63-year-old male was admitted to accident and emergency 2 days after discharge following an apparently uncomplicated MI. He complained of rapidly worsening shortness of breath over the previous 48 hours but no further chest pain. He was tachypnoeic and had a regular pulse of 110/minute, which proved to be sinus tachycardia. The jugular venous pressure was raised and a pan-systolic murmur was noted, maximal at the left sternal edge. Which of the following is the most likely diagnosis?

    A.   Mitral incompetence
    B.   Ventricular septal defect
    C.   Aortic stenosis
    D.   Dressler's syndrome
    E.   Further myocardial infarction

19. Hypertension (2)

A 57-year-old male is admitted complaining of headaches and blurring of vision. His blood pressure is found to be 240/150 mmHg and he has bilateral papilloedema, but is fully orientated and coherent. He had been known to be hypertensive for about five years and his blood pressure control had been good on three drugs. However, he had decided to stop all medication two months before this event. Which of the following would be your preferred parenteral medication at this point?

    A. Glyceryl trinitrate
    B. Hydralazine
    C. Labetalol
    D. Sodium nitroprusside
    E. Phentolamine

20. Mid-systolic murmur

A 16-year-old male is referred for assessment of hypertension. On average, his blood pressure is 165/85 mmHg, with radiofemoral delay. There is a mid-systolic murmur maximal at the aortic area, and radiating to the back. Clinical findings and the ECG are compatible with left ventricular hypertrophy. What is the most likely underlying pathology?

    A. Hypertrophic obstructive cardiomyopathy
    B. Congenital aortic stenosis
    C. Coarctation of the aorta
    D. Patent ductus ateriosus
    E. Atrial septal defect

21. Ventral septal defect

A 16-year-old boy is diagnosed with a small ventricular septal defect, having been screened by echocardiography because of a family history of hypertrophic obstructive cardiomyopathy. He is entirely asymptomatic, plays several sports regularly and has no growth retardation. The echocardiogram also confirms a small left to right shunt, with pulmonary to systemic flow ratio only just above one. Which of the following is the most likely to be a significant complication of his condition?

    A. Pulmonary hypertension
    B. Heart failure
    C. Dysrhythmias
    D. Endocarditis
    E. Shunt reversal (right to left flow)

22. Microscopic haematuria

A 52 year-old woman has been treated for several years with amlodipine and lisinopril for what has been presumed to be primary hypertension. She is seen by her GP having complained of persistent left loin pain. Her BP is 150/95 mmHg. She is tender in the left loin and both kidneys appear to be enlarged. On urine dipstick testing, there is microscopic haematuria. Which of the following is likely to be the most appropriate investigation at this point?

A. Urinary tract ultrasound
B. Abdominal and pelvic computed tomography (CT) scan
C. Microscopy of the urine (microbial and cytological)
D. Renal biopsy
E. Intravenous urogram

23. Retrosternal chest pain

A 61-year-old man presents with a 2-hour history of moderately severe retrosternal chest pain, which does not radiate and is not affected by respiration or posture. He complains of general malaise and nausea, but has not vomited. His ECG shows ST segment depression and T wave inversion in the inferior leads. Troponin levels are not elevated. He has already been given oxygen, aspirin and intravenous GTN; he is an occasional user of sublingual GTN and takes regular bisoprolol for stable angina. What would be the most appropriate next step in his management?

A. IV low-molecular weight heparin
B. Thrombolysis with alteplase
C. IV nicardapine
D. Angiography with stenting
E. Oral clopidogrel

24. Pulmonary embolism management

A 41-year-old woman is referred for assessment after suffering a second pulmonary embolus within a year. She has not been travelling recently, has not had any surgery, does not smoke and does not take the oral contraceptive pill. She is not currently on any medication as the diagnosis is retrospective and she is now asymptomatic. What should be the next step in her management?

A. Initiation of warfarin therapy
B. ECG
C. Thrombophilia screen
D. Insertion of inferior vena cava filter
E. Duplex scan of lower limb veins and pelvic utrasound

25. Mid-diastolic murmur

A 32-year-old woman attends her GP for a routine medical examination and is noted to have a mid-diastolic murmur with an opening snap. Her blood pressure is 118/71 mmHg and the pulse is regular at 66 beats per minute. She is entirely asymptomatic and chest x-ray and ECG are normal. What would be the most appropriate investigation at this point?

A. Echocardiography
B. Anti-streptolysin O titre
C. Cardiac catheterization
D. Thallium radionuclide scanning
E. Colour Doppler scanning

26. Severe chest pain

A 46-year-old man develops sudden severe central chest pain after lifting heavy cases while moving house. The pain radiates to the back and both shoulders but not to either arm. His BP is 155/90 mmHg, pulse rate is 92 beats per minute and the ECG is normal. He is distressed and sweaty, but not nauseated. What would you consider the most likely diagnosis?

A. Pneumothorax
B. MI
C. Pulmonary embolism
D. Aortic dissection
E. Musculoskeletal pain

27. Decrescendo diastolic murmur

A 49-year-old woman presents with increasing shortness of breath on exertion developing over the past three months. She has no chest pain or cough, and has noticed no ankle swelling. On examination, blood pressure is 158/61 mmHg, pulse is regular at 88 beats per minute and there are crackles at both lung bases. There is a decrescendo diastolic murmur at the left sternal edge. What is the most likely diagnosis?

A. Aortic regurgitation
B. Aortic stenosis
C. Mitral regurgitation
D. Mitral stenosis
E. Tricuspid regurgitation

28. Supraventricular tachycardia

A 21-year-old man is on his way home from a party when he experiences the sudden onset of rapid palpitations. He feels uncomfortable but not short of breath and has no chest pain. He goes to the nearest accident and emergency department, where he is found to have a supraventricular tachycardia (SVT) at a rate of 170/minute. Carotid sinus massage produced transient reversion to sinus rhythm, after which the tachycardia resumed. What would be the next step in your management?

    A. Repeat carotid sinus massage
    B. IV verapamil
    C. IV propranolol
    D. IV adenosine
    E. Synchronized DC cardioversion

29. Chest pain (3)

A 44-year-old woman attends her local accident and emergency department with a history of at least six months of frequent central chest pain in the early morning or during the night. She had no chest pain on exertion. This had been a particularly severe attack, lasting over 2 hours. Her pulse rate is 84/minute in sinus rhythm, and blood pressure is 134/86 mmHg. The ECG shows anterior ST segment elevation, but troponin levels do not rise. Subsequent coronary angiography is normal. What is the most likely diagnosis?

    A. MI
    B. Stable angina
    C. Unstable angina
    D. Anxiety
    E. Variant angina

30. Shortness of breath (2)

A previously fit 19-year-old man presents with unusual shortness of breath on exertion. At times, this is also associated with central chest pain. On examination there is a loud mid-systolic murmur at the left sternal edge. Heart rate and blood pressure are normal and there is no oedema. The ECG shows left axis deviation and the voltage criteria for left ventricular hypertrophy and the echocardiogram reveals a significant thickened interventricular septum, with delayed ventricular filling during diastole. There is a family history of sudden death below the age of 50. Which of the following would be your initial therapy?

    A. Digoxin
    B. Long-acting nitrates
    C. Beta-blockers
    D. Rate-limiting calcium channel blockers
    E. Partial excision of the septum

31. Hypertension (3)

A 44-year-old woman presents with episodes of headaches, associated with anxiety, sweating and a slow pulse rate. At the time of her initial consultation, her blood pressure was 150/95 mmHg seated, but 24 hour ambulatory monitoring shows a peak of 215/130 mmHg, associated with the symptoms described above. Which of the following would be your initial diagnostic procedure?

A. Magnetic resonance imaging (MRI) scans of the abdomen and pelvis
B. Measurement of random plasma catecholamines
C. Measurement of urinary metanephrines over several 24 hour periods
D. Glucose tolerance test
E. Pharmacological provocation using clonidine

32. Chest pain (4)

A 56-year-old man presents to the accident and emergency department with a 2-hour history of central chest pain radiating to the left arm. He is anxious, nauseated and sweaty. His pulse rate is 120/minute in sinus rhythm and the ECG reveals ST elevation in leads II, III and aVF. The troponin level is significantly raised. This is certainly acute MI. Which is the most likely coronary vessel to be occluded?

A. Circumflex artery
B. Left anterior descending artery
C. Right coronary artery
D. Left main coronary artery
E. Posterior descending artery

33. Constrictive pericarditis

A 45-year-old woman complains of increasing shortness of breath on exertion, as well as orthopnoea, for the previous 3–4 months. She had apparently recovered from pericarditis about a year earlier. On ECG there is low voltage, especially in the limb leads, and the chest x-ray shows pericardial calcification. The presumptive diagnosis is constrictive pericarditis. Which of the following physical signs would be consistent with this?

A. Increased jugular distention on inspiration
B. Third heart sound
C. Fourth heart sound
D. Rales at both lung bases
E. Loud first and second heart sounds

34. Visual disturbance

A 71-year-old man is being treated for congestive heart failure with a combination of drugs. He complains of nausea and anorexia, and has been puzzled by observing yellow rings around lights. His pulse rate is 53/minute and irregular and blood pressure is 128/61 mmHg. Which of the following medications is likely to be responsible for these symptoms?

    A. Lisinopril
    B. Spironolactone
    C. Digoxin
    D. Furosemide
    E. Bisoprolol

35. Weight loss

A 29-year-old woman goes to see her GP complaining of fatigue and palpitations. She says she has also lost weight, though without dieting. On examination, her pulse rate is approximately 120/min and irregularly irregular. Her blood pressure is 142/89 mmHg and her body mass index is 19. There are no added cardiac sounds. The ECG confirms the diagnosis of atrial fibrillation. What would you suggest as the most useful next investigation.

    A. Thyroid function tests (TSH, free T4)
    B. ECG
    C. Chest x-ray
    D. Full blood count
    E. Fasting blood sugar

36. Postmyocardial infarction (2)

A 58-year-old man has made an excellent functional recovery after an anterior MI. He is entirely asymptomatic and there is no abnormality on physical examination. His blood pressure is 134/78 mmHg and he is undertaking a cardiac rehabilitation programme. Which of the following would you not recommend as part of his secondary prevention planning?

    A. Aspirin
    B. Lisinopril
    C. Simvastatin
    D. Bisoprolol
    E. Omega-3 fatty acids

37. Mitral valve prolapse complication

A 25-year-old woman with known mitral valve prolapse develops a low grade fever, malaise and night sweats within a couple of weeks of a major dental procedure. Examination reveals a pulse rate of 110/minute, which is regular, tender vasculitic lesions on the finger pulps and microscopic haematuria. Which investigation is most likely to provide a definitive diagnosis?

A. Full blood count
B. ECG
C. Autoantibody screen
D. Blood culture
E. Coronary angiography

38. Mitral valve prolapse

An asymptomatic 31-year-old woman has been referred for cardiological assessment. After her ECG she was told that she had mitral valve prolapse and would like further information on this condition. Which of the following statements is correct?

A. Beta-blocker therapy is indicated
B. Angiotensin-converting enzyme (ACE) inhibitor therapy is indicated
C. One or both leaflets of the mitral valve are pushed back into the left atrium during systole
D. Significant mitral regurgitation will eventually develop
E. Exercise should be restricted

39. Paroxysmal atrial fibrillation

A 69-year-old woman complains of intermittent palpitations, lasting several hours, which then stop spontaneously. She also suffers from asthma. Holter monitoring confirms paroxysmal atrial fibrillation. Which of the following statements is correct regarding the management of this patient?

A. Digoxin effectively prevents recurrence of the arrhythmia
B. Anticoagulation is not necessary
C. Sotalol may be effective
D. Amiodarone should be avoided
E. Flecainide orally may be an effective as-needed treatment to abort an attack

40. Hypertension management

A 57-year-old man is reviewed in a hypertension clinic, where it is found that his blood pressure is 165/105 mmHg despite standard doses of amlodipine, perindopril, doxazosin and bendroflumethiazide. Electrolytes and physical examination have been, and remain, normal. Which of the following would be your next stage in his management?

    A. Arrange for his medication to be given under direct observation
    B. Add spironolactone to his medication
    C. Arrange urinary catecholamine assays
    D. Request an adrenal CT scan
    E. Add verapamil to his medication

ANSWERS

Myocardial infarction

1 D   Time equates to muscle. Judging from the urgency, this male presented with an ST elevation MI (STEMI) which is an indication for urgent primary percutaneous coronary intervention (PCI). Compare this to a non-ST elevation MI (NSTEMI) which indicates ischaemia rather than infarction and PCI should be carried out within 48 hours (answers A and C). The angiogram shows that the left circumflex artery is occluded, resulting in a lateral infarct. This area is represented by leads V5–6 (**D**). V1–4 represents the territory of the left anterior descending artery. If the entire left mainstem had been occluded, changes would have shown throughout leads V1–6 (**B**).

Leads II, III and aVF (C and E) point to an inferior infarct and involvement of the right anterior descending artery (see Figure 1.1 below).

(a)

(b)

(c)

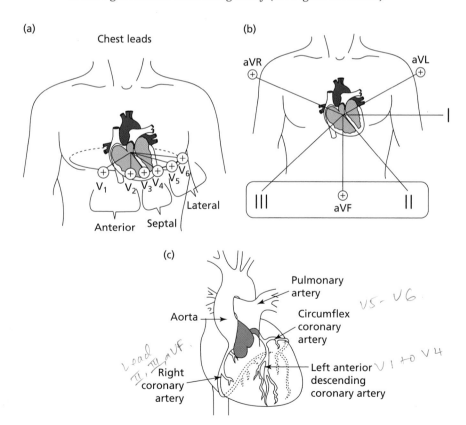

Fig. 1.1 (a,b) Chest leads. (c) Anatomy of coronary arteries (from Koppel and Naparus (2008) *Thinking Medicine: Structure your knowledge for success in medical exams*, Cavaye, with permission).

The location of the changes tells you which part of the heart is affected as shown in the diagrams. These depict:

1   the position of the chest leads and the parts of the heart they investigate;

2   the position of the limb leads and the parts of the heart they investigate;

3   the anatomy of the coronary arteries.

Putting all of these together will allow you to pinpoint the location of the lesion.

Leads	Area	Supplied by
V1–2	Anterior	LCA: Diagonal branch of LAD
V3–4	Septal	LCA: Septal branch of LAD
V5–6	Lateral	LCA: Left circumflex artery
V1–6	Anterolateral	LCA: Left main stem disease
II, III, aVF	Inferior	RCA: Posterior descending branch

Heart failure

2 D   Aortic stenosis will first result in left ventricular failure as a result of increased ventricular pressure as the ventricle tries to pump blood across a narrowed valve. Initially the pressure load will cause a backlog of blood into the lungs, resulting in pulmonary oedema – the first sign of which will be bibasal crepitations (D) before enough fluid accumulates as pleural effusions visible on chest x-ray (A). Earlier signs of pulmonary oedema include upper lobe blood diversion and Kerley B lines as fluid infiltrates the interstitium. If the backlog continues back into the right heart, eventually signs of right-sided heart failure will be evident including raised JVP (B) and bilateral pedal oedema (C). Atrial fibrillation (E) may coexist with aortic stenosis, however it is more commonly associated as a result of mitral stenosis as the enlarged atrium disrupts the normal electrical pathways.

Valve lesion signs

3 B   A murmur heard loudest on inspiration (A) points to a right-sided valve lesion. The right intercostal space midclavicular line (C) is the anatomical landmark for the aortic valve. The mitral area is over the apex. A murmur louder with the patient in the left lateral position (B) (as opposed to leaning forward) is associated with mitral lesions. If heard, you should determine whether the murmur radiates to the axilla. Corrigan's sign (D) (visibly exaggerated pulsating carotids) is one of the many signs of a hyperdynamic circulation associated with aortic regurgitation (including de Mussets, Traubes, Quinkes, Duroziez and a whole host of others). A narrow pulse pressure (E) is a sign of aortic stenosis.

CHAD2 score

4 E Ideally this patient should be started on antihypertensives, a beta blocker and a statin. There is no indication for hypoglycaemics at present. There is no indication that this is acute atrial fibrillation and she does not seem to be compromised in a female of this age, cardioversion (C) is unlikely to be successful. She should be rate-controlled but the beta blockade is more appropriate in light of her ischaemic heart disease. Whether to start anticoagulation (A) is a decision that has to be tailor-made for each individual patient. The CHAD2 score is a quick and dirty but very useful way of predicting risk of subsequent stroke as a result of atrial fibrillation and helps guide the prescription of prophylactic antiplatelets or anticoagulants. Other factors, such as ease of taking and monitoring warfarin, risk of falls and important risk factors, such as vascular disease, should be taken into account.

C	Congestive heart failure	1
H	Hypertension: blood pressure consistently above 140/90 mmHg (or treated hypertension on medication)	1
A	Age ≥75 years	1
D	Diabetes mellitus	1
S2	Previous stroke or TIA	2

A score of 0 is low risk (2 per cent of patients/year will have a stroke without treatment), aspirin is considered adequate. A score of 1 is moderate risk (3 per cent annual stroke risk) and either warfarin or aspirin (D) is indicated according to the individual. A score of two or above (>4 per cent annual stroke risk) is classified as high risk and warfarin (E) should be started unless there are clear contraindications. A patient with a full-house of risk factors (scores 6) has an almost 20 per cent chance of stroke/year.

Chest pain

5 C Acute coronary syndrome is a spectrum of cardiac ischaemia-infarction determined by the presence of two out of three factors: chest pain, ECG changes and cardiac enzyme rise. Depending on these results, patients will fall into one of the following categories: unstable angina, NSTEMI or STEMI. Inverted T waves (A) and ST depression (B) are signs of ischaemia. ST elevation, Q waves and raised troponin are indicative of infarction. Initially, 'ST elevation' or 'non ST elevation' ECG changes are used to stratify each patient's risk as the results of blood tests for troponin levels (E) (which should be carried out 12 hours after the pain started) are not known and Q waves have not had time to develop. ST elevation (C) is a very good predictor of imminent infarction (positive troponin). However, if this patient is treated quickly enough with thrombolysis or primary PCI, infarction can be avoided. A patient with STEMI who goes on to have negative troponin is termed to have had an 'aborted MI'. Q waves (D) (indicating full-thickness MI) take time to develop, so 'Q wave' or 'non Q wave' MI is a diagnosis given on discharge.

		ECG: ST elevation	
		+	−
Troponin	+	STEMI	NSTEMI
	−	Aborted MI	Unstable angina

Shortness of breath

6 E   This patient is most likely suffering from a pulmonary embolism (E), defined as an occlusion of the pulmonary vasculature by a thrombus causing an area of lung that is ventilated but not perfused. Patients most often complain of shortness of breath, pleuritic chest pain and haemoptysis. Clinical signs can include a pleural rub, coarse crackles and atrial fibrillation. In massive pulmonary embolism there can be a raised JVP, respiratory rate, heart rate and hypotension. The Geneva scoring system (see below) is useful for predicting the risk of a pulmonary embolism: a score of ≤3 (mild), 4–10 (moderate) and ≥11 (high). Muscular strain (A) typically occurs on movement and is not associated with shortness of breath or leg pain and there is usually an indicator of injury or a preceding stressor. Heart failure (B) is unlikely due to the acute presentation of symptoms which tend to occur more insidiously and can be associated with bilateral leg oedema, murmurs, orthopnoea or hepatomegaly, among others. A pneumothorax (C) can present with a similar pleuritic chest pain that occurs in an embolism, however, there is no association with limb pain and a respiratory examination is likely to reveal hyper-resonance. Angina (D) is typically described as a dull or crushing chest pain in the centre of the chest, patients have risk factors such as diabetes, hyperlipidaemia, obesity, smoking and hypertension.

Measurement	Score
≥65 years	1
Previous DVT or PE	3
Surgery or fracture ≤4 weeks	2
Malignancy	2
Unilateral leg pain	3
Unilateral oedema	4
Haemoptysis	2
Heart rate: 75–94	3
Heart rate: >95	5

Murmurs

7 A   This patient is suffering from a mitral valve prolapse (Barlow syndrome, click murmur syndrome) (A). A mid-systolic click followed by a late systolic murmur is heard at the apex as the thickened mitral valve leaflet is displaced into the left atrium during systole. An Austin Flint murmur (B) produces a low pitched, mid-diastolic rumble at the apex. Classically, mitral valve displacement as well as aortic turbulence due to regurgitation qualifies as an Austin Flint murmur. A patent ductus arteriosus (C) produces a constant machinery murmur. A Graham Steell murmur (D) is typically heard best at the left sternal edge, second intercostals space during inspiration. A high pitched early diastolic murmur is heard associated with pulmonary hypertension. A Carey Coombs murmur (E) is a short, mid-diastolic rumble heard best at the apex due to turbulent blood flow over a thickened mitral valve, most often due to rheumatic fever.

Chest pain

8 C   All of the answer options can present as central chest pain, however the patient describes a very typical description of an aortic dissection (C), usually a severe, tearing pain that radiates toward the back though this can be to the jaw depending on the location of the dissection. An MI (A) is typically described as severe, crushing chest pain with an acute onset, this patient has been suffering from a 3-day history of chest pain which makes an infarction unlikely. Although myocardial ischaemia (B), i.e. angina, can occur for a longer period of time they tend not radiate to the back but more toward the jaw, arms or epigastrum, and again are described as crushing in nature rather than tearing. A pulmonary embolism (D) typically presents with pleuritic chest pain, cough and haemoptysis which are not present in this patient, or preceding risk factors such as long haul travel or surgery. Pneumonia (E) is associated with fever and productive coughing.

Chest pain management

9 D   NICE guideline protocols state that in a patient with suspected MI, pain relief in the form of GTN spray or morphine should be administered. Since the patient has had an adequate response to GTN spray, further pain relief in the form of morphine (B) is unnecessary. In patients who are not allergic, 300 mg of aspirin is recommended and ideally should be given in the ambulance. However, if the patient is allergic to aspirin (A) it should not be given since an anaphylactic reaction would compromise the patient's airway and does not overrule the harm from a possible MI. Although heparin (C) and warfarin (E) would provide good anticoagulant cover, they are slower to act and current guidance advises clopidogrel monotherapy (D) in those patients allergic to aspirin.

Ventricular tachyarrhythmia

10 B This patient is suffering from a life-threatening ventricular tachyarrhythmia of which there are two types, sustained ventricular tachycardia and ventricular fibrillation. In ventricular fibrillation (B) the patient is pulseless and cardioversion is required. A sustained ventricular tachycardia (C) is usually recognized by cannon 'a' waves on JVP and broad QRS complexes if an ECG is available. If stable, patients can be cardioverted with amiodarone, if unstable, electrocardioversion is required. Torsades de pointes (A) presents with irregular QRS complexes and prolonged QT interval, a non-sustained ventricular tachycardia (D) is defined by more than five consecutive heart beats within 30 seconds, while a normal heart ventricular tachycardia (E) is a benign tachyarrhythmia. Answers (A), (D) and (E) are not shockable rhythms.

Jugular venous pressure

11 D The JVP provides clinicians with information regarding right atrial pressures and filling. It mainly consists of five wave forms:

1   a wave – representing atrial systole;

2   c wave – representing closure of the tricuspid valve (this wave is not usually visible);

3   x descent – representing a fall in atrial pressure during ventricular systole;

4   v wave – representing atrial filling against a closed tricuspid valve;

5   y descent – representing the opening of the tricuspid valve.

In atrial fibrillation, the 'a waves' are absent (D) due to dysfunctional atrial systole. A raised JVP with normal waveform pattern (A) is usually seen in fluid overload and right heart failure. Large v waves (B) are usually seen in patients with tricuspid regurgitation. Cannon 'a waves' (C) are seen in patients with complete heart block, single chamber ventricular pacing, ventricular arrhythmias and ventricular ectopics. Large 'a waves' (E) can be seen in pulmonary hypertension and pulmonary stenosis.

Heart failure

12 A Cardiomegaly (B), bilateral pleural effusions (C), alveolar oedema (D) and Kerley B lines (E) (representing interstitial oedema) are all features that can be seen in a chest x-ray in patients with congestive cardiac failure. Upper lobe diversion is usually seen on chest x-ray and not lower lobe diversion (A).

First degree heart block

13 D The PR interval is usually measured from the start of the P-wave to the start of the QRS and the normal range lies within 0.12–0.2s (i.e. 120–200ms). In first degree heart block, the PR interval is prolonged, greater than 0.2 s (200 ms) (D). Shortened PR interval (i.e <120 s or <0.12 s) (E) results from fast AV conduction, usually down an accessory pathway seen in Wolff–Parkinson–White syndrome.

Mitral stenosis

14 C Malar flush (A), atrial fibrillation (B), a tapping apex beat (D) and right ventricular heave (E), which occurs secondary to pulmonary hypertension, are all clinical signs associated with mitral stenosis. On auscultation of the praecordium, a mid-diastolic murmur (±opening snap, representing a mobile valve) is heard rather than a pan-systolic murmur (C) which is usually heard in mitral regurgitation, tricuspid regurgitation and ventricular septal defects.

Hypertension

15 B ACE inhibitors (e.g. lisinopril (B)) commonly cause a dry cough in some patients. If this occurs, patients are usually taken off the ACEI and started on either an ARB (e.g. irbesartan, losartan, telmisartan) or different class of antihypertensive. Amlodipine (A), bendroflumethiazide (C), frusemide (D) and atenolol (E) do not commonly cause a dry cough as a side effect.

Palpitations

16 B The onset of the arrhythmia is recent, and there is a good chance of successful cardioversion (B) at this point without the need for anticoagulation. Conservative management (E) is also reasonable, though the patient is in some discomfort. 'Chemical' cardioversion (D) may be somewhat less likely to succeed than DC cardioversion but may be preferred by the patient. Digoxin (A) may eventually control resting, but not ambulant heart rate, but would probably take several days before it did so. Option (C) is certainly suitable in cases of persistent or permanent atrial fibrillation where it is decided to opt for rate control.

Murmurs

17 B This is a classical presentation of aortic stenosis, with syncope following a period of increasing shortness of breath on exertion and angina, with relatively narrow pulse pressure and ECG (or echo) indications of left ventricular hypertrophy. The answer is therefore (B). (A) is the murmur of mitral stenosis (with opening snap and loud P2), (C) of aortic regurgitation, (D) of mitral regurgitation and (E) of tricuspid regurgitation. Aortic stenosis is by far the most common valvular lesion likely to be seen in general medicine.

Postmyocardial infarction (1)

18 B Ventricular septal defect (B) is the most likely diagnosis and this is potentially a very serious complication which will need endovascular or surgical intervention. The murmur is not where one would expect to locate it for mitral incompetence (A), and there is also the finding of raised jugular venous pressure in this case. Aortic stenosis (C) would have quite different clinical findings, including the murmur, Dressler's syndrome (D) is a type of possibly autoimmune pericarditis and there is nothing pointing to another myocardial infarction (E).

Hypertension

19 D It is generally agreed that in situations where relatively rapid blood pressure lowering is indicated, sodium nitroprusside (D) is the most effective and reliable drug. However, it can only be used safely if there are facilities for continuous intra-arterial blood pressure monitoring, since it can produce very rapid drops in blood pressure which can lead to acute cerebral, cardiac or optic hypoperfusion. GTN (A), hydralazine (B) and labetalol (C) have also been used in hypertensive emergencies but are less reliable, GTN is the drug of second choice. They may be preferred if intensive monitoring is not available. Phentolamine (E) is used in phaeochromocytoma-caused hypertensive crises. It should be noted that the evidence base for the management of hypertensive emergencies is still under review.

Mid-systolic murmur

20 C Coarctation of the aorta (C) is the only diagnosis compatible with the hypertension present here. The other features are also characteristic of this condition. Bruits over the intercostal spaces with notching of the lower margins of the ribs may also be apparent.

Ventral septal defect

21 D Large ventricular septal defects (VSDs) may indeed be associated with pulmonary hypertension (A), heart failure (B) and shunt reversal (E), but a small defect is unlikely to lead to these problems and, in general, VSDs are not associated with dysrhythmias (C). Endocarditis (D) is, however, a persistent hazard. Routine antibiotic prophylaxis for dental procedures is no longer recommended.

Microscopic haematuria

22 A The picture strongly suggests polycystic kidney disease. The least invasive productive investigation is likely to be urinary tract ultrasound (A). The CT scan (B) is also useful, but is more costly and involves exposure to radiation without yielding more diagnostic information in this case than high-quality ultrasound. Intravenous urogram (E) would show filling defects without defining their nature. Urine microscopy (C) will yield no additional data. Renal biopsy (D) is unjustifiable. Ultrasound screening of first-degree relatives could be discussed with them as most cases are inherited as autosomal dominant traits. Unfortunately, even excellent blood pressure control does not slow the deterioration in renal function which usually accompanies this condition, though of course it is still indicated for other reasons.

Retrosternal chest pain

23 A IV low-molecular weight heparin (A) should almost always form part of the immediate management of an acute coronary syndrome, such as in this case. If the patient were not already on a beta-blocker this would also be given. At this point it would be classified as unstable angina as there is no evidence of actual tissue damage. Thrombolysis (B) probably worsens outcomes in this situation. In the absence of actual thrombus, calcium channel blockers (C) have no proven benefit and at this stage clopidogrel (E) is not indicated, although it would be if stenting (D) is carried out. If the facilities are available, that would be the next step after anticoagulation.

Pulmonary embolism management

24 C As the history strongly suggests a thrombophilic trait, e.g. the presence of factor V Leiden, the correct option is a thrombophilia screen (C). This should be completed as rapidly as possible before starting warfarin (A) therapy, which would prevent a proper screen. In fact, a duplex scan (E) would probably be carried out at the same time as the screening, to exclude the presence of thrombus and of pelvic masses. An ECG (B) is irrelevant, while an inferior vena cava filter (D) may be considered later if anticoagulation is ineffective or not tolerated.

Mid-diastolic murmur

25 A This is typical mitral stenosis and the correct answer is echocardiography (A). Colour Doppler scanning (E) would almost certainly follow to assess flow and pressure. Cardiac catheterization (C) may be performed prior to surgery, while thallium radionuclide scanning (D) is not relevant. The antistreptolysin O titre (B) can confirm streptococcal infection and the presumed rheumatic fever responsible for the lesion, but only around the time it occurs. It would yield no useful information years later, as would be the case here.

Severe chest pain

26 D The most likely diagnosis, and the one that must be most urgently excluded, is an aortic dissection (D). The location does not indicate a pneumothorax

(A), the symptoms and ECG are against an MI (B) and the pain seems too severe for a pulmonary embolus (C), or pain of musculoskeletal origin (E). Chest x-ray may show widening of the aorta, and CT and MRI scans may be diagnostic. If confirmed, BP reduction and dampening of the aortic systolic wave by beta-blockade is indicated and urgent surgical intervention should be considered.

Decrescendo diastolic murmur

27 A This is a typical clinical scenario for an aortic regurgitation (A), with early cardiac failure. Note the wide pulse pressure, and it is also usual for the pulse to be rapidly collapsing. The only lesion producing a diastolic murmur, among those listed, is of course mitral stenosis (D). No other valve abnormality (B), (C) or (E) produces a wide pulse pressure as seen here, but remember that in older people, almost always over the age of 60, similarly wide or even wider pulse pressures may be noted. This would be due to isolated systolic hypertension, i.e. systolic pressure >140 mmHg and diastolic ≤90 mmHg.

Supraventricular tachycardia

28 D IV adenosine (D) has a very high likelihood of success, with rapid onset and offset. It may cause very brief chest pain (which is not ischaemic) and very occasionally bronchospasm. Verapamil (B) and beta-blockers (C) may also be effective but have a longer duration of action which is unnecessary here, may cause excessive bradycardia, and are in any case less effective than adenosine. If the patient has severe haemodynamic compromise, DC cardioversion (E) could be considered but would be excessive here. Carotid sinus massage (A) is likely to remain ineffective. SVT is common in young people and may be associated with excessive nicotine, caffeine and alcohol and patients should be advised about this, although they may not take much notice!

Chest pain

29 E Variant angina, sometimes called Prinzmetal's angina (E), of which this is a typical presentation. Its mechanism is controversial and even its existence has been questioned. The general view is that it is due to vasospasm in small coronary arteries and this is likely to respond to the effects of nitrates and calcium channel blockers such as verapamil. Beta-blockers are not effective and in theory could make it worse by aggravating vasoconstriction, but whether this actually happens is also controversial.

Shortness of breath

30 C The diagnosis here is hypertrophic obstructive cardiomyopathy, which is associated with the risk of sudden death. The best answer is beta-blockers

(C), closely followed by rate-limiting calcium channel blockers (D). These drugs slow the heart and improve diastolic relaxation. Nitrates (B) do the opposite while digoxin (A) may increase contractility and thereby worsen the outflow obstruction. Surgery (E) may ultimately be indicated.

Hypertension

31 C Although there is some debate on this issue, the general consensus is that the best answer is option (C), which is highly sensitive and specific, with levels as much as ten-fold greater than normal. Option (B) may be normal between episodes, option (D) may well be abnormal but would not be diagnostic, and option (E) is not recommended or necessary. Option (A) will be essential once the diagnosis is definite or highly probable.

Chest pain

32 C The answer is right coronary artery (C). This is the artery that supplies the inferior and posterior aspects of the left ventricle. The circumflex artery (A) would affect the anterolateral territory (leads I, aVL, V5–6). The left anterior descending artery (B) supplies the septum (leads V1–V4). The left main coronary artery (D) would include the circumflex artery and left anterior descending artery territory. The posterior descending artery (E) affects a limited portion of the posterior wall, and is associated with tall R waves in V1–2.

Constrictive pericarditis

33 A The answer is (A) (Kussmaul's sign). Third heart sounds (B) and fourth heart sounds (C) are associated with heart failure, but not pericardial diseases. Lung signs are less likely than 'right sided' ones, such as ascites and peripheral oedema. The first and second heart sounds are usually reduced as the pericardial wall is thickened and sound transmission is reduced.

Visual disturbance

34 C These symptoms are characteristic of digoxin (C) (cardiac glycosides). The yellow-tinged vision (xanthopsia) is particular to these drugs. The slow pulse, with probable ectopics, together with the subjective symptoms, suggests toxicity and plasma digoxin should be measured, with lowering of the dosage or withdrawal of the drug, which is not considered first-line therapy in any case in the management of congestive heart failure.

Weight loss

35 A This clinical picture strongly suggests thyrotoxicosis and therefore the correct answer is TFTs (A). This is probably the most common cause of atrial fibrillation in a young person, particularly in the absence of valve disease. No doubt an ECG (B) will be carried out to exclude this but there are no physical signs to suggest an abnormality: the mitral valve is the one most likely to be associated with atrial fibrillation, probably at least in part because of stretching of the left atrium. It is certain that full blood count (D) and fasting blood sugar (E) will be carried out routinely, while a chest x-ray (C) may form part of the search for a retrosternal goitre if there is any indication of this.

Postmyocardial infarction (2)

36 E There is strong clinical trial evidence for the other four classes of drugs (A–D), although it is not clear how long the duration of therapy should be in each case. This benefit is applicable to normotensive patients with 'normal' LDL levels, although what constitutes normal in this case is controversial. Targets are likely to be reduced in the near future. One clinical trial did appear to shown additional benefit for the omega-3 fatty acids (E) but this was in a population where few were receiving statins. Subsequent data have not supported their routine use.

Mitral valve prolapse complication

37 D The diagnosis here is subacute bacterial endocarditis, probably due to *Streptococcus viridans*. The definitive diagnosis is by blood culture (D) although echocardiography (B) will show vegetations on affected heart valves. Although the lesions described are vasculitic (as are the painless Janeway lesions and the Roth spots in the retina), in this case they are due to antigen–antibody complexes triggered by infection. The issue of routine prophylaxis for patients with valvular disease prior to dental procedures is controversial; in the UK, it is no longer recommended.

Mitral valve prolapse

38 C There is no indication for ACE inhibitor therapy (B), while beta-blockers (A) may be used for management of arrhythmias if these occur. Mitral regurgitation (D) is unlikely to occur, although it is a possibility. There is no need to limit exercise (E) in an asymptomatic patient. As mentioned elsewhere, endocarditis is a persistent risk, with the need for antibiotic prophylaxis a topic of current debate.

Paroxysmal atrial fibrillation

39 E Oral flecainide (E) is now widely recommended to avoid continuous therapy. Propafenone is used in a similar way. Digoxin (A) is not effective in this situation; sotalol (C) may be used but should be avoided because of this patient's asthma. Amiodarone (D) is effective, but has numerous serious adverse reactions including pulmonary fibrosis, liver damage, peripheral neuropathy and abnormal thyroid function. Anticoagulation (B) is very important to prevent strokes, although in low-risk patients aspirin may be adequate. In patients where drug therapy is ineffective or poorly tolerated, ablation therapy can have a high success rate.

Hypertension management

40 A Poor adherence to therapy (A) is probably the most common cause of apparent resistance to hypertensive therapy. In cases where this occurs despite good adherence, spironolactone (B) is often highly effective, although it is not clear why. Verapamil (E) is very occasionally added to a dihydropyridine in severe hypertension. If he is already a patient of the hypertension clinic, one can presume that he has been screened for possible secondary causes (C and D), so this is very likely to be primary hypertension.

SECTION 2: RESPIRATORY

Questions

QUESTIONS

1. Breathlessness

You see a 68-year-old man in clinic, with a 40 (cigarette) pack year history, who has been experiencing breathlessness on exertion and a productive cough of white sputum over the last four months. You assess his spirometry results which reveal an FEV_1/FVC of 51 per cent with minimal reversibility after a 2-week trial of oral steroids. Cardiological investigations are normal. Which of the following is the most likely diagnosis?

A. Asthma
B. Chronic obstructive pulmonary disease (COPD)
C. Left ventricular failure
D. Chronic bronchitis
E. Lung fibrosis

2. Assessment of pneumonia

A 67-year-old woman is admitted to accident and emergency with pyrexia (38.1°C) and a cough productive of green sputum. The observations show a pulse rate of 101, BP 80/60 and respiratory rate of 32. She is alert and orientated in space and time. Blood results reveal a WCC of 21, urea of 8.5 and chest x-ray shows a patch of consolidation in the lower zone of the right lung. She is treated for severe community-acquired pneumonia. Which of the following is the correct calculated CURB-65 score?

A. 6
B. 8
C. 4
D. 0
E. 1

3. Organisms in atypical pneumonia

Which of the following organisms would typically be found in a patient with atypical community-acquired pneumonia?

A. *Staphylococcus aureus*
B. *Pseudomonas* spp.
C. *Streptococcus pneumonia*
D. *Legionella pneumophilia*
E. *Haemophilus influenza*

4. Interpretation of arterial blood gases (1)

You are asked to interpret an arterial blood gas of a 76-year-old patient who was admitted to accident and emergency with an acute onset of breathlessness and low oxygen saturations. The test was taken on room air and read as follows: pH 7.37, PO_2 7.8, PCO_2 4.1, HCO_3 24, SO_2 89 per cent. Choose the most likely clinical interpretation from these arterial blood gas results:

    A. Compensated respiratory acidosis
    B. Type 1 respiratory failure
    C. Compensated respiratory alkalosis
    D. Type 2 respiratory failure
    E. None of the above

5. Shortness of breath (1)

A 54-year-old woman is seen in clinic with a history of weight loss, loss of appetite and shortnesss of breath. Her respiratory rate is 19 and oxygen saturations (on room air) range between 93 and 95 per cent. On examination, there is reduced air entry and dullness to percussion on the lower to midzones of the right lung. There is also reduced chest expansion on the right. From the list below, select the most likely diagnosis:

    A. Right middle lobe pneumonia
    B. Pulmonary embolism
    C. Right-sided pleural effusion
    D. Right-sided bronchial carcinoma
    E. Right lower lobe pneumonia

6. Diagnostics in respiratory medicine (1)

A 45-year-old woman with unexpected weight loss, loss of appetite and shortness of breath presents to you in clinic. On examination, there is reduced air entry and dullness to percussion in the right lung. A pleural tap is performed and the aspirate samples sent for analysis. You are told that the results reveal a protein content of >30 g/L. From the list below, select the most likely diagnosis:

    A. Bronchogenic carcinoma
    B. Congestive cardiac failure
    C. Liver cirrhosis
    D. Nephrotic syndrome
    E. Meig's syndrome

7. Diagnostics in respiratory medicine (2)

You are discussing a patient with your registrar who has become acutely short of breath on the ward. After performing an arterial blood gas, you have high clinical suspicion that the patient has a pulmonary embolism. Which of the following is the investigation of choice for detecting pulmonary embolism?

A. Magnetic resonance imaging (MRI) of the chest
B. High-resolution CT chest (HRCT)
C. Chest x-ray
D. Ventilation/perfusion scan (V/Q scan)
E. CT pulmonary angiogram (CT-Pa)

8. Management of asthma

A 28-year-old man has been newly diagnosed with asthma. He has never been admitted to hospital with an asthma exacerbation and experiences symptoms once or twice a week. You discuss the treatment options with him. His peak expiratory flow reading is currently 85 per cent of the normal predicted value expected for his age and height. Which of the following is the most appropriate first step in treatment?

A. Short-acting beta-2 agonist inhaler
B. Long-acting beta-2 agonist inhaler
C. Low-dose steroid inhaler
D. Leukotriene receptor antagonists
E. High-dose steroid inhaler

9. Investigations

You see a 46-year-old man who has presented to accident and emergency with an acute onset of shortness of breath. Your registrar has high clinical suspicion that the patient is suffering from a pulmonary embolism and tells you that the patient's ECG has changes pointing to the suspected diagnosis. From the list below, which of the following ECG changes are classically seen?

A. Inverted T-waves in lead I, tall/tented T-waves in lead III and flattened T-waves in lead III
B. Deep S-wave in lead I, pathological Q-wave in lead III and inverted T-waves in lead III
C. Flattened T-wave in lead I, inverted T-wave in lead III, and deep S-wave in lead III
D. No changes in lead I, deep S-wave in lead III
E. Deep S-wave in lead I with no changes in lead III

10. Interpretation of arterial blood gases (2)

Which of the following arterial blood gas results, taken on room air, would you expect to see in a 67-year-old patient who has been suffering with COPD for two years and is not on home oxygen?

    A. pH 7.35, PO_2 11, PCO_2 5.3, HCO_3 24, SO_2 98 per cent
    B. pH 7.47, PO_2 12, PCO_2 5.1, HCO_3 30, SO_2 97 per cent
    C. pH 7.44, PO_2 8.3, PCO_2 6.7, HCO_3 28, SO_2 93 per cent
    D. pH 7.31, PO_2 10.2, PCO_2 6.8, HCO_3 25, SO_2 95 per cent
    E. pH 7.30, PO_2 11.5, PCO_2 5.2, HCO_3 18, SO_2 96 per cent

11. Bronchiectasis

You see a 46-year-old woman on your ward who has been diagnosed with bronchiectasis following a three-month history of a mucopurulent cough. Which of the following from the list below is not a cause of bronchiectasis?

    A. Kartagener's syndrome
    B. Cystic fibrosis
    C. Pneumonia
    D. Left ventricular failure
    E. Bronchogenic carcinoma

12. Finger clubbing

A 30-year-old man presents to your clinic with a cough and finger clubbing. From the list below, which of these answers is not a respiratory cause of finger clubbing?

    A. Empyema
    B. Mesothelioma
    C. Bronchogenic carcinoma
    D. Cystic fibrosis
    E. COPD

13. Lung tumours

A 55-year-old woman, who has never smoked, presents to you on the ward with a history of weight loss, decreased appetite and finger clubbing. You are told that her chest x-ray revealed opacity in the hilar region of the right lung suggesting a bronchogenic carcinoma. She is currently awaiting a CT-chest with bronchoscopy to follow. From the list below, select the most likely diagnosis:

    A. Squamous cell carcinoma of the lung
    B. Adenocarcinoma of the lung
    C. Small cell carcinoma of the lung
    D. Large cell carcinoma of lung
    E. Carcinoid tumour of the lung

14. Shortness of breath (2)

You see a 28-year-old man, with no past medical history, in accident and emergency who developed an acute onset of pleuritic chest pain and shortness of breath while playing football. On examination, oxygen saturations are 93 per cent on room air, respiratory rate 20 and temperature is 37.1°C. There is decreased expansion of the chest on the left side, hyper-resonant to percussion and reduced air entry on the left. The most likely diagnosis is:

A. Left-sided pneumothorax
B. Left-sided pneumonia
C. Left-sided pleural effusion
D. Lung fibrosis
E. Traumatic chest injury

15. Investigating shortness of breath

You are asked to request imaging for a patient with a suspected pneumothorax who you have just examined in accident and emergency. Which of the following would be the most appropriate first step imaging modality?

A. CT-chest
B. Ultrasound chest
C. Chest x-ray
D. V/Q scan
E. CT-PA

16. Management of pulmonary emboli

A 68-year-old woman has presented with acute onset shortness of breath 24 hours after a long haul flight. Her blood results show a raised D-dimer level and the arterial blood gas shows a $PO2$ of 8.3 kPa and PCO_2 of 5.4 kPa. Your consultant suspects a pulmonary embolism and the patient needs to be started on treatment while a CT-PA is awaited. From the list below, please select the most appropriate treatment regime.

A. Commence loading with warfarin and aim for an international normalized ratio (INR) between 2 and 3
B. Thromboembolic deterrent stockings
C. Aspirin 75 mg daily
D. Prophylactic dose subcutaneous low molecular weight heparin + loading with warfarin and aim for INR between 2 and 3
E. Treatment dose subcutaneous low molecular weight heparin + loading with warfarin and aim for INR between 2 and 3

17. Pancoast's tumour

You see a 67-year-old man who has been referred to the chest clinic following a three-month history of weight loss and signs which may suggest a Pancoast's tumour. Which of the following symptoms from the list below is not associated with a Pancoast's tumour?

    A. Hoarse voice
    B. Miosis
    C. Anhydrosis
    D. Exopthalmos
    E. Ptosis

18. Cough

A 50-year-old Afro-Caribbean man, with no past medical history, presents with a four-month history of dry cough and shortness of breath on exertion. The patient's GP referred him to the chest clinic after performing blood tests which revealed a raised erythrocyte sedimentation rate (ESR) and serum angiotensin-converting enzyme (ACE) level. You review the patient's chest x-ray which reveals bilateral hilar lyphadenopathy. From the list below, select the most likely diagnosis:

    A. Rheumatoid arthritis
    B. Systemic lupus erythematosus (SLE)
    C. Sarcoidosis
    D. Idiopathic pulmonary fibrosis
    E. Bronchogenic carcinoma

19. Cor pulmonale

A 67-year-old man presents with dyspnoea and fatigue with signs of a raised jugular venous pressure (JVP), hepatomegaly and peripheral oedema. The patient has a longstanding history of COPD. You suspect cor pulmonale. Which of the following is not a cause of cor pulmonale?

    A. Pulmonary fibrosis
    B. Primary pulmonary hypertension
    C. Myasthenia gravis
    D. COPD
    E. Multiple sclerosis

20. Chest x-ray interpretation

You are told by your registrar that a 69-year-old man has been admitted to the chest ward with dyspnoea, cyanosis and finger clubbing. His chest x-ray shows bilateral lower zone reticulo-nodular shadowing. From the list below, which is the most likely diagnosis?

A. Bronchiectasis
B. Pulmonary fibrosis
C. Bronchogenic carcinoma
D. Bronchitis
E. COPD

21. Asthma

A 25-year-old woman is admitted to accident and emergency with a severe exacerbation of asthma. On examination, her respiratory rate is 30, oxygen saturations are 95 per cent on 15 L O_2 and temperature is 37.2°C. As you feel the peripheral pulse, the volume falls as the patient inspires. Which of the following explains this clinical sign?

A. Increased left atrial filling pressures on inspiration
B. Decreased right ventricular filling pressures on inspiration
C. Peripheral vasodilation
D. Decreased right atrial filling pressures on inspiration
E. Decreased left atrial filling pressures on inspiration

22. Management of community-acquired pneumonia

A 55-year-old man, who has never smoked and with no past medical history, has been diagnosed with right basal community-acquired pneumonia. There are minimal changes on his chest x-ray and bloods reveal a neutrophil count of 8.2 and a C-reactive protein (CRP) of 15. He has no drug allergies. Although he has a productive cough of green sputum, his respiratory rate is 16, oxygen saturations are 97 per cent on room air and his temperature is 37.4°C. You are asked to place him on treatment. Which of the following treatment options would be appropriate for this patient?

A. Oral amoxicillin
B. Oral erythromycin
C. Intravenous ertapenem
D. Intravenous ertapenem with a macrolide (e.g. clarithromycin)
E. Intravenous tazocin

23. Complications of pneumonia

A 56-year-old woman who has recently been discharged from your ward, with oral antibiotics for right basal community-acquired pneumonia, is re-admitted with transient pyrexia and shortness of breath. She is found to have a right-sided pleural effusion which is drained and some pleural aspirate sent for analysis. The results reveal an empyema. Which of the following, from the pleural aspirate analysis, would typically be found in a patient with an empyema?

A. pH >7.2, ↑ LDH, ↑ glucose
B. pH <7.2, ↑ LDH, ↑ glucose
C. pH >7.2, ↓ LDH, ↓ glucose
D. pH <7.2, ↑ LDH, ↓ glucose
E. pH <7.2, ↔ LDH, ↔ glucose

24. Cystic fibrosis (1)

You are told that a patient in clinic has been diagnosed with cystic fibrosis using the sodium chloride sweat test. Which of the following results from the latter test would indicate a positive diagnosis of cystic fibrosis?

A. Sodium chloride <40 mmol/L
B. Sodium chloride >60 mmol/L
C. Sodium chloride >50 mmol/L
D. Sodium chloride <60 mmol/L
E. Sodium chloride <30 mmol/L

25. Cystic fibrosis (2)

Which of the following organisms, responsible for causing chronic pneumonia, is most commonly found in patients with longstanding cystic fibrosis?

A. *L. pneumophilia*
B. *S. pneumonia*
C. *Burkholderia cepacia*
D. *Pseudomonas aeruginosa*
E. *H. influenza*

26. Carcinogen exposure

From, the list below, which of the following carcinomas of the lung is highly associated with exposure to asbestos?

A. Adenocarcinoma
B. Small cell carcinoma
C. Squamous cell carcinoma
D. Malignant mesothelioma
E. Large cell carcinoma

27. Shortness of breath (3)

You see a 67-year-old man who has presented with a four-month history of progressive shortness of breath, initially on exertion but now also at rest. Associated symptoms include a dry cough. His past medical history includes atrial fibrillation, hypertension and hypercholesterolaemia. On examination, oxygen saturations are 92 per cent on room air, respiratory rate is 19 and the patient is apyrexial. On auscultation of the chest you hear bibasal fine inspiratory crackles. You review the patient's medication history. Which of the following drugs from the patient's list is most likely to cause the symptoms experienced by the patient?

A. Amlodipine
B. Aspirin
C. Amiodarone
D. Simvastatin
E. Alendronate

28. Hypersensitivity pneumonitis

You see a 70-year-old man diagnosed with hypersensitivity pneumonitis following a four-month history of shortness of breath at rest and cyanosis. Which of the following does not fall under the category of hypersensitivity pneumonitis?

A. Coal worker's lung
B. Pigeon fancier's lung
C. Mushroom picker's lung
D. Farmer's lung
E. Malt worker's lung

29. Pyrexia

A 44-year-old plumber has a 4-day history of fever and generalized myalgia. Two days ago he developed a dry cough coupled with mild dyspnoea and has been feeling very lethargic. On examination his temperature is 38.5°C, respiratory rate 20, oxygen saturations ranging between 93 and 96 per cent on room air and auscultation of the chest reveals bibasal crackles. Bloods show a raised white cell count of 18.2 and neutrophil count of 11.0, CRP of 90 and a raised ALT of 261 and ALP 96. Chest x-ray reveals bibasal consolidation. The patient is treated with antibiotics for bibasal pneumonia. From the list below, select the most likely organism responsible for the pneumonia:

A. *Pseudomonas* spp.
B. *S. pneumoniae*
C. *Mycoplasma pneumoniae*
D. *L. pneumophilia*
E. *S. aureus*

30. Treatment of aspergillosis

Which of the drugs below would be the most appropriate to treat pulmonary *Aspergillus* spp. infection?

    A. Amoxicillin
    B. Erythromycin
    C. Amphotericin B
    D. Flucloxacillin
    E. Fluconazole

31. Acute management of chronic obstructive pulmonary disease

A 68-year-old woman is admitted to accident and emergency with shortness of breath and cough. She has been a smoker for 25 years, smoking on average 20 cigarettes a day, and is a known COPD patient with home oxygen. The observations read a pulse rate of 101, blood pressure of 100/60, respiratory rate of 20, oxygen saturations of 88 per cent on air and temperature of 37.2°C. On auscultation you hear bilateral expiratory wheeze. She is prescribed nebulizers (salbutamol 5 mg + ipratropium 500 µg) with oxygen and chest x-ray requested. Intravenous access has been established and bloods sent for analysis. From the list below, select the most appropriate next step in this patient's management plan.

    A. Arterial blood gas sampling
    B. Peak flow assessment
    C. Urine dip ± microscopy and sensitivity
    D. Start non-invasive ventilation (e.g. BIPAP)
    E. Obtain sputum for microscopy, culture and sensitivity (MC&S)

32. Hyponatraemia

During the consultant ward round, you see a 78-year-old woman who is being investigated for hyponatraemia, weight loss and haemoptysis. A mass lesion was detected on a CT-chest scan which has been biopsied and sent for histological analysis. Your consultant has a high suspicion that the patient may have bronchogenic carcinoma. From the list below, select the most likely type of bronchogenic carcinoma that would explain the above patient's symptoms:

    A. Large cell carcinoma
    B. Small cell carcinoma
    C. Adenocarcinoma
    D. Squamous cell carcinoma
    E. Alveolar cell carcinoma

33. Severity of chronic obstructive pulmonary disease

The severity of COPD is assessed using post bronchodilator spirometery analysis. From the list below, select the values that you would expect to see in a patient with moderate COPD.

A. FEV_1/FVC <0.7, FEV_1 per cent predicted 30–49 per cent
B. FEV_1/FVC <0.7, FEV_1 per cent predicted ≥80 per cent
C. FEV_1/FVC <0.7, FEV_1 per cent predicted <30 per cent
D. FEV_1/FVC <0.7, FEV_1 per cent predicted 50–79 per cent
E. FEV_1/FVC <0.7, FEV_1 per cent predicted 60–70 per cent

34. Management of stable chronic obstructive pulmonary disease

A 58-year-old man with known COPD, diagnosed eight months ago, attends your clinic with persistent shortness of breath despite stopping smoking and using his salbutamol inhaler (given to him at the time of diagnosis), which he finds he is using more frequently. You assess the patient's lung function tests that have been recorded just before he saw you in clinic on this occasion. His FEV_1 = 65 per cent of the predicted value. Oxygen saturations are 95 per cent on room air, respiratory rate in 18, and his temperature is 37.1°C. From the list below, select the next most appropriate step in this patient's management.

A. 40 mg daily oral prednisolone for 5 days
B. Start long-term oxygen therapy
C. Start inhaled corticosteroid therapy
D. Add oral theophylline therapy
E. Add a long-acting β_2 agonist inhaler

35. Exacerbation of asthma

A 58-year-old man is admitted with a mild exacerbation of asthma. He suffers with hypertension which is controlled with medication. He was given 5 mg salbutamol and 500 μg ipratropium nebulizers, on route to hospital, by paramedics and has received 'back to back' salbutamol 5 mg nebulizers since admission to accident and emergency. The patient was then sent to the acute medical unit where he was given regular nebulizers along with his regular antihypertension medication. Before he was discharged, his serum potassium reading was 2.9. Select, from the list below, the drug which is most likely to have caused the hypokalaemia.

A. Ipratropium
B. Ramipril
C. Salbutamol
D. Amlodipine
E. Paracetamol

36. Haemoptysis

A 56-year-old man attends your clinic with a three-month history of a productive cough with blood-tinged sputum, following his return from India. Associated symptoms include lethargy, night sweats and decreased appetite. He is normally fit and healthy with no past medical history. On examination, the patient's chest has good air entry bilaterally with no added sounds and his temperature is 37.3°C. A sputum sample sent from the patient's GP reveals a growth of acid fast bacilli. From the list below, which is the most likely diagnosis?

A. Pulmonary embolism
B. Tuberculosis
C. Bronchitis
D. Pneumonia
E. Bronchogenic carcinoma

37. Management of respiratory disease

Your clinic patient has been diagnosed with pulmonary tuberculosis (TB) following a three-month history of haemoptysis and fever. The patient is due to start on treatment and you are asked by your registrar which of the following regimes is the most suitable. The patient has no known drug allergies and, in addition, liver function tests and urea and electrolytes results are all within normal ranges. From the list below, which of the following answers is the most appropriate and recommended treatment regimen for this patient?

A. Three months of isoniazid, rifampicin, ethambutol and pyrazinamide, followed by three months of isoniazid and rifamipicin
B. Four months of isoniazid and rifampicin, followed by two months of isoniazid, rifampicin, ethambutol and pyrazinamide
C. Six months of isoniazid, rifampicin, ethambutol and pyrazinamide
D. Six months of isoniazid and rifampicin
E. Two months of isoniazid, rifampicin, ethambutol and pyrazinamide, followed by four months of isoniazid and rifampicin

38. Side effects of tuberculosis treatment

A 45-year-old man with diabetes, diagnosed with pulmonary TB who started treatment two months ago, presents to you with a week's history of pins and needles in his hands and feet with associated numbness. He tells you that his symptoms started since he stopped taking the vitamins given to him at the start of his TB treatment. From the list below, which of the following drugs is responsible for the symptoms described by the patient?

A. Pyrazinamide
B. Rifampicin
C. Ethambutol
D. Isoniazid
E. None of the above

39. Acute respiratory distress syndrome

A 37-year-old woman is admitted to accident and emergency with severe facial burns. Despite prompt management, she develops acute respiratory distress syndrome (ARDS). Which of the following is not associated with the diagnostic criteria for ARDS?

    A. Bilateral infiltrates on chest x-ray
    B. Acute onset
    C. Pulmonary capillary wedge pressure >19
    D. Refractory hypoxaemia (P_aO_2:FiO_2 <200)
    E. Lack of clinical congestive heart failure

40. Pyrexia and tachypnoea

You see a 76-year-old woman in accident and emergency who has been admitted with a 1-day history of shortness of breath and pyrexia (38.4°C). The patient's past medical history includes hypertension, stroke and insulin-dependent diabetes. She has no known drug allergies. The nursing staff report that the patient vomited after her lunchtime meal yesterday. On examination the patient's respiratory rate is 26, oxygen saturations 93 per cent on room air. On auscultation of the chest, you hear right basal crackles. You suspect that this patient is suffering from aspiration pneumonia. From the list below, which is the most appropriate antibiotic regimen for this patient?

    A. Intravenous cefuroxime and metronidazole
    B. Oral amoxillicin and metronidazole
    C. Intravenous clarithromycin
    D. Intravenous cefuroxime
    E. Oral co-amoxiclav

ANSWERS

Breathlessness

1 B The patients symptom history coupled with the spirometry results indicate that he has an obstructive defect. Spirometry is typically used to measure functional lung volumes. The ratio of the forced expiratory volume in one second (FEV_1) to the forced vital capacity (FVC), provides a reliable approximation of severity of airflow obstruction; the normal being 80 per cent. An FEV_1/FVC ratio of less than 80 per cent indicates an obstructive defect seen in COPD and asthma while a ratio of greater than 80 per cent is representative of a restrictive defect seen in lung fibrosis (E). The spirometry results coupled with minimal reversibility points the diagnosis to COPD (B) rather than asthma (A), where reversibility of the FEV_1/FVC ratio is usually seen. Chronic bronchitis (D) can be defined as cough productive of sputum for three months of two successive years which does not corroborate with the onset of symptoms. Left ventricular failure (C) is obviously incorrect due to the fact that cardiological tests have been mentioned as normal.

Assessment of pneumonia

2 C The CURB-65 (C – confusion, U – urea >7 mmol/L, R – respiratory rate >30, B – blood pressure of less than 90 systolic or less than 60 diastolic and 65 – age of 65 or above) criteria is a clinical prediction rule validated and recommended by the British Thoracic Society for assessing the severity of community-acquired pneumonia. The score ranges from 0 to 5 and a score of 1 or 0 can be given if each of the above risk factors are present or not, respectively. A score between 0 and 1 indicates that the patient may be treated as an outpatient. Patients with a score of 2 may be considered for a short stay in hospital with outpatient follow up. Scores between 3 and 5 indicate severe pneumonia and hospitalization with the possibility of escalation to intensive care being required. The CURB-65 criteria is regarded as a prognostic score and should not be used as a stand-alone tool for assessing the severity of pneumonia. For example, there are patients over the age of 65 who have a baseline urea of >7 mmol/L which puts the CURB-65 score at 2. Therefore the tool should be used in the context of the clinical situation, existing co-morbidities and social circumstances of the patient.

The mortality risk can also be approximated using this score:

CURB-65 score	Mortality risk (%)
0–1	<5
2–3	<10
4–5	15–30

This patient has a CURB-65 score of 4 (C), indicating a severe pneumonia and a mortality risk of 15–50 per cent.

Organisms in atypical pneumonia

3 D From the list of answers above, *H. influenzae* (E) and *S. pneumoniae* (C) are organisms which are usually responsible for community-acquired pneumonia. *S. aureus* (A) and *Pseudomonas* spp. (B) are usually found in patients with hospital-acquired pneumonia. *L. pneumophilia* (D), along with *Chlamydia* spp. and *Mycoplasma pneumoniae*, are the atypical pneumonia-causing organisms. A urinary antigen test is routinely used for the detection of *Legionella* spp. Serological tests can be used for the detection of *Mycoplasma* and *Chlamydia* spp. and also *Legionella* spp.

Interpretation of arterial blood gases (1)

4 B Type 1 respiratory failure (B) is defined as a PO_2 <8 kPa (hypoxia) with a normal or low PCO_2. The primary cause is a ventilation/perfusion mismatch of which some of the common causes include pneumonia, pulmonary oedema, pulmonary embolism, asthma, emphysema, fibrosing alveolitis and acute respiratory distress syndrome (ARDS). Type 2 respiratory (D) failure is defined as a PO_2 <8 kPa (hypoxia) with a PCO_2 >6.5 kPa (hypercapnia) and is caused by alveolar hypoventilation, with or without V/Q mismatch, of which some of the causes are pulmonary disease (pneumonia, COPD, asthma, obstructive sleep apnoea), reduced respiratory drive (sedative drugs, CNS tumour, trauma), neuromuscular disease (cervical cord lesion, diaphragmatic paralysis, myasthenia gravis, Guillain–Barré syndrome) and thoracic wall disease (flail chest, kyphoscoliosis). Compensated respiratory acidosis (A) and compensated respiratory alkalosis (C) would cause the HCO_3 to be elevated or low respectively, which is not the case here.

Shortness of breath (1)

5 C The fact that there is reduced air entry, dullness to percussion in the lower and midzones of the right lung and reduced chest expansion, indicates that there is most likely to be a pleural effusion (C) from the list of answers above. 'Stony dullness' is usually used to describe the presence of a pleural effusion but, in clinical practice, distinguishing between dullness and stony dullness can be quite challenging for even the most experienced clinicians. Pulmonary embolism (B) does not usually present with any chest signs. Pneumonia (A and E) and bronchial carcinoma (D) can lead to a secondary pleural effusion, but during the initial stages will present with bronchial breathing over the affected area of the lung.

Diagnostics in respiratory medicine (1)

6 A Pleural effusions can be categorized into transudates and exudates according to their protein content. Transudates (protein content <30 g/L) occur as a result of increased venous pressure (cardiac failure (B), restrictive pericarditis, fluid overload), hypoproteinaemia (cirrhosis (C), nephrotic syndrome (D), malabsorption) hypothyroidism and Meig's syndrome (E) (right pleural effusion coupled with ovarian fibroma). Exudates occur as a result of increased capillary permeability secondary to infection (pneumonia, tuberculosis), inflammation (pulmonary infarction, rheumatoid arthritis, SLE) or malignancy (bronhogenic carcinoma, secondary metastases, lymphoma, mesothelioma, lymphangitis carcinomatosis). From the history, the most likely answer is bronchogenic carcinoma (A).

Diagnostics in respiratory medicine (2)

7 E CT-Pa (E) is regarded as the investigation/diagnostic tool of choice for the detection of pulmonary embolisms (being the most readily available, sensitive and specific test). CT-Pa is able to detect PEs down to the 5th order pulmonary arteries and is readily obtainable out of hospital hours. Although V/Q scans (D) have high sensitivity/specificity, they are unlikely to be available out of hours and results are reported as low, moderate or high probability. Low probability V/Q scan results may require follow up with CT-Pa for exclusion/diagnosing PEs. Chest x-rays (C) may be normal or may show decreased vascular markings, atelectasis or a small pleural effusion. An occasional late sign on chest x-ray may be a homogenous wedge-shaped area of pulmonary infarction in the lung periphery. High resolution CT-chest (B) may not accurately detail the pulmonary vasculature but will confirm atelectasis and pleural effusion. MRI chest (A) is not used for the exclusion/diagnosis of PEs due to inaccurate imaging of pulmonary vasculature, lengthy scan times and difficulty obtaining a scan out of hours.

Management of asthma

8 A The British Thoracic Society has introduced a five step approach in the management of chronic asthma (2008 guidelines). Step 1: The use of short-acting beta-2 agonists in mild intermittent asthma. Step 2: If the patient is using beta-2 agonists three times a week or more or is symptomatic or has required oral corticosteroids in the last two years, then regular preventer therapy is required with an inhaled steroid (C) (e.g. 400 µg beclomethasone inhaler twice a day). The dose of steroid inhaler should be titrated according to disease severity. Step 3: Add-on therapy is usually instituted if the patient is symptomatic despite being on steroid inhalers. Long-acting beta-2 agonists (B) (e.g. salmeterol) can be used and the dose of steroid inhaler can be increased (E) if there is still poor asthma control. Step 4: If control remains inadequate despite additions used in step 3, the use of leukotriene receptor antagonists (D) (e.g. montelukast), theophyllines or slow release beta-2 agonist tablets is advised. Step 5: If control remains poor, then the addition of oral low dose steroids can be used.

This patient has been newly diagnosed and coupled with the fact that he experiences symptoms once or twice, at most, a week, puts him into the mild intermittent asthma category. Thus the introduction of short-acting beta-2 agonists (A) is the most appropriate answer here.

Investigations

9 B Although rare, the '$S_1Q_3T_3$' (B) (deep S-wave in lead I, pathological Q-wave in lead III, and inverted T-waves in lead III) pattern may be seen in patients with pulmonary embolism. More commonly, sinus tachycardia is usually observed. Right axis deviation, right bundle branch block, right ventricular strain patterns (inverted T-waves in V_1–V_4) or atrial fibrillation (new onset) have also been seen in patients with pulmonary embolism.

Interpretation of arterial blood gases (2)

10 C Patients with longstanding COPD rely on hypoxic drive in order to drive respiration. This occurs due to the fact that the respiratory centre in the brain is relatively insensitive to carbon dioxide. This is why oxygen therapy should be used cautiously in patients with COPD; giving too much oxygen may cause a decrease in respiratory drive and hence patient deterioration. Typically, patients with COPD usually exhibit a type-2 respiratory failure picture (see Question 4) in terms of arterial blood gas parameters, caused by alveolar hypoventilation, with or without V/Q mismatch. The longstanding hypercapnia results in a respiratory acidosis which over a long period of time is compensated by the kidneys retaining more bicarbonate (HCO_3) in order to normalize the pH levels. From the answers, 'C' would therefore be the most appropriate selection.

Bronchiectasis

11 D Bronchiectasis is defined as chronic infection of the bronchi and bronchioles leading to permanent dilatation of these airways. The main organisms involved in this condition are *H. influenzae, S. pneumoniae, S. aureus* and *P. aeruginosa*. Answers A–C and E are all known causes of bronchiectasis. The causes can be divided into: (1) Congenital: cystic fibrosis, Young's syndrome, primary ciliary dyskinesia, Kartagner's syndrome; and (2) Acquired: Post-infection with measles, pertussis, bronchiolitis, pneumonia, TB and HIV. Other acquired causes include bronchial obstruction secondary to tumours or foreign bodies, allergic bronchopulmonary aspergillosis (ABPA), hypogammaglobulinaemia, rheumatois arthritis, ulcerative colitis and idiopathic.

Finger clubbing

12 E The respiratory causes of clubbing include bronchogenic carcinoma (C), empyema (A), mesothelioma (B), cystic fibrosis (D), lung abscess, fibrosing alveolitis and bronchiectasis.

In patients with COPD, the signs that may be seen in the hands are carbon dioxide retention tremor, peripheral cyanosis and tar staining in the fingertips.

Lung tumours

13 B Bronchogenic carcinomas can be divided into non-small cell and small cell carcinomas (C). Non-small cell lung carcinomas (NSCLC) can be further divided into subtypes: squamous cell carcinoma (A), adenocarcinoma (B), large cell carcinoma (D), carcinoid tumours and unspecified (E), which is the least common of the NSCLC subtypes. The category of adenocarcinomas can be further divided into 'not otherwise specified adenocarcinoma' and bronchioloalveolar carcinoma. Most cases of lung cancers are associated with smoking. The adenocarcinomas are the most common form of lung cancer in patients who have never smoked; with the bronchioloalveolar subtype being more common in females who have never smoked.

Although answers A–E are all possibilities, the key information provided above is the fact that the patient has never smoked, making the adenocarcinoma (B) the most likely answer in this scenario.

Shortness of breath (2)

14 A Hyper-resonance coupled with pleuritic chest pain and an acute onset from the history strongly points to a diagnosis of pneumothorax. Pneumothoraces are usually spontaneous in young thin men and tend to occur due to subpleural bulla rupture. Some other causes include asthma, COPD, TB, pneumonia, connective tissue disorders (e.g. Marfan's syndrome, Ehlers–Danlos syndrome), trauma, iatrogenic (e.g. pleural aspiration/biopsy, percutaneous liver biopsy, etc.)

There is no history of cough and, in addition, the patient is afebrile with no bronchial breathing over the chest wall to suggest pneumonia (B). With pleural effusion (C) there would be dullness to percussion and reduced air entry on the affected side; there would also be a more chronic onset of symptoms from the history. Lung fibrosis (D) would not typically present with signs of hyper-resonance and furthermore, disease is usually bilateral with air entry. Fine inspiratory crackles are heard on auscultation.

Although pneumothoraces can develop from chest trauma, there is no history of this from the question stem, making a traumatic chest injury (E) unlikely.

Investigating shortness of breath

15 C Although CT-chest (A) would give an accurate confirmation of pneumothorax, it would not be the most appropriate first step in imaging modality. A simple chest x-ray (C) would suffice in identifying a pneumothorax. V/Q scanning (D) and CT-PA are usually requested for the assessment of pulmonary emboli. An ultrasound of the chest (B) is better at assessing pleural effusions and are increasingly used in guiding chest drain insertions.

Small pneumothoraces (small rim of air around the lung) do not usually require treatment with a chest drain if the patient is not short of breath, has good oxygen saturations, does not have a history of previous pneumothoraces and no existing lung disease. A repeat chest x-ray will be required in 7–10 days to assess whether the pneumothorax is resolving.

Large pneumothoraces (lung collapsed half-way towards heart border) require aspiration with a chest drain. Chest x-rays post chest drain insertion and after 24 hours are usually taken to assess correct chest drain placement and resolution of pneumothorax, respectively.

Complete pneumothoraces (airless lung, separate from diaphragm) will warrant the same treatment as moderate pneumothoraces (see above).

Management of pulmonary emboli

16 E Once pulmonary embolism is suspected, anti-coagulation must be commenced with treatment dose subcutaneous low molecular weight heparin (e.g. Dalteparin) and warfarin loading (E). Once the INR has stabilized, usually between a therapeutic range of 2–3, the low molecular weight heparin may be stopped and the patient is to continue on warfarin for a minimum of three months. If this is a first presentation of pulmonary embolism, treatment usually ranges from three to six months. If there is a recurrent history of pulmonary embolism, the patient will usually stay on warfarin for life. Patients who have pulmonary emboli secondary to a malignant process (e.g. ovarian carcinoma, bronchogenic carcinoma) will usually be on life-long treatment dose low molecular weight heparin as studies have shown improved anti-coagulation when compared to warfarin.

Therefore, answers A–D are incorrect here.

Pancoast's tumour

17 D Pancoast's tumours are defined as tumours arising from the lung apex either on the left or right side. As the tumour grows it can compress structures such as the brachiocephalic vein, subclavian artery, recurrent laryngeal nerve (causing voice hoarseness (A)), vagus nerve, phrenic nerve or compression of the sympathetic ganglion resulting in a group of symptoms known as Horner's syndrome (miosis (B) – pupil constriction, enopthalmos – sunken eye, ptosis (E) – drooping eyelid and ipsilateral anhydrosis (C) – loss of sweating due to compression of sympathetic supply (thoracic outlet) to the face).

Exopthalmos (D) is defined as the appearance of protruding eye and is seen in patients with Grave's disease.

Cough

18 C Sarcoidosis (C) is a multisystemic granulomatous disorder of unknown aetiology which commonly affects adults, with an increased prevalence in the Afro-Caribbean population compared to Caucasians. Usually discovered during incidental findings on chest x-ray, patients with sarcoidosis (20–40 per cent) are usually asymptomatic. Acute presentations include erythema nodosum (painful, erythematous, raised lesions on shin fronts with/without arm/thigh involvement) with/without polyarthralgia.

Ninety per cent of patients with pulmonary disease will have abnormal chest x-rays with bilateral hilar lymphadenopathy. Other signs on chest x-ray include pulmonary infiltrates or fibrosis. Patients may present with dry cough, progressive dyspnoea, reduced exercise tolerance and chest pain. In some patients with pulmonary sarcoidosis (10–20 per cent), symptoms progress leading to a decline in lung function.

Some of the non-pulmonary manifestations of sarcoidosis include lymphadenopathy, hepatomegaly, splenomegaly, uveitis, conjunctivitis, lacrimal and parotid gland enlargement.

Blood tests may reveal a raised ESR, lymphopenia, deranged LFTs, elevated serum ACE and raised immunoglobulins. Twenty-four hour urine collections may reveal hypercalciuria.

Tissue biopsy (of lung, liver, lymph nodes, skin nodules or lacrimal glands) is usually diagnostic, with histology revealing non-caseating granulomata.

Patients with bilateral hilar lymphadenopathy without systemic manifestations do not require corticosteroid treatment. Acute presentations usually require bed rest, NSAIDS and possibly corticosteroid therapy.

Corticosteroid treatment is usually indicated in patients with parenchymal lung disease, uveitis, hypercalcaemia, neurological/cardiac involvement. In severe disease, intravenous corticosteroid therapy or immune suppressants may be required.

Cor pulmonale

19 E Cor pulmonale is defined as right heart failure caused by chronic pulmonary hypertension. Patients usually present with dyspnoea, fatigue/syncope. Signs include cyanosis, tachycardia, raised JVP, right ventricular heave, loud P2 + pansystolic murmur, early diastolic (Graham Steel murmur), hepatomegaly and oedema.

Causes can be categorized into: (1) Lung disease: severe/chronic asthma, COPD (D), bronchiectasis, pulmonary fibrosis (A), lung resection;

(2) Pulmonary vascular disease: pulmonary emboli, pulmonary vasculitis, primary pulmonary hypertension (B), acute respiratory distress syndrome, sickle-cell disease, parasite infestation; (3) Thoracic cage abnormality: kyphosis, scoliosis, thoracoplasty; (4) Neuromuscular disease: myasthenia gravis (C), poliomyelitis, motor neurone disease; (5) Hypoventilation: sleep apnoea, enlarged adenoids in children and cerebrovascular disease.

Therefore, from the list it is obvious that multiple sclerosis is not one of the many causes of cor pulmonale.

Chest x-ray interpretation

20 B Classically, answers A and C–E do not produce bilateral reticulo-nodular shadowing on a chest x-ray. In addition, only the diseases mentioned in answers A–C produce clubbing as one of the clinical signs. This pattern of opacification occurs in the spectrum of fibrosing lung disease (B). In advanced fibrotic lung disease, honeycombing of the lung may be seen. Fibrosis of the lung usually starts at the bases and spreads superiorly to the upper zones of the lung as disease progresses.

Asthma

21 E As the patient inspires, at high respiratory rates, with air flow compromise due to the narrowing of airways that occurs in acute asthma exacerbations, this results in a sudden increase in negative intrathoracic pressure which causes dilatation of the pulmonary vasculature. This effect causes pooling of blood in the lungs which results in diminished pulmonary venous return to the left atrium (decreased left atrial filling (E)), hence reducing stroke volume, causing the blood pressure to drop and hence the volume of the pulse thus falls in response. In addition, an increase in negative intrathoracic pressure also causes increased venous return to the right atrium which leads to expansion of the right side of the heart resulting in compromised filling of the left side of the heart.

Management of community-acquired pneumonia

22 A From the history we can see that this patient has a CURB-65 score of 0 putting him into a good prognostic category. Second, he is normally fit and well and has no past medical history. Therefore, he is in the category of non-severe pneumonia and does not require hospitalization. Hence, oral antibiotic therapy is preferred. From the list, amoxicillin (A) would be preferred over erythromycin (B) as it covers the most common organism (*S. pneumoniae*) and has a broad spectrum of action while the macrolide will cover for atypical organisms (e.g. legionella, mycoplasma, etc.). In some centres, amoxicillin with a macrolide may be given if there is any reason to suspect atypical pneumonia (e.g. patient works with air conditioners, or has just come back from holiday and living in an air-conditioned room, plumber dealing with water tanks, etc.). Intravenous tazocin (E) and ertapenem (C + D) are not always used across all hospital trusts; antibiotic protocols vary and it is important to check the hospital trust policy for updated guidelines.

Complications of pneumonia

23 D Empyema can be defined as pus in the pleural space which can occur in patients with resolving pneumonia. Associated symptoms include transient fever, shortness of breath and pleural effusion on the side of the resolving pneumonia. Management includes ultrasound-guided chest drain insertion coupled with antibiotic therapy. The pleural aspirate obtained during the chest drain insertion may appear turbid and (yellow) straw in colour. Empyema falls into the category of exudates, hence protein content is >30 g/L.

The pH of pleural fluid is used to ascertain pleural infection. The normal pH of pleural fluid is approximately 7.6. A pleural pH of <7.2 with a normal blood pH is usually found in:

- pleural infections;
- empyema;
- TB;
- malignancy;
- oesophageal rupture.

Light's criteria states that pleural fluid can be categorized as an exudate if one or more of the following exist: (1) The pleural fluid protein divided by serum protein >0.5; (2) Pleural fluid LDH divided by serum LDH >0.6 and (3) Pleural fluid LDH is more than two-thirds the upper limits of normal serum LDH.

A low glucose level (<3.3 mmol/L) is usually seen in the following conditions:

- empyema;
- rheumatoid arthritis;
- SLE;
- TB;
- malignancy;
- oesophageal rupture.

Therefore, from the answers above, **D** is the most appropriate.

Cystic fibrosis (1)

24 B Cystic fibrosis is an autosomal recessive condition that arises due to mutations in the cystic fibrosis transmembrane conductance regulator (CTFR) gene found on chromosome 7. Cystic fibrosis tends to affect Caucasians with one in every 2000 live births. Mutations within this gene lead to increased chloride secretion and sodium absorption respectively, resulting in mucus accumulation and plugging of the airways leading to chronic infections and bronchiectasis. Neonates present with failure to thrive, meconium ileus and rectal prolapse. Presenting clinical features in children and young adults can be categorized into: (1) Respiratory: cough, wheeze, recurrent infections, bronchiectasis, pneumothorax, haemoptysis, respiratory failure, cor pulmonale; (2) Gastrointestinal: pancreatic insufficiency leading to diabetes mellitus and/or steatorrhoea, distal intestinal obstruction syndrome which is the equivalent of meconium ileus in neonates, gallstones, cirrhosis. Other features include male infertility, osteoporosis, arthritis, vasculitis, hypertrophic pulmonary osteoathropathy (HPOA), nasal polyps and sinusitis.

Diagnosis is usually made using the sodium chloride sweat test. A positive test for cystic fibrosis usually indicates a reading of >60 mmol/L (B) (chloride levels being greater than sodium). Genetic testing can also reveal common mutations in the CFTR gene. Faecal elastase can be measured to assess exocrine pancreatic dysfunction.

Management is based on the affected symptoms and can be listed as: (1) Respiratory: postural drainage, bronchodilators, IV/PO antibiotics (for infective exacerbations and prophylaxis); (2) Gastrointestinal: pancreatic enzyme replacement, fat-soluble vitamin replacement therapy, ursodeoxycholic acid treatment if impaired liver function exists. Gene therapy, which entails transferring the CFTR gene to the lungs using liposomes and adenovirus vectors. Although promising, gene therapy still carries problems concerning efficiency and target delivery of the CFTR gene.

Cystic fibrosis (2)

25 D Mucus build-up coupled with decreased mucociliary clearance results in clogging of the airways and an inflammation-rich environment which predisposes patients with cystic fibrosis to chronic lower respiratory tract infections (LRTIs). The three most common organisms responsible for causing LRTIs in cystic fibrosis are *S. aureus, H. influenza* and *P. aeruginosa* (D). In the early stages of the condition, *S. aureus* and *H. influenza* colonize and infect the lung parenchyma. With time and chronicity of disease, *P. aeruginosa* and *Burkholderia cepacia* (C) predominate with 80 per cent of patients harbouring the former and 3.5 per cent the latter, respectively.

Carcinogen exposure

26 D Asbestos exposure is considered to be a strong predisposing (occupational) factor to the development of malignant mesothelioma (D). Approximately 90 per cent of patients with malignant mesothelioma report a previous history of asbestos exposure. The latter is a rare form of cancer which develops from the mesothelial cells from the pleural lining. It can also develop from the peritoneum, the heart and pericardium but this is relatively less common. There is a latent period of approximately 40–45 years between the time of exposure and development of the condition. Patients may present with weight loss, cough, dyspnoea, finger clubbing and pleural effusions (recurrent). With secondary metastases, lymphadenopathy, hepatomegaly, bony pain and tenderness, abdominal pain and bowel obstruction with peritoneal malignant mesothelioma can occur. Diagnosis is usually histological (pleural biopsy with Abrams' needle or during thoracoscopy) and cytological analysis can be performed via pleural aspiration.

Shortness of breath (3)

27 C This patient has signs and symptoms of worsening pulmonary fibrosis secondary to amiodarone treatment. Amiodarone along with bleomycin, bulsulfan, nitrofurantoin, methotrexate and sulfasalazine are drugs that can cause pulmonary fibrosis with long-term use. Amlodipine (A), aspirin (B), simvastatin (D) and alendronate (E) have not been documented to cause pulmonary fibrosis.

Hypersensitivity pneumonitis

28 A Hypersensitivity pneumonitis, also known as extrinsic allergic alveolitis (EAA), occurs as a result of inhalation of organic allergens such as fungal spores or avian proteins which initiates a hypersensitivity reaction. Individuals are commonly exposed to the allergens by their occupation or hobbies. In the acute phase of the hypersensitivity reaction, alveolar infiltration occurs with inflammatory cells (e.g. monocytes and macrophages/giant cells) giving rise to poorly formed non-caseating interstitial granulomas. In the chronic phase, well-formed granulomas and obliterative bronchiolitis may ensue. The chronic inflammatory process causes alvelor destruction (honeycombing of the lung) which is associated with fibrosis. The main causes include: farmer's lung (D) – from mouldy hay (*Thermophilic actinomycetes, Aspergillus* spp., *Saccharopolyspora rectivirgula, Micropolyspora faeni*); bird/pigeon fancier's lung (B) – feathers and bird droppings (avian proteins); mushroom picker's lung (C) – from mushroom compost (*T. actinomycetes*); malt worker's lung (E) – from mouldy barley (*Aspergillus clavatus*) and bagassosis – from mouldy bagasse (*T. actinomycetes*). Four to six hours post allergen exposure, the patient may experience fever, rigors, dry cough and dyspnoea. With disease progression, increasing dyspnoea, weight loss, exertional dyspnoea, type-1 respiratory failure and cor pulmonale may occur.

A full blood count may reveal a neutrophilia, and ESR may be raised. Chest x-ray may show upper zone fibrosis and honeycombing. Lung function tests will show a restrictive lung defect. Acute allergen exposure management entails removing the allergen, oxygen therapy, intravenous and oral steroid treatment. Chronic disease management involves allergen avoidance and long-term oral steroid therapy. Coal worker's lung (A), along with asbestosis, silicosis, berylliosis, anthracosis, etc., falls under the category of pneumoconiosis (occupational lung disease/restrictive lung disease caused by inhalation of dust often in mines). Patients with pneumoconiosis usually develop pulmonary fibrosis.

Pyrexia

29 D This patient is suffering from a bibasal pneumonia caused by atypical *L. pneumophilia* (D). The first clue in the question is given away by the patient's occupation; *Legionella* spp. tend to colonize in water tanks kept at <60°C. Patients may initially experience flu-like symptoms of fever, malaise and myalgia followed by a dry cough and sometimes dyspnoea. Other symptoms include anorexia, diarrhoea and vomiting, hepatitis, renal failure, confusion and coma. The patient also has deranged LFTs which is the second clue in the question. Blood tests may also show lymphopenia and hyponatraemia. Urine analysis may reveal microscopic haematuria and diagnosis is usually made using legionella urinary antigen testing or serology (see answer to question 3). Treatment comprises of high-dose macrolide therapy. *Mycoplasma* spp. (C) pneumonia tends to present similarly to *Legionella* spp. pneumonia and occurs in epidemics about every four years. Chest x-ray may show bilateral patchy consolidation. Patients may suffer from autoimmune haemolytic anaemia from the build-up cold agglutinins. *S. pneumoniae* (B) is the most common organism responsible for most community-acquired pneumonia presentations. Again, the history from the questions does not make this option the likely causative organism and treatment is usually penicillin-based or with macrolides for penicillin allergic patients. *S. aureus* (E) may occur in the young, elderly, intravenous drug users and patients with underlying diseases such as leukaemia or lymphoma cystic fibrosis. It may cause bilateral cavitating bronchopneumonia and may be treated with flucloxacillin. *Pseudomonas* spp. (A) is usually found in nosocomial pneumoniae and in patients with bronchiectasis and cystic fibrosis. *Pseudomonas* infections can be treated with ciprofloxacin, carbopenems or cephalosporins.

Treatment of aspergillosis

30 C From the answers, amoxicillin (A), erythromycin (B) and flucloxacillin (D) are all antibacterial agents and do not target fungal infections. Therefore the only possible answers are C and E. Fluconzaole (E), although a widely used antifungal, is not effective against *Aspergillus* spp. Amphotericin B, along with other antifungals such as voriconazole, itraconazole and caspofungin, is effective in treating *Aspergillus* infections which can affect the lung in five ways: (1) Type-1 hypersensitivity reaction causing atopic asthma through inhalation of fungal spores; (2) Allergic bronchopulmonary aspergillosis (ABPA) which results from a type-3 hypersensitivity reaction to *A. fumigates*; (3) Aspergilloma (mycetoma) which is a fungus ball within a pre-existing cavity, often caused by tuberculosis and sarcoidosis; (4) Invasive aspergillosis which occurs in immunocompromised patients, SLE, burns and after broad-spectrum antibiotic therapy; and (5) Hypersensitive pneumonitis (see question 28).

Acute management of chronic obstructive pulmonary disease

31 A This patient is suffering from an exacerbation of COPD and, due to the inefficiency of gas exchange due to underlying disease, will be unable to maintain and expel adequate oxygen saturations and carbon dioxide, respectively. Performing arterial blood gas (ABG) sampling (A) is the most appropriate step here; this will enable the physician to assess the levels of oxygen (PO_2) and carbon dioxide (PCO_2), as well as the acid-base status which will determine whether the patient requires non-invasive or invasive ventilation in the intensive care unit. Performing ABGs on admission and after treatment are also useful in determining whether the initial treatment given in the acute setting has made an improvement. Peak flow assessment (B), urine analysis (C) and sputum analysis (E), although important tests, do not need to be carried out initially. Non-invasive ventilation (D) would be considered following full clinical assessment of the patient coupled with his/her acid base status from the findings of the ABG.

Hyponatraemia

32 B Small cell carcinomas (B) are thought to originate from the neuroendocrine cells of the bronchus and express neuroendocrine markers which may lead to ectopic hormone production (e.g. ADH and ACTH), resulting in the paraneoplastic syndromes. The patient has a likely diagnosis of syndrome of inappropriate ADH secretion (SIADH). This results in a dilutional hyponatraemia. Twenty-four hour urine collection will reveal high urine sodium concentration and high urine osmolality. Symptoms of weight loss and haemoptysis can be seen in most types of bronchogenic carcinoma but the presenting hyponatraemia makes small cell carcinoma (B) the most appropriate answer here.

Severity of chronic obstructive pulmonary disease

33 D With reference to the NICE guidelines 2010, COPD can be divided into mild, moderate, severe and very severe. The values are obtained with post bronchodilator spirometry and are as follow:

Mild COPD: FEV_1/FVC <0.7, FEV_1 % predicted ≥80 per cent (B)

Moderate COPD: FEV_1/FVC <0.7, FEV_1 % predicted 50–79 per cent (D)

Severe COPD: FEV_1/FVC <0.7, FEV_1 % predicted 30–49 per cent (A)

Very severe COPD: FEV_1/FVC <0.7, FEV_1 % predicted <30 per cent (C)

Very severe COPD can also be seen in patients with FEV_1 % predicted <50 per cent with respiratory failure.

Management of stable chronic obstructive pulmonary disease

34 E This patient was diagnosed with COPD eight months ago and was started on a short-acting β_2 agonist inhaler. With reference to the NICE guidelines in managing stable COPD, this patient can either have a long-acting β_2 agonist (LABA) inhaler (e.g. salmeterol) or a long-acting muscarinic antagonist (LAMA) inhaler (e.g. tiotropium). Therefore, from the list, **E** is the most appropriate answer.

Inhaled therapy is usually started when the patient is diagnosed with COPD and is breathless and/or has exercise limitation. Either a short-acting β_2 agonist (SABA) inhaler (e.g. salbutamol) or short-acting muscarinic antagonist (SAMA) inhaler (e.g. ipratropium) can be used initially.

If the patient experiences frequent exacerbations or persistent breathlessness, despite being on either a SABA or SAMA, two pathways can be taken:

- If the FEV_1 ≥50 per cent
    - either a LABA inhaler can be added (this can coexist with the SABA)
    - or a LAMA inhaler can be used – the LAMA will replace the SAMA in this case
- If the FEV_1 <50 per cent
    - either the addition of a LABA + inhaled corticosteroid (ICS) in a combination inhaler (e.g. salmeterol + fluticasone)
    - or the addition of a LAMA inhaler – again the SAMA inhaler should be stopped.

If the patient remains breathless or experiences persistent exacerbations:

- ICS (C) therapy can be added as a combination inhaler if LABA inhaler was added before. If the patient remains breathless and experiences exacerbations, a LAMA inhaler can be offered.
- If a LAMA was added before, addition of a LABA + ICS can be considered
- A LAMA inhaler can be offered if the patient is already on a LABA + ICS.

Oral therapy:

- Oral corticosteroid (A) maintenance therapy is not advised in COPD, although patients with advanced COPD may require low-dose oral corticosteroid therapy to prevent exacerbations. Osteoporosis prophylaxis should be considered.

- Theophylline therapy (D) is offered to patients who cannot use inhalers or after trials of short- and long-acting bronchodilators. Theophylline can be used in combination with β_2 agonists and muscarinic antagonists.

- Mucolytic therapy (e.g. carbocysteine) can be considered in people with a chronic productive cough.

Oxygen (i.e. long-term oxygen therapy) (B) therapy should be assessed in patients who have any of the following:

- very severe airflow obstruction (e.g. FEV_1 <30 per cent predicted);
- cyanosis;
- polycythaemia;
- peripheral odema;
- raised JVP;
- oxygen saturations less than or equal to 92 per cent on room air.

For further clarification on COPD management, consult the latest guidelines from NICE or the BTS.

Exacerbation of asthma

35 C The correct answer here is salbutamol (C). Regular nebulized salbutamol is commonly associated with hypokalaemia. Ipratropium is not documented to cause electrolyte disturbances. Ramipril (B) is reported to causes hyperkalaemia rather than hypokalaemia. Amlodipine (D) and paracetamol (E) are also not known to cause hypokalaemia. This patient will require potassium supplementation either via intravenous infusion or oral administration.

Haemoptysis

36 B Although answers A–E can all cause haemoptysis, the clue in this question points towards the sputum analysis report which shows a growth of acid fast bacilli seen in tuberculosis (TB) (B) which can be categorized into pulmonary (75 per cent of cases) and extrapulmonary (25 per cent of cases). The gram-positive aerobic bacterium (*Mycobacterium tuberculosis*) is usually airborne, transmitted by people suffering from active pulmonary

TB (e.g. via coughing, sneezing, speaking, spitting, etc.), sharing of needles among intravenous drug users, within high-risk racial or ethnic minority populations and people suffering from immunocompromised conditions. Most people (90 per cent) infected with the bacterium are asymptomatic (latent TB) with an approximately 10–15 per cent lifetime chance that the latent infection will progress to full blown TB. Once the mycobacteria reach the alveoli (primary TB), replication of the bacteria occur with formation of a Ghon focus (granuloma formation), which is usually located in the upper or lower lobes of the lung. Granuloma formation occurs (aggregation of macrophages, T- and B-lymphocytes and fibroblasts) in an attempt to kill the mycobacteria but this is not always efficient, especially with dormant bacteria. The bacteria can spread via the lymphatic system or bloodstream to other organs causing secondary TB (refer to Section 11, Infectious diseases, for further reading). Symptoms of primary pulmonary TB include chronic cough, haemoptysis, pyrexia, night sweats, loss of appetite, weight loss and lethargy. Chest x-ray may show a 'coin lesion' in the upper or lower lobes of the lung, sputum analysis may show growths of mycobacterium but can sometimes be difficult to culture *in vitro* and may take from 4 to 12 weeks. Interferon gamma release assays (IGRAs) can also be performed where the detection of interferon gamma release, from the blood, is tested against certain mycobacterial proteins. Tuberculin skin tests, although widely performed, produce false negatives and therefore making the IGRAs more favourable in diagnostic capability due to the reduced number of false negatives. Bronchoscopy can also be performed with BAL specimens sent to the laboratory for culture and sensitivity.

Management of respiratory disease

37 E NICE guidelines (March 2006; Clinical diagnosis and management of tuberculosis and measures for its prevention and control) recommend a standard regimen of six months which includes:

- The use of four drugs initially (e.g. isoniazid, rifampicin, ethambutol and pyrazinamide) for a total of two months.

- This is then followed by four months treatment with isoniazid and rifampicin.

This regimen is viewed as first choice daily dosing and given in fixed-dose combination tablets. This standard regimen is usually used for fully drug-susceptible TB at all sites except for the CNS, all ages (children and adults) and patients with negative or positive HIV status.

Second-line drugs (e.g. amikacin, capreomycin, cycloserine, azithromycin, clarithromycin, moxifloxain and levofloxacin) are used in special situations such as bacterial resistance and drug intolerance.

For further information, please consult the NICE guidelines mentioned above.

Side effects of tuberculosis treatment

38 D This patient is suffering from peripheral neuropathy secondary to isoniazid
(D) administration. Isoniazid is associated with depletion of vitamin B_6
(pyridoxine) and therefore results in peripheral neuropathy. Other side
effects include rash, deranged liver function (due to the fact that this drug
is metabolized in the liver by acetylation and dehydrazination and
converted to ammonia compounds which can cause hepatitis), CNS effects
and sideroblastic anaemia.

The common side effects of pyrazinamide (A) (a pro-drug that inhibits
growth of *M. tuberculosis*) include arthralgia, hepatoxicity, gastrointestinal
disturbances, rash, pruritus and sideroblastic anaemia.

Side effects of rifampicin (B) (a cytochrome P450 inducer) include
hepatoxicity, fever, gastrointestinal disturbances, rash and can also cause
the urine and tears to become an orange–red colour which is considered a
benign side effect.

The side effects associated with ethambutol (C) (a bacteriostatic drug that
inhibits the formation of the cell wall in *M. tuberculosis*) include optic
neuritis, red–green colour blindness, peripheral neuropathy and vertical
nystagmus.

Although ethambutol could also be a possible answer here, the clue given
in the question points to the patient having stopped taking his vitamins
which are usually given in conjunction with isoniazid treatment.

Acute respiratory distress syndrome

39 C ARDS, or acute lung injury, is caused either by direct injury to the lung
(e.g. trauma, iatrogenic, etc.) or secondary to severe systemic illness.
Damage to the lung results in the release of acute phase proteins and other
inflammatory mediators which give rise to increased capillary permeability
and noncardiogenic pulmonary oedema which is often associated with
multiorgan failure.

Causes can be divided into: (1) Pulmonary (e.g. pneumonia, gastric
aspiration, inhalation of smoke/soot, trauma, contusions and vasculitis);
and (2) extrapulmonary (e.g. septic/haemorrhagic shock, multiple
transfusions, DIC and pancreatitis).

Clinical features include cyanosis, tachypnoea, tachycardia, peripheral
vasodilation and bilateral fine inspiratory crackles.

A diagnosis of ARDS is made if all four of the following criteria exist:

1 acute onset (B);

2 bilateral infiltrates present n chest X-ray (A);

3   pulmonary capillary wedge pressure of $<19\,$mmHg or lack of clinical congestive heart failure (E);

4   refractory hypoxaemia with $P_aO_2{:}FiO_2<200$ (D) for ARDS.

A total intrathoracic compliance of $<30\,$mL/cm H_2O may also exist.

Management is ITU based and involves supportive therapy and treating the underlying cause.

Pyrexia and tachypnoea

40 A It is very important to consider the use of a broad spectrum antibiotic coupled with another agent that will cover for anaerobic bacteria from the oral flora and gastric contents (e.g. *Bacteroides* spp., *Prevotella* spp., *Fusobacterium* spp., etc.). In addition, this patient is systemically unwell and the use of intravenous antibiotics would be more appropriate in the initial stages of treatment. From the list above, the use of intravenous cefuroxime and metronidazole (A) is therefore the most appropriate answer. Intravenous clarithromycin (C) treatment would be indicated if the patient had a penicillin allergy and, by itself, may not be enough to cover the range of aerobic and anaerobic bacteria. Refer to your local hospital trust for relevant antibiotic protocol prescribing, as these differ from one hospital to the next.

SECTION 3: GASTROINTESTINAL

QUESTIONS

1. Dysphagia

A 47-year-old woman presents to your clinic with a three-month history of dysphagia. There is no history of drastic weight loss and the patient experiences symptoms when swallowing solids but not liquids. Which of the following is not an obstructive cause of dysphagia?

A. Pharyngeal carcinoma
B. Oesophageal web
C. Retrosternal goitre
D. Peptic stricture
E. Achalasia

2. Abdominal pain (1)

You see a 47-year-old man in clinic with a three-month history of epigastric dull abdominal pain. He states that the pain is worse in the mornings and is relieved after meals. On direct questioning, there is no history of weight loss and the patient's bowel habits are normal. On examination, his abdomen is soft and experiences moderate discomfort on palpation of the epigastric region. The most likely diagnosis is:

A. Gastric ulcer
B. Gastro-oesophageal reflux disease (GORD)
C. Duodenal ulcer
D. Gastric carcinoma
E. Gastritis

3. Management of peptic ulcer disease

A 55-year-old woman is referred by her GP for upper gastrointestinal (GI) endoscopy following a four-month history of epigastric pain despite treatment with antacids and proton pump inhibitors (PPIs). The results demonstrate a duodenal ulcer coupled with a positive campylobacter-like organism (CLO) test. The patient has no past medical history and has no known drug allergies. The most appropriate treatment is:

A. Seven-day course of twice daily omeprazole 20 mg, 1 g amoxicillin and 500 mg clarithromycin
B. Seven-day course of twice daily omeprazole 20 mg
C. Seven-day course of twice daily omeprazole 20 mg and 1 g amoxicillin
D. Seven-day course of twice daily omeprazole 20 mg and 500 mg clarithromycin
E. Seven-day course of twice daily 1 g amoxicillin and 500 mg clarithromycin

4. Peptic ulcer disease

Which of the following is the most common cause of duodenal ulcers?

    A. NSAIDs
    B. *Helicobacter pylori*
    C. Alcohol abuse
    D. Chronic corticosteroid therapy
    E. Zollinger–Ellison syndrome

5. Investigation of gastro-oesophageal reflux disease

You see a 48-year-old lorry driver, who presents to you with a three-month history of heartburn after meals which has not been settling with antacids and PPIs. You suspect that the patient has a hiatus hernia. The most appropriate investigation for diagnosing a hiatus hernia is:

    A. Computer tomography (CT) scan
    B. Chest x-ray
    C. Upper GI endoscopy
    D. Barium meal
    E. Ultrasound

6. Complications of gastro-oesophageal reflux disease

You see a 56-year-old man who was admitted for an elective upper GI endoscopy due to longstanding GORD which has failed to improve on antacids and PPIs. Your registrar suspects that this patient may have Barrett's oesophagus and asks you to define what this is. The most appropriate description of Barrett's oesophagus is:

    A. Metaplasia of the squamous epithelium of the lower third of the oesophagus to columnar epithelium
    B. Metaplasia of the columnar epithelium of the upper third of the oesophagus to squamous epithelium
    C. Metaplasia of the columnar epithelium of the lower third of the oesophagus to squamous epithelium
    D. Metaplasia of the squamous epithelium of the upper third of the oesophagus to columnar epithelium
    E. Metaplasia of the squamous epithelium of the middle third of the oesophagus to columnar epithelium

7. Diarrhoea (1)

You see a 25-year-old woman who presents with a 24-hour history of watery diarrhoea. She states that she has opened her bowels 11 times since her onset of symptoms. Associated symptoms include nausea and vomiting with abdominal cramps and pain which started in the evening following a barbeque meal in the afternoon that day. The patient is alert and orientated and her observations include a pulse rate of 69, blood pressure of 124/75 and temperature of 37.1°C. On examination, her abdomen is soft, there is marked tenderness in the epigastric region and bowel sounds are hyperactive. The patient is normally fit and well with no past medical history. The most likely diagnosis is:

- A. Irritable bowel syndrome
- B. Gastroenteritis
- C. Ulcerative colitis
- D. Laxative abuse
- E. Crohn's disease

8. Management of diarrhoea

A 35-year-old woman presents with a 24-hour history of profuse, watery diarrhoea. She has opened her bowels nine times since the onset of her symptoms. You diagnose gastroenteritis after learning that the patient and her family all ate at a new restaurant and the rest of her family have had similar problems. The most appropriate management is:

- A. Oral rehydration advice and discharge home
- B. Oral antibiotic therapy and discharge home
- C. Admission for intravenous fluid rehydration
- D. Admission for intravenous antibiotic therapy
- E. No treatment required

9. Investigation of diarrhoea

A 56-year-old man presents with a 2-week history of diarrhoea which has not settled following an episode of 'food poisoning'. Which of the following would be the most appropriate investigation?

- A. Full blood count
- B. Urea and electrolytes
- C. Stool sample for microscopy, culture and sensitivities
- D. Abdominal x-ray
- E. Liver function tests

10. Diarrhoea (2)

You are questioned by your registrar regarding bacteria responsible for causing blood-stained diarrhoea. From the list below, select the organism which is not responsible for causing blood-stained diarrhoea.

    A. *Campylobacter* spp.
    B. *Salmonella* spp.
    C. *Escherichia coli*
    D. *Shigella* spp.
    E. *Staphylococcus* spp.

11. Hepatomegaly

A 69-year-old man present with a 2-week history of abdominal pain which has worsened over the last few days. On examination, the patient is jaundiced and the abdomen is distended with tenderness in the epigastric region. In addition, there is a smooth hepatomegaly and shifting dullness. Which of the following is a cause of hepatomegaly?

    A. Iron deficiency anaemia
    B. Budd–Chiari syndrome
    C. Ulcerative colitis
    D. Crohn's disease
    E. Left-sided heart failure

12. Jaundice (1)

You see a 19-year-old Caucasian man in your clinic who presents with a history of transient jaundice. On direct questioning, you ascertain that the jaundice is noticeable after periods of increased physical activity and subsides after a few days. The patient has no other symptoms and physical examination is unremarkable. Full blood count is normal (with a normal reticulocyte count) and liver function tests reveal a bilirubin of 37 μmol/L. The most appropriate management is:

    A. Reassure and discharge
    B. Start on a course of oral steroids
    C. Request abdominal ultrasound
    D. Request MRCP
    E. Refer to Haematology

13. Jaundice (2)

You see a 54-year-old woman, referred to accident and emergency through her GP, with a week's history of jaundice and right upper quadrant abdominal pain. Associated symptoms include dark urine and pale stools. There is no history of weight loss and the patient does not consume alcohol. Her liver function tests reveal a bilirubin of 40 μmol/L, ALT of 40 iu/L, AST 50 iu/L and ALP of 350 iu/L. The most likely diagnosis is:

    A. Gallstones
    B. Viral hepatitis
    C. Alcoholic hepatitis
    D. Carcinoma of the head of the pancreas
    E. Autoimmune hepatitis

14. Investigation of jaundice

You are asked by your registrar to request an imaging investigation for a 49-year-old woman with jaundice and abdominal pain. She has a past medical history of gallstones and you suspect this is a recurrence of the same problem. The most appropriate imaging investigation is:

    A. Abdominal x-ray
    B. Abdominal ultrasound
    C. Abdominal CT
    D. Magnetic resonance imaging (MRI)
    E. Endoscopic retrograde cholangiopancreatography (ERCP)

15. Drug-induced cholestasis

You see a 47-year-old woman who presents with a 3-day history of jaundice. You assess her liver function tests (LFTs) and see that the ALP iu/L is raised at 350 iu/L, AST 45 iu/L, ALT 50 iu/L and bilirubin 50 iu/L. The patient feels well in herself, although she has noticed that her urine has become quite dark and her stools quite pale. You assess her medication history. Which of the following drugs from the patient's medication history may be responsible for the cholestasis?

    A. Co-amoxiclav
    B. Bendroflumethiazide
    C. Ramipril
    D. Amlodipine
    E. Aspirin

16. Constipation

During your on-call, you are bleeped to see an 80-year-old woman on the ward who has not opened her bowels for the last 4 days. She is not known to have a history of constipation. On examination, her observations are within normal range, the abdomen is soft and there is mild discomfort at the left iliac fossa. Bowel sounds are present and on PR examination, the rectum is empty. You consult your registrar who asks you to prescribe an osmotic laxative. What is the most appropriate treatment?

    A. Ispaghula husk
    B. Docusate sodium
    C. Lactulose
    D. Senna
    E. Methylcellulose

17. Finger clubbing

Which of the following gastroenterological conditions would give rise to finger clubbing?

    A. Hepatocellular carcinoma
    B. Ulcerative colitis
    C. Irritable bowel syndrome
    D. Duodenal ulcer
    E. Pancreatic carcinoma

18. Abdominal pain (2)

You see an 80-year-old man who presents to accident and emergency with epigastric pain. The pain started 3 days ago and today he noticed that the colour of his stools has changed to a 'tarry-black' colour. Associated symptoms include nausea and lethargy. The patient is a smoker of 20 cigarettes a day and has recently finished eradication treatment for a duodenal ulcer. The patient is alert and orientated with a pulse rate of 99 and blood pressure of 98/69, respiratory rate of 18, oxygen saturations of 98 per cent on room air and temperature of 37.2°C. On examination, the abdomen is soft with marked tenderness in the epigastric region and bowel sounds are present. The rectum is empty, on PR examination, with some traces of malaena. The patient has been started on high flow oxygen and has been given some oral analgesia. The most appropriate next step in managing this patient is:

    A. Keep nil by mouth and arrange endoscopy
    B. Request an erect chest x-ray
    C. Intravenous pantoprazole
    D. ECG
    E. Intravenous cannulation and fluids

19. Causes of upper gastrointestinal bleeding

You see a 75-year-old man with an acute episode of haematemesis, who was admitted the night before and is awaiting an upper GI endoscopy. You are asked on the ward round about the common causes of upper GI bleeding. From the list below, which of the following is the most common cause of upper GI bleeding?

A. Mallory–Weiss tear
B. Peptic ulcers
C. Oesophageal varices
D. Drug induced
E. Malignancy

20. Management of oesophageal varices

A 60-year-old man with alcoholic liver disease was admitted with an upper GI bleed secondary to oesophageal varices. The patient undergoes endoscopic variceal banding and is discharged after 2 weeks in-hospital stay. Which of the following medications would act as prophylaxis in preventing a rebleed from his oesophageal varices?

A. Frusemide
B. Amlodipine
C. Ramipril
D. Propranolol
E. Irbesartan

21. Jaundice (3)

A 46-year-old woman presents to your clinic with a week's history of jaundice. Her past medical history includes longstanding atrial fibrillation and hypertension. Physical examination reveals hepatomegaly. You assess her liver function which shows a bilirubin of 41 iu/L, AST 111 iu/L, ALT 55 iu/L and ALP 98 iu/L. There is no history of travel. You have a look at the patient's medication history. Which of the following drugs below is likely to have caused the derangement in the patient's liver function?

A. Aspirin
B. Ramipril
C. Amiodarone
D. Bendroflumethiazide
E. Amlodipine

22. Clinical signs of chronic liver disease

A 67-year-old man presents feeling unwell and complaining of general malaise. He mentions a long history of alcohol abuse and his past medical history shows deranged liver function tests. Which of the following clinical signs does not form part of chronic liver disease?

    A. Finger clubbing
    B. Palmer erythema
    C. Spider naevia
    D. Koilonychia
    E. Jaundice

23. Alcoholic liver disease

You see a 56-year-old man in your clinic with suspected alcoholic liver disease. Liver function tests reveal a bilirubin of 36 iu/L, AST of 150 iu/L, ALT 75 iu/L and ALP 100 iu/L. Which of the following blood test parameters would support a diagnosis of alcoholic-related liver disease?

    A. Normal mean cell volume (MCV)
    B. Low MCV
    C. Normal mean cell haemoglobin (MCH)
    D. Low MCH
    E. Raised MCV

24. Deranged liver function

You see a 52-year-old woman with rheumatoid arthritis in your clinic. She was referred by her GP after her ALP levels were found to be abnormally high at 300 iu/L. In addition, she was also found to be serum anti-mitochondrial antibody (AMA) positive. The most likely diagnosis is:

    A. Primary biliary cirrhosis
    B. Wilson's disease
    C. Heriditary haemochromotosis
    D. Primary sclerosing cholangitis
    E. Alcoholic liver disease

25. Ascites

A 47-year-old man presents complaining of weight gain, on examination there is an abdominal distension with a fluid thrill. Which of following is not a cause of ascites secondary to venous hypertension?

    A. Congestive heart failure
    B. Cirrhosis
    C. Constrictive pericarditis
    D. Budd–Chiari syndrome
    E. Nephrotic syndrome

26. α_1-antitrypsin deficiency

A 56-year-old man, diagnosed with emphysema, presents with a one-month history of jaundice and ascites. Your registrar suspects that this patient may have liver disease secondary to α_1-antitrypsin deficiency. Select the most likely mode of inheritance from the list below:

   A. Autosomal dominant
   B. X-linked dominant
   C. Autosomal recessive
   D. Polygenic
   E. None of the above

27. Chronic liver disease

You see a 56-year-old woman who presents with a two-month history of jaundice. Associated symptoms include lethargy and polyarthralgia. Her LFTs reveal a bilirubin of 46 iu/L, AST 200, ALT 175, ALP 104. On examination, the patient is jaundiced and has finger clubbing. There are several spider naevi on the front and back of the trunk. Her abdomen is soft and there is a smooth hepatomegaly. Prior to her onset of symptoms, the patient has been fit and well. Viral serology is normal and anti-soluble liver antigen (SLA) is detected. You decide to start this patient on treatment. The most appropriate treatment is:

   A. Liver transplantation
   B. Methotrexate
   C. Prednisolone
   D. Cyclosporin
   E. Antivirals

28. Primary sclerosing cholangitis

You are told by your registrar that one of your inpatients has been diagnosed with primary sclerosing cholangitis (PSC). Your registrar suspects that the patient may have an associated condition. Primary sclerosing cholangitis is associated with which of the following diseases?

   A. Thyroid disease
   B. Systemic sclerosis
   C. Rheumatoid arthritis
   D. Ulcerative colitis
   E. Irritable bowel syndrome

29. Complications of primary sclerosing cholangitis

A 68-year-old man presents to his GP with signs of drastic weight loss. He is known to have PSC. The GP suspects an underlying malignancy. Which of the following tumours would a patient with primary sclerosing cholangitis be more at risk of developing?

    A. Hepatocellular carcinoma
    B. Cholangiocarcinoma
    C. Hepatic fibroma
    D. Hepatic haemangioma
    E. Pancreatic carcinoma

30. Liver tumours

During a ward round, you are questioned about tumours that may arise from the liver parenchyma. Which of the following liver tumours is considered to be benign?

    A. Angiosarcoma
    B. Fibrosarcoma
    C. Adenoma
    D. Hepatoblastoma
    E. Leiyomyosarcoma

31. Hepatocellular carcinoma

A patient on your ward is diagnosed with hepatocellular carcinoma. You are asked to perform a tumour marker level on this patient. Which of the following tumour markers are elevated in hepatocellular carcinoma?

    A. α-fetoprotein
    B. Carcinoembryonic antigen (CEA)
    C. CA 15-3
    D. HcG
    E. CA 125

32. Jaundice (4)

A 64-year-old woman attends your clinic with a 2-week history of jaundice. Over the last three months the patient has lost 10 kg. Associated symptoms include decreased appetite, dark urine and pale stools. On examination, the patient is jaundiced, her abdomen is soft and you can palpate a painless mass in the right upper quadrant. From the list of answers below, select the initial most appropriate investigation that you would request for this patient:

    A. Abdominal x-ray
    B. Abdominal CT
    C. MRI of the abdomen
    D. Abdominal ultrasound
    E. ERCP

33. Rectal biopsy

A 28-year-old man undergoes a sigmoidoscopy for longstanding diarrhoea and weight loss. On visualization of the rectum, the mucosa appears inflamed and friable. A rectal biopsy is taken and the histology shows mucosal ulcers with inflammatory infiltrate, crypt abscesses with goblet cell depletion. From the list of answers below, which is the most likely diagnosis describing the histology report?

- A. Crohn's disease
- B. Pseudomembranous colitis
- C. Irritable bowel syndrome
- D. Ulcerative colitis
- E. No diagnosis – the report is inconclusive

34. Severity of ulcerative colitis

You are told by your registrar that one of the clinic patients has been admitted with a 'flare up' of ulcerative colitis (UC) which he reports as being severe. From the list of answers below, select the parameters which are likely to reflect a severe flare up of ulcerative colitis:

- A. Fewer than four bowel motions per day with large amounts of rectal bleeding
- B. Between four and six bowel motions per day with large amounts of rectal bleeding
- C. More than four bowel motions per day with large amounts of rectal bleeding
- D. More than five bowel motions per day with large amounts of rectal bleeding
- E. More than six bowel motions per day with large amounts of rectal bleeding

35. Investigating inflammatory bowel disease

You read a report which was handwritten in a patient's medical notes who you suspect has inflammatory bowel disease. The report reads, '... there is cobblestoning of the terminal ileum with the appearance of rose thorn ulcers. These findings are suggestive of Crohn's disease'. Select the most likely investigation that this report was derived from:

- A. Colonoscopy
- B. Sigmoidoscopy
- C. Barium follow through
- D. Abdominal CT
- E. Abdominal ultrasound

36. Management of ulcerative colitis

You are asked to see a 29-year-old woman diagnosed with ulcerative colitis 18 months ago. Over the last 4 days she has been experiencing slight abdominal cramps, opening her bowels approximately 4–5 times a day and has been passing small amounts of blood per rectum. The patient is alert and orientated and on examination her pulse is 67, blood pressure 127/70, temperature 37.3°C and her abdomen is soft with mild central tenderness. PR examination is nil of note. Blood tests reveal haemoglobin of 13.5 g/dL and a CRP of 9 mg/L. The most appropriate management plan for this patient is:

    A.   Admission to hospital for intravenous fluid therapy and steroids
    B.   Oral steroid therapy + oral 5-ASA + steroid enemas + discharge
    C.   Admission and refer to surgeons for further assessment
    D.   Oral steroid therapy and discharge home
    E.   Reassurance and discharge home with no treatment required

37. Crohn's disease

A 29-year-old anxious man is diagnosed with mild Crohn's disease. Due to time constraints, the patient was asked to come back for a follow-up appointment to discuss Crohn's disease in more detail. The patient returns with a list of complications he researched on the internet. Which of the following are not associated with Crohn's disease?

    A.   Cigarette smoking reduces incidence
    B.   Fistulae formation
    C.   Abscess formation
    D.   Non-caseating granuloma formation
    E.   Associated with transmural inflammation

38. Vitamin B$_{12}$ deficiency

You see a 40-year-old woman who was diagnosed with Crohn's disease ten years ago. Due to a severe attack of Crohn's which failed to respond to medical therapy, she had a small bowel resection. Your registrar tells you that she is at risk of developing vitamin B$_{12}$ deficiency as a result of her surgery. Which part of the small bowel is responsible for the absorption of vitamin B$_{12}$?

    A.   Jejunum
    B.   Proximal ileum
    C.   Duodenum
    D.   Terminal ileum
    E.   None of the above

39. Diarrhoea (3)

A 47-year-old woman has been experiencing a four-month history of diarrhoea and bloating. Associated symptoms include lethargy and weight loss. Full blood count reveals haemoglobin of 9.3 d/gL and MCV 70 fL. Which of the following investigations would be helpful in the patient's diagnosis?

   A. Anti-mitochondrial antibodies
   B. Anti-smooth muscle antibodies
   C. Anti-tissue transglutaminase antibodies
   D. Anti-nuclear antibodies
   E. Anti-neutrophil cytoplasmic antibodies

40. Weight loss

A 65-year-old man attends your clinic with a three-month history of weight loss of approximately 9 kg despite a normal appetite. A full blood count reveals that his haemoglobin is 9.0 g/dL (previous haemoglobin was 13.5 g/dL one year ago) and the MCV is 71 fL. Abdominal examination is unremarkable and per rectum exam is nil of note. The patient states that he has normal bowel habits and has been feeling quite tired lately. The most appropriate management is:

   A. Reassure and discharge
   B. Arrange an upper and lower GI endoscopy
   C. Prescribe iron tablet supplementation
   D. Arrange an abdominal ultrasound
   E. Arrange an abdominal x-ray

ANSWERS

Dysphagia

1 E Answers A–D are all termed obstructive causes of dysphagia. The causes can be categorized into:

- Obstructive
  - Oesophageal carcinoma
  - Peptic strictures (D)
  - Oesophageal web/ring (B)
  - Gastric carcinoma
  - Pharyngeal carcinoma (A)
  - Extrinsic pressure from, for example, lung carcinoma, retrosternal goitre (C)
- Oesophageal motility disorders
  - Achalasia (E)
  - Systemic sclerosis
  - Stroke
  - Myasthenia gravis
  - Neurological degenerative conditions, e.g. motor neurone disease, Parkinson's disease
- Others
  - Oesophagitis
  - Pharyngeal pouch
  - Oesophageal candidiasis

Abdominal pain

2 C Although all of the answers may present with abdominal pain, the key to the answer is in the history. Duodenal ulcers (C), which are four times more common than gastric ulcers, classically present with abdominal pain which is usually relieved after meals or drinking milk. Gastric ulcers (A) on the other hand present with abdominal pain which tends to worsen after meals. In either duodenal/gastric ulcers, weight loss may be an associated symptom, but this is usually more common in gastric ulcers. Patients who suffer from GORD (B) usually experience retrosternal discomfort ('heartburn') after meals and on lying flat. In addition, abdominal discomfort and pain in patients with gastritis (E) usually occurs after meals. Gastric carcinomas (D) tend to present with abdominal pain and drastic weight loss (e.g. 2–3 stone weight loss in the space of three months).

Management of peptic ulcer disease

3 A This patient has been diagnosed with a duodenal ulcer secondary to *H. pylori* infection. The CLO test (also known as the rapid urease test) is positive, confirming the presence of the bacterium. A 7-day course of 'triple therapy' (PPI + two antibiotics) is recommended for patients with duodenal ulcers positive for *H. pylori*. The eradication therapy regimen is based on twice daily dosing and, as well as aiming to clear the *H. pylori* infection with the antibiotics, the PPI is used to enhance the healing of the ulcer. Therefore in this scenario, (A) is the most appropriate from the list. For patients who are allergic to penicillin, clarithromycin and metronidazole can be used instead.

Peptic ulcer disease

4 B The most common causative agent that gives rise to approximately 90 per cent of duodenal ulcers is infection with *H. pylori* (B) (a helical-shaped gram-negative microaerophilic bacterium). The bacteria favours low pH environments and, with the help of its flagella, moves to the epithelial lining of the stomach and duodenum. The bacterium produces ammonia and proteases which break down the epithelial linings of the stomach and duodenal mucosa causing ulceration. Non-steroidal anti-inflammatory drugs (NSAIDs) (A), alcohol abuse (C), chronic corticosteroid therapy (D) and Zollinger–Ellison syndrome (E) (increase in gastrin production, from e.g. a gastrinoma, which stimulates the parietal cells of the stomach to produce excess hydrochloric acid leading to peptic ulceration) are all less common causes of peptic ulceration.

Investigation of gastro-oesophageal reflux disease

5 D All the above investigations have been shown to be useful in the diagnosis of a hiatus hernia. However, upper GI barium meals/swallows (D) have been shown to be the most definitive modality in diagnosing hiatus hernias. Chest x-rays (B) may be normal, but in some cases may show an air fluid level above the level of the left hemi-diaphragm. Upper GI endoscopy (C) is commonly used to assess symptoms of dyspepsia and has not been shown to be as sensitive as barium studies in the detection of hiatus hernias. In the UK, CT scanning (A) is not routinely used for the investigation of hiatus hernias, but the latter are incidentally detected on scanning of the abdomen for the investigation of other pathology. Compared to the barium study, CT scanning delivers relatively high levels of radiation. Positive results obtained with ultrasound scanning (E) may lead to inconsistent and false-positive/negative results due to the operator-associated variability regarding technical experience.

Complications of gastro-oesophageal reflux disease

6 A Barrett's oesophagus occurs as a result of chronic inflammation of the oesophagus, usually secondary to GORD. Typically, the lower third of the oesophagus is affected whereby the squamous cells are subjected to longstanding acid reflux from the stomach. This gives rise to chronic inflammation of the lower third of the oesophagus and results in metaplastic change of the squamous cells to columnar type which is thought to be an adaptive mechanism in withstanding the erosive action of the stomach acid. This metaplasia is described as a premalignant state and increases the risk of adenocarcinoma of the oesophagus. Diagnosis is made via upper GI endoscopy and biopsy.

Diarrhoea

7 B The history of the acute onset of diarrhoea coupled with nausea and vomiting a few hours after a meal is highly suggestive of a clinical diagnosis of gastroenteritis (B). Irritable bowel syndrome (A) sufferers usually experience chronic diarrhoea alternating with constipation. There is no history of blood-stained or mucus-based diarrhoea, which is usually seen in inflammatory bowel disease (C and E) (ulcerative/Crohn's colitis). With regard to the clinical scenario, the patient has no past medical history which therefore makes laxative abuse (D) very unlikely.

Management of diarrhoea

8 A Gastroenteritis is usually a self-limiting disease that often does not require pharmacological therapy. The mainstay of treatment is to advise patients to increase oral fluid intake (A) to compensate for the water lost from diarrhoea and vomiting. However, in some circumstances, where severe dehydration secondary to profuse diarrhoea exists (leading to confusion and hypotension) patients may warrant admission for intravenous fluid rehydration (C). Antibiotic therapy (B) and (D) is usually not indicated for gastroenteritis unless a bacterial organism has been isolated. The fact that the patient's observations are within the normal range and she is not systemically unwell, the most appropriate answer here would be to advise the patient on oral fluid rehydration followed by discharge.

Investigation of diarrhoea

9 C The most appropriate investigation for this patient would be to obtain a stool sample (C), especially if there is a history of travel. Performing tests such as full blood count (A), urea and electrolytes (B), abdominal x-ray (D) and liver function tests (**E**) would not change the management of this patient and hence in this scenario would not be indicated. A stool sample would enable the physician to isolate the causative organism (if present), which would consequently determine if antibiotic therapy is required.

Diarrhoea

10 E All of the organisms listed are known to cause diarrhoea in patients with gastroenteritis. From the list of answers, Campylobacter (**A**), *Salmonella* (**B**), *E. coli* (**C**) and *Shigella* (**D**) are bacteria known to cause bloody diarrhoea.

Hepatomegaly

11 B From the answers above, Budd–Chiari syndrome (**B**) (which presents with a triad of symptoms: acute abdominal pain, hepatomegaly and ascites), is the most likely cause of hepatomegaly. The condition results from hepatic vein outflow obstruction of which:

- there is no known cause in 50 per cent of sufferers;
- of the remaining 50 per cent of patients diagnosed with Budd–Chiari syndrome, 75 per cent of these are due to thrombosis of the hepatic vein (primary Budd–Chiari syndrome) and 25 per cent are due to external compression of the hepatic vein (secondary Budd–Chiari syndrome).

The causes of hepatomegaly can be classified according to:

1 Maligancy: primary (e.g. HCC) or secondary.

2 Hepatic congestion secondary to: right heart failure, Budd–Chiari syndrome.

3 Infection: hepatitis (secondary to viruses, malaria, shistosomiasis, amoebic abscess, hydatid cyst), infectious mononucleosis.

4 Haematological: leukaemia, lymphoma, myeloproliferative disorders, such as myelofibrosis, sickle-cell disease, haemolytic anaemias.

5 Anatomical: Riedel's lobe.

6 Other causes include early cirrhosis, fatty liver, porphyria, amyloidosis, Gaucher's disease.

Jaundice

12 A This patient has Gilbert's syndrome, an autosomal recessive (although some heterozygous cases have been reported in the Asian population) disorder characterized by unconjugated hyperbilirubinaemia. Genetic mutations in the gene responsible for coding for the enzyme uridine-diphosphoglucuronate glucuronosyltransferase results in decreased conjugation of bilirubin. Patients usually present in their adolescence with asymptomatic jaundice which is noticed after fasting, intercurrent illness (e.g. viral URTI), exercising or lack of sleep. In addition, exposure to certain drugs (e.g. chemotherapy) may precipitate jaundice. No treatment is usually required for Gilbert's syndrome. Therefore, from the answers, (A) is the most appropriate. The fact that the reticulocyte count is normal indicates that there is no haemolysis and hence there would be no need to refer to a haematologist (E) or start a course of oral steroids (B). Requesting an MRCP (D) or abdominal ultrasound (C) would not reveal any positive findings and is therefore not required.

Jaundice

13 A From the history, it is clear that the patient is suffering conjugated hyperbilirubinaemia with symptoms of jaundice coupled with dark urine and pale stools. The liver function tests support a diagnosis of cholestasis – bilirubin of 40 μmol/L, with an unparalleled rise in ALP (350 iu/L). AST and ALT are mildly elevated in comparison. Therefore, from the list of possible answers, gallstones (A) are the most likely diagnosis. With viral (B), alcoholic hepatitis (C) and autoimmune hepatitis (E) one would expect elevation in ALT and AST enzymes due to hepatocellular damage. There is no history of weight loss which makes pancreatic carcinoma (D) unlikely.

Investigation of jaundice

14 B The most appropriate imaging modality for the investigation of gallstones is abdominal ultrasound (B). This remains the imaging modality of choice. It is highly sensitive (gallstones are echogenic and will usually cast a 'shadow' on US), fast, non-invasive, free from radiation exposure and is relatively cheap compared to CT and MRI. Although patients who are admitted via accident and emergency with an acute abdomen will usually have an abdominal x-ray (A), this investigation is not done in attempting to detect gallstones as only 10 per cent are radiopaque. CT scanning (C) has been shown to be less sensitive than ultrasound scanning in the detection of gallstones and, in addition, delivers a very large quantity of radiation which can be avoided in this case. MRI (D) is not routinely performed for gallstone detection as it is costly, time consuming and, again, not as sensitive as ultrasound scanning. ERCP (E) is useful in the detection of gallstones within the common bile duct, but cannot clearly identify stones within the gallbladder and, being quite an invasive procedure, would not be recommended as first-line imaging in this scenario.

Drug induced cholestasis

15 A Drugs which are known to cause cholestasis include:

- Clavulanic acid
- Penicillins

- Oestrogens

- Erythromycin

- Chlorpromazine

Therefore, (A) would be the most likely drug to cause cholestasis. The drugs mentioned in answers B–E are not known to cause cholestasis.

Constipation

16 C Osmotic laxatives work by retaining fluid within the bowel. Examples include lactulose (C) (a semi-synthetic dissacharide which produces an osmotic diarrhoea), magnesium salts which are used when rapid bowel evacuation is required, sodium salts and phosphate enemas which are also used for rapid bowel evacuation. Senna (D) and docusate sodium (B), along with bisacodyl, are stimulant laxatives which work by increasing intestinal motility. Stimulant laxatives are not indicated in intestinal obstruction and should not be used for a long duration of time as this may give rise to colonic atony and hypokalaemia. Other forms of stimulant laxatives are the rectal stimulants such as glycerin suppositories. Ispaghula husk (A) and methylcellulose (E) are examples of bulking agents which increase faecal mass resulting in an increase in peristalsis. They are usually mixed with water before ingestion and are contraindicated in patients with intestinal obstruction, faecal impaction and swallowing difficulty.

Finger clubbing

17 B Inflammatory bowel disease (e.g. ulcerative colitis and Crohn's disease) is a known gastroenterological cause of finger clubbing along with liver cirrhosis, primary biliary cirrhosis, oesophageal leiyomyoma, coeliac disease and achalasia. Therefore, (B) is the most likely answer here.

Abdominal pain

18 E The patient's symptoms of epigastric pain and malaena point to a diagnosis of an upper GI bleed which can also present with haematemesis. The cause could possibly be due to a (recurrent) bleeding duodenal ulcer. The initial assessment/management of any acute medical condition should follow the 'ABC' (airway, breathing and circulation) route. Answers A–E are all steps in managing an upper GI bleed but, in this question, the most appropriate next step in management would be to insert two large bore cannulae and commence IV fluids (E). In addition, although not mentioned in the answer, taking blood for investigations (e.g. FBC, U&Es, coagulation screen, group and save, amylase and liver function tests) would also be performed when the cannulae are inserted. Once the patient has been stabilized haemodynamically (with IV fluids or blood if required in cases of severe anaemia), he/she is usually placed nil by mouth and an upper GI endoscopy is arranged to identify, and treat, any sites of bleeding. The Rockall score can be used to assess: (1) Risk of rebleeding/mortality pre-endoscopy; and (2) Risk of rebleeding/mortality post-endoscopy.

Causes of upper gastrointestinal bleeding

19 B Approximately 80 per cent of upper GI bleeds have known identifiable causes, some of which include:

- peptic ulcers – approximately 35–50 per cent of bleeds (B);
- Mallory–Weis tears – 15 per cent (A);
- oesophagitis – 5–15 per cent;
- gastritis and gastric erosions – 5–15 per cent;
- oesophageal varices – 5–10 per cent (C);
- drugs (e.g. NSAIDs, steroids, anticoagulants) – 5 per cent (D);
- upper GI malignancy – 5 per cent (E);
- rarer causes (<5 per cent):
  - Dieulafoy's lesion;
  - angiodysplasia;
  - haemobilia;
  - aorto-enteric fistula.

Management of oesophageal varices

20 D Oesophageal varices arise as a result of portal hypertension (>10 mmHg) which leads to dilated collateral veins at sites of portosystemic anastomsis (e.g. the lower oesophagus). The causes of portal hypertension can be divided into: (1) Pre-hepatic: portal-vein thrombosis, splenic vein thrombosis; (2) Hepatic: cirrhosis (accounts for 80 per cent of causes of portal hypertension), shistosomiasis (most common cause worldwide), sarcoidosis, myeloproliferative disease, congenital hepatic fibrosis; and (3) Post-hepatic: Budd–Chiari syndrome, right heart failure, constrictive pericarditis, veno-occlusive disease. Once portal pressures are >12 mmHg, variceal bleeding may develop. Prophylaxis for the prevention of variceal bleeding can be divided into: (1) Primary: non-selective β-blockade (e.g. propranolol) and/or endoscopic banding ligation; (2) Secondary (i.e. after an initial variceal bleed: non-selective β-blockade, endoscopic banding ligation, transjugular intrahepatic portosystemic shunting (TIPPS) for varices resistant to banding or surgical shunts if TIPPS is not possible.

Therefore, (**D**) is the most appropriate medication for prophylaxis in the prevention of variceal rebleeding.

Jaundice

21 C   This patient is suffering from drug-induced liver cirrhosis secondary to chronic amiodarone therapy. Amiodarone (**C**) along with other drugs, such as methyldopa and methotrexate, are known to induce liver cirrhosis. Liver cirrhosis is characterized, histologically, by a loss of the normal hepatic architecture coupled with bridging fibrosis and nodular regeneration. The causes of liver cirrhosis include chronic alcoholism, non-alcholic steatohepatitis, chronic hepatitis B and C infections, autoimmune conditions (e.g. auto-immune hepatitis, primary biliary cirrhosis, primary sclerosing cholangitis), genetic disorders (e.g. haemochromatosis, Wilson's disease), cryptogenic (in approximately 20 per cent), Budd–Chiari syndrome. In some cases, patients do not present with clinical signs although LFTs may show derangement. Some patients may show signs of chronic liver disease such as leuconychia, clubbing, palmar erythema, hyperdynamic circulation, Dupuytren's contracture, spider naevi, xanthelasma, gynaecomastia, atrophic testes, loss of body hair, hepatomegaly (occurs in initial stages then shrinks in late disease).

Investigations include:

- blood: FBC, LFTs, clotting studies (there is a decline in synthetic function of the liver leading to an elevated INR), iron studies, hepatitis serology, immunoglobulins, autoantibodies, AFP, caeruloplasmin , α_1-antitrypsin;

- liver ultrasound and duplex;

- MRI;

- ascitic tap for MC&S (spontaneous bacterial peritonitis (SBP)), protein content, LDH, glucose, cell count and biochemistry;

- liver biopsy – confirms diagnosis.

Complications of liver cirrhosis include: (1) Hepatic failure leading to conditions such as coagulopathy, encephalopathy, hypoalbuminaemia, sepsis and hypoglycaemia; (2) Portal hypertension leading to ascites, splenomegaly, oesophageal varices and other portosystemic shunts; (3) Increased risk of hepatocellular carcinoma. Management is targeted towards stopping/removing the underlying causative factor and to treat symptoms (e.g. cholestyramine can be used for pruritus, interferon-α treatment for HCV-induced cirrhosis, penicillamine for Wilson's disease). Ascites can be managed through fluid restriction, low salt diet, diuretics (e.g. spironolactone). If SBP is suspected (i.e. on a clinical basis before the

MC&S results of the ascitic tap are obtained), antibiotic treatment should commence.

Definitive treatment for liver cirrhosis is liver transplantation which increases the five-year survival from 20 to 70 per cent in end-stage disease.

Clinical signs of chronic liver disease

22 D Finger clubbing (A), palmar erythema (B), spider naevi (C) and jaundice (E) are all known clinical signs of chronic liver disease. Others include bruising and liver flap (secondary to hepatic encephalopathy). Koilonychia (D) refers to spooning of the nails and occurs in iron deficiency anaemia. It is leuconychia (whitening of the nails due to hypoalbuminaemia which can occur due to chronic liver disease, nephrotic syndrome, malnutrition) that is seen in chronic liver disease.

Alcoholic liver disease

23 E Macrocytosis, i.e. an elevated MCV (>96 fL) of which the causes can be seen in:

- megaloblastic anaemia secondary to vitamin B_{12} and folic acid deficiency;

- chronic alcoholism and/or alcoholic liver disease (most common causes of all causes of macrocytosis), pregnancy, hypothyroidism, reticulocytosis, aplastic anaemia, myelodysplastic syndromes and can also be caused by drugs that inhibit DNA synthesis (e.g. azathioprine);

an elevated MCV would suggest, along with the deranged LFTs, and support a diagnosis of alcoholic liver disease.

Therefore answers A–D are incorrect.

Deranged liver function

24 A This patient is suffering from primary biliary cirrhosis (PBC) (A) which is characterized by chronic granulomatous inflammation leading to damage of interlobular bile ducts. This chronic inflammatory process leads to cholestasis, cirrhosis and portal hypertension. The cause of PBC is thought to be of autoimmune origin (women being more affected than men) and is associated with various autoimmune conditions. Patients are often asymptomatic and diagnosis is usually made when abnormal LFTs are detected with an abnormal rise in serum ALP. Symptoms include lethargy and pruritus which can occur before the presentation of jaundice. Signs include jaundice, xanthelasma, xanthomata, skin pigmentation, splenomegaly and hepatomegaly. Investigations include blood tests: (1) LFTs (raised ALP, γ-GT, with mildly elevated AST and ALT. In late disease there is a raised bilirubin level and low levels of albumin with an increase in the prothrombin time); (2) Ninety-eight per cent of patients with PBC are anti-mitochondrial antibody (AMA) positive. ANA, SMA and ANCA autoantibodies may also be present but at low titres; (3) IgM (usually raised); (4) Raised levels of TSH and cholesterol may be present. Performing radiological imaging, such as ultrasound, will exclude extrahepatic cholestasis and liver biopsy will confirm granulomas (not specific to PBC) surrounding the bile ducts, progressing to cirrhosis.

Treatment is divided into:

- symptomatic – for symptoms of pruritus (e.g. colestyramine) , diarrhoea (e.g. codeine phosphate) and osteoporosis (e.g. bisphosphonates);

- specific – vitamin A, D, K supplementation, ursodeoxycholic acid for improving jaundice and ascites;

- liver transplantation for end-stage liver disease.

Wilson's disease (B) is an autosomal recessive disorder (of gene on chromosome 13 that codes for copper transporting ATPase) resulting in toxic accumulation of copper in the liver and central nervous system. Twenty-four hour urinary copper excretion is high ($>100\,\mu g/24\,h$ with normal levels being $<40\,\mu g$) with low copper and caeruloplasmin levels. Diagnosis can be confirmed by genetic testing and liver biopsy. Patients present with signs of liver disease. Kayser–Fleischer rings are pathognomonic (copper deposits in iris). Hereditary haemochromatosis (C) is an inherited condition characterized by a disorder in iron metabolism. There is increased intestinal iron absorption which is deposited in multiple organs such as the liver, heart, pancreas, etc. LFTS are usually elevated with raised ferritin and serum iron levels, and low total iron-binding capacity (TIBC). Diagnosis can be confirmed with HFE (mutation in HFE gene is responsible for hereditary haemochromatosis) genotyping and liver biopsy. Patients are initially asymptomatic then eventually experience arthralgia and tiredness with slate-grey skin pigmentation with late disease progression. Iron deposition also occurs in the pancreas leading to impaired insulin secretion and eventually diabetes (also known as bronze diabetes). Primary sclerosing cholangitis (D) is a condition of unknown cause which is defined by non-malignant, non-bacterial inflammation, fibrosis and strictures of the intra- and extrahepatic bile ducts. It is serum AMA negative but ANA, SMA and ANCA may be positive. Diagnosis is made with MRCP and liver biopsy. Patients are initially asymptomatic and may present with jaundice, pruritus, abdominal pain and fatigue. Alcoholic liver disease (E) is incorrect here as there is no mention, in the clinical scenario, of raised AST/ALT levels which would signify hepatocellular damage.

Ascites

25 E Ascites can be described as the pathological accumulation of fluid in the abdominal cavity. Ascites occur secondary to:

- conditions leading to venous hypertension (e.g. cirrhosis, congestive heart failure, constrictive pericarditis, Budd–Chiari syndrome, portal vein thrombosis);
- hypoalbuminaemia (e.g. nephrotic syndrome, malnutrition);
- malignant disease (e.g. secondary metastases of carcinomas of breast, ovary, colon);
- infections (e.g. tuberculosis);
- others (e.g. pancreatic disease, ovarian disease, myxoedema).

Answers A–D are all known causes of ascites that occur secondary to venous hypertension. Nephrotic syndrome (E), however, leads to ascites secondary to hypoalbuminaemia.

α_1-antitrypsin deficiency

26 C α_1-antitrypsin deficiency is an autosomal recessive disorder (C), which results from single amino acid substitutions at positions 264 and 342 on chromosome 14. α_1-antitrypsin is a serine protease, synthesized in the liver, required in controlling inflammatory cascades. The lack of this serine protease results in emphysema (75 per cent), chronic liver disease and hepatocellular carcinoma, asthma, pancreatitis, gallstones, Wegener's granulomatosis.

Patients with liver disease secondary to α_1-antitrypsin deficiency usually present with dyspnoea (from emphysema), liver cirrhosis, cholestatic jaundice. Investigations include: serum α_1-antitrypsin levels, liver biopsy, genetic phenotyping and DNA analysis at prenatal diagnosis. Management involves quitting smoking, augmentation therapy with α_1-antitrypsin pooled from human plasma and liver transplantation is the treatment of choice in decompensated cirrhosis.

Chronic liver disease

27 C This patient has symptoms of chronic liver disease secondary to auto-immune hepatitis (AIH) which is indicated from the history (no history of excessive alcohol consumption), negative viral serology and positive SLA autoantibody. AIH is an inflammatory liver disease of unknown cause which is characterized by suppressor T-cell defects which are directed against hepatocyte surface antigens. Three types of AIH have been identified according to the various autoantibodies detected (e.g. Type-1: anti-smooth muscle antibodies, antinuclear antibodies; type-2:

anti-liver/kidney microsomal type 1 antibodies; and type-3: antibodies against soluble liver antigen or liver–pancreas antigen). AIH is known to affect women (young and middle-aged) with 25 per cent presenting with acute hepatitis and signs of autoimmune disease (e.g. polyarthralgia, glomerulonephritis, pernicious anaemia, PSC). The remaining patients are asymptomatic and are diagnosed when signs of chronic liver disease develop. Investigations include: (1) Blood: LFTs, immunoglobulins (e.g. IgG), auto-antibodies (see above) and FBC (may show low WCC and platelets); (2) liver biopsy may reveal mononuclear infiltration, fibrosis or cirrhosis; and (3) MRCP to exclude PSC. Management involves: (1) Symptomatic treatment for chronic liver disease; (2) immunosuppressant therapy: Corticosteroid therapy (e.g. prednisolone) or steroid-sparing agent such as azathioprine can be used; and (3) liver transplantation is indicated for decompensated liver cirrhosis or failure to respond to medical treatment.

Primary sclerosing cholangitis

28 D Eighty to 100 per cent of patients with PSC will have ulcerative colitis (D). On the other hand, 3 per cent of patients with ulcerative colitis will have PSC. Thyroid disease (A), systemic sclerosis (B) and rheumatoid arthritis (C) are associated with primary biliary cirrhosis.

Complications of primary sclerosing cholangitis

29 B Twenty to 30 per cent of patients diagnosed with PSC are more likely to develop cholangiocarcinoma, which is defined as a malignancy of the biliary tree. Other causes include flukes (in the East), congenital biliary cysts and N-nitroso toxins. Patients may present with fever, abdominal pain with or without ascites, and jaundice. LFTs show raised bilirubin with highly elevated ALP. Ultrasound scanning may be performed to detect lesions and ERCP and biopsy is diagnostic. Seventy per cent of cholangiocarcinomas cannot be surgically resected. Of those treated through the surgical route (hepatectomy and extrahepatic bile duct excision and caudate lobe resection), 76 per cent recur. For tumours that cannot be surgically treated, palliative stenting may be conducted to improve quality of life. Hepatocellular carcinoma (A) is a malignant tumour of hepatocytes and accounts for approximately 90 per cent of primary liver tumours. Causes include viral hepatitis, cirrhosis (related to alcohol, PBC, haemochromotosis), aflatoxin, parasites such as *Clonorchis sinensis* and anabolic steroids. Hepatic fibroma (C) and haemangiomas (D) are benign liver tumours which do not usually require treatment. They are not related with PSC. Pancreatic carcinoma (E), although a possible answer, is unlikely here as patients with PSC do not have an increased chance of developing this condition.

Liver tumours

30 C Benign primary liver tumours include:

- haemangiomas (most common);

- adenomas (C);

- cysts;

- focal nodular hyperplasia;

- fibromas;

- leiyomyomas.

The malignant primary liver tumours include:

- hepatocellular carcinoma (accounts for 90 per cent of primary liver tumours);

- cholangiocarcinoma;

- angiosarcoma (A);

- hepatoblastoma (D);

- fibrosarcoma (B);

- leiyomyosarcoma (E).

Hepatocellular carcinoma

31 A Fifty to 80 per cent of hepatocellular carcinomas are associated with high serum levels of α-fetoprotein (AFP), a tumour marker, which is also linked to, and elevated in, testicular carcinomas. Serum levels of AFP can be monitored either post-surgical resection (if the tumour is solitary) or post chemotherapy; falling or rising levels post treatment could be indicative of disease remission or progression, respectively. CEA (B) is primarily linked with colorectal carcinoma. CA 15-3 (C) is linked with breast carcinoma. HcG(D) and CA 125 (E) are usually associated with ovarian carcinoma.

Jaundice

32 D The patient is exhibiting Courvoisier's law which states that a palpable gallbladder in the presence of painless jaundice is unlikely due to gallstones. In this scenario, it is likely that the patient's symptoms of painless jaundice, dark urine and pale stools coupled with drastic weight loss point to a diagnosis of carcinoma of the head of the pancreas. Risk factors include smoking, chronic excessive alcohol consumption, diabetes mellitus, high fat diet and chronic pancreatitis. Patients usually present with symptoms of painless cholestatic jaundice, weight loss, diabetes or acute pancreatitis. Some rare features include thrombophlebitis migrans, hypercalcaemia, portal hypertension and nephrosis. Signs include jaundice, palpable gallbladder, epigastric mass, hepatomegaly, splenomegaly, lymphadenopathy and ascites. Investigations include blood tests (FBC, LFTs), imaging modalities such as abdominal ultrasound and abdominal CT (B) (which can also be used for guided biopsies of lesions and staging before surgical intervention), ERCP (E) (may be able to localize site of obstruction leading to cholestasis) and endoscopic sonography (has been shown to be the most accurate diagnostic and staging tool). Referring to the question, the most appropriate answer would be to initially request an abdominal ultrasound (B) which would provide non-invasive imaging of the pancreas.   (D)

Rectal biopsy

33 D The most likely diagnosis is ulcerative colitis (UC) (D) based on the histological results of the rectal biopsy. The findings of inflammatory infiltrates coupled with mucosal ulcers, goblet cell depletion and crypt abscesses are highly suggestive of a diagnosis of UC. UC is described as a relapsing and remitting inflammatory bowel disorder of the colonic mucosa. The condition usually starts at the rectum (proctitis in 50 per cent) and spreads proximally, in a continuous fashion, to affect parts of the colon (e.g. left-sided colitis in 30 per cent) or the entire colonic tract (pancolitis in 20 per cent). UC tends not to spread beyond the ileocaecal valve but may cause a condition called 'backwash ileitis'. Histologically, Crohn's disease (A) is characterized by transmural, non-caseating granulomatous inflammation, coupled with fissuring ulcers, lymphoid aggregates and neutrophil infiltrates. Crohn's disease can affect any part of the GI tract from the mouth to the anus (but favours the terminal ileum in 50 per cent) and is also characterized by skip lesions (unaffected bowel between areas of active disease) whereas in UC, disease spreads from the rectum to the ileocaecal valve in a continuous fashion depending on the stage of disease. Pseudomembranous colitis (PC) (B) is characterized by the formation of an adherent inflammatory membrane (the pseudomembrane) overlying sites of muscosal injury within the colon. The histology of PC is described as small surface erosions of the superficial colonic crypts coupled with overlying accumulation of neutrophils, fibrin, mucus and necrotic epithelial cells forming a 'summit lesion'. The toxins (toxin A and B) produced by the gram-positive anaerobic bacillus, *Clostridum difficile*, are meant to be the cause of PC.

There is normal histology of the bowel in irritable bowel syndrome (C).

Severity of ulcerative colitis

34 E Using the Truelove and Witts criteria, which asseses the severity of UC, patients with UC opening their bowels greater than six times a day, and passing large amounts of blood per rectum, are considered to have severe UC. The other parameters that are recognized under the severe UC category are body temperature >37.8°C, a pulse rate >90 beats per minute, a haemoglobin <10.5 g/dl and an ESR >30 mm/h.

Moderate UC is defined as opening bowels between four and six times a day and passing moderate amounts of blood per rectum, body temperature between 37.1 and 37.8°C, a pulse rate between 70 and 90 beats per minute and haemoglobin between 10.5 and 11 g/dL.

Mild UC is classified as experiencing fewer than four bowel motions per day and passing small amounts, if not no blood, per rectum, normal body temperature, pulse rate <70, haemoglobin of >11 g/dL and an ESR of <30 mm/h.

Investigating inflammatory bowel disease

35 C The appearance of 'cobblestoning' and 'rose thorn ulcers' are radiological descriptions, seen in Crohn's disease, obtained from barium follow-through (C) investigations of the ileum. Lower GI endoscopy is preferred in establishing a diagnosis of IBD (either Crohn's or UC) because the operator is allowed direct visualization of the bowel and biopsies may be taken; skip lesions can be seen on direct visualization but the appearance of 'rose thorn ulcers' have only been described in barium radiography studies.

Management of ulcerative colitis

36 B From the patient's symptoms and signs, it is evident that she is experiencing a moderate flare-up of UC (Truelove and Witts criteria in the assessment of severity of UC). Treatment of UC flare-ups is targeted at inducing and maintaining remission. In this question, the patient, although experiencing mild abdominal cramps, frequent bowel motions and passing small amounts of blood per rectum, is systemically well. In addition, her haemoglobin levels are within normal range and her CRP is <10 mg/dL. Therefore, based on the information from the patient's history coupled with the blood test results, hospital admission would not be warranted. This patient can be treated as an outpatient and followed up either in clinic or by her GP. In terms of treatment regimens for moderate UC, patients are usually started on a course of steroids (e.g. 40 mg of prednisolone), which is decreased on a weekly basis coupled with twice daily 5-ASA (e.g. mesalazine) and topical treatment of per rectum steroid foams (e.g. hydrocortisone). If symptoms do not resolve in 10–14 days, the patient is usually treated as severe UC. For mild UC, the aim of treatment again is to induce and maintain remission. This involves commencing a tapering dose of oral steroids with a 5-ASA. In some patients with distal disease, the use of steroid foams per rectum has shown to be of benefit. If symptoms improve, 5-ASA foams can be used instead of steroid foams. However, if symptoms do not improve in 10–14 days, the patient is usually treated as moderate UC. In severe UC, patients are usually admitted for intravenous fluid and steroid (e.g. IV hydrocortisone) therapy. Rectal steroids are also given. Patients are monitored closely and are examined on a twice daily basis to assess for abdominal distension, bowel sounds and abdominal tenderness. Worsening of these signs may be suggestive of toxic dilatation of the colon which would require surgical intervention due to the high risk of bowel perforation.

Therefore, (B) is the most appropriate management plan.

Crohn's disease

37 A Answers B–E are all facts that are associated with Crohn's disease, whereas cigarette smoking has been reported to increase the incidence of Crohn's disease but has found to be protective in UC; 70–80 per cent of non-smokers have UC compared to 50–60 per cent of patients who are smokers with Crohn's disease.

Vitamin B$_{12}$ deficiency

38 D The terminal ileum is responsible for the absorption of vitamin B$_{12}$. If this vitamin is not supplemented, the patient will experience symptoms of glossitis, neuropathy, macrocytic anaemia. The proximal ileum is responsible for absorption of vitamin B$_2$ and vitamin C. The jejunum is responsible for the absorption of vitamin D, folic acid and nicotinamide. The duodenum is responsible for the absorption of the minerals calcium and iron.

Diarrhoea

39 C The patient is suffering from coeliac disease which is a T-cell mediated autoimmune disease of the small bowel characterized by intolerance to alcohol-soluble proteins in wheat, barley, rye and oats (also known as prolamin) leading to villous atrophy and malabsorption.

Patients may present with steatorrhoea, diarrhoea, abdominal pain and bloating, nausea and vomiting, signs of microcytic anaemia (secondary to iron deficiency) or macrocytic anaemia (secondary to vitamin B$_{12}$ or folate deficiency), weight loss, failure to thrive in children.

Diagnosis is made by:

- testing for antibodies: α-gliadin, tissue transglutaminase and anti-endomysial (an IgA antibody which is 95 per cent specific for coeliac disease unless the patient is IgA deficient);

- duodenal biopsy which can be performed at upper GI endoscopy.

Aim of treatment is to completely avoid gluten-containing food.

From the list of answers, (C) is therefore the correct answer.

Weight loss

40 B This patient is suffering from iron deficiency anaemia which could potentially be secondary to an upper or lower GI malignancy. The fact that there has been drastic weight loss despite no change in appetite suggests a cachectic process. In addition, there has been a 4.5 g/dL drop in the patient's haemoglobin. Tying in these clinical findings, ruling out a malignancy should be the priority. Therefore, from the list of answers above, the most appropriate plan of management would be to arrange an upper and lower GI endoscopy (B).

SECTION 4: RENAL

QUESTIONS

1. Haematuria (1)

A 21-year-old man presents with painless haematuria which he has noticed in the last 3 days. He suffers from type 1 diabetes which is well controlled, but is otherwise fit and healthy. The patient has recently recovered from a mild throat infection. Urine dipstick analysis reveals blood and protein in the urine. The most likely diagnosis is:

A. Henoch–Schonlein purpura
B. Benign prostate hypertrophy
C. IgA nephropathy
D. Diabetic nephropathy
E. Urinary tract infection (UTI)

2. Hyponatraemia

A 74-year-old type 2 diabetic woman undergoes a bowel resection for cancer of the colon. She is well prior to the operation with well–controlled diabetes and no other underlying disease. The operation is successful and the patient is given postoperative insulin and IV dextrose. Two days after the operation she becomes very agitated.

Sodium	124	(135–145)
Potassium	3.3	(3.5–5.0)
Urea	3.1	(3.0–7.0)
Glucose	7.2	(2.5–6.0)
Serum osmolality	265	(275–295)
Urine osmolality	150	

The most likely cause of the hyponatraemia is:

A. Addison's disease
B. Syndrome of inappropriate anti-diuretic hormone (SIADH)
C. Diabetic nephropathy
D. Excess insulin
E. Water overload

3. Fever

A 16-year-old boy presents with a low-grade fever which started 1 week ago. The patient also reports feeling fatigued and indicates pain in his joints. His parents mention that he has been visiting the toilet more often than usual. A urine dipstick shows trace proteins, while a blood test shows raised eosinophils. The most likely diagnosis is:

    A. Acute tubulointerstitial nephritis
    B. Renal failure
    C. Diabetes mellitus
    D. UTI
    E. Reactive arthritis

4. Pitting oedema

A 58-year-old African man presents with pitting oedema of his ankles. He suffers from recently diagnosed hypertension, but is otherwise healthy. Blood results show low albumin and a urine dipstick is positive for protein. The most appropriate initial treatment is:

    A. High protein diet
    B. Diuretics
    C. Prophylactic anticoagulation
    D. ACE inhibitor
    E. Bed rest

5. Flank pain

A 33-year-old woman presents to accident and emergency with severe right flank pain. The pain started 3 hours ago and is not constant, occasionally moving towards her right iliac fossa. The patient also feels nauseous and has a low-grade fever. The most appropriate investigation is:

    A. Abdominal x-ray
    B. Magnetic resonance imaging (MRI) scan
    C. Intravenous urography
    D. Computed tomography (CT) scan
    E. Abdominal ultrasound (US) scan

6. Dysuria

A 42-year-old diabetic Asian male complains of dysuria, increased urinary frequency and general malaise for the past six months. In the last few days, he has noticed blood in the urine. Examination of the urine shows the presence of neutrophils with no organisms detected on urine culture. The most likely diagnosis is:

- A. Tuberculosis
- B. Renal cell cancer
- C. Diabetic nephropathy
- D. Bladder cancer
- E. Nephritic syndrome

7. Periorbital oedema

A 17-year-old patient is referred by his GP after presenting with periorbital oedema. The patient noticed the oedematous eyes 3 days ago, but reports feeling unwell since a throat infection 3 weeks ago with nausea and vomiting in the last week. A urine dipstick is positive for protein and blood while serum creatinine and urea are mildly deranged. The most likely diagnosis is:

- A. Nephrotic syndrome
- B. Nephritic syndrome
- C. Renal failure
- D. Glomerulonephritis
- E. Von Grawitz tumour

8. Urinary tract infection in pregnancy

A 28-year-old woman patient who is 13 weeks pregnant presents for an antenatal clinic appointment. The patient feels embarrassed when asked to provide a urine sample and produces enough for a urine dipstick test only which is positive for leukocytes and nitrites. The patient denies any symptoms. The most appropriate treatment is:

- A. Trimethoprim
- B. Quinolone
- C. Tetracycline
- D. Cephalexin
- E. Ampicillin

9. Distress

A 32-year-old builder presents in accident and emergency in a distressed state. He reports suffering from chest pain for the last 2 weeks, the pain is sharp and only occurs when he moves heavy objects. He has a family history of cardiovascular disease and is worried about a heart attack. His blood gas findings are as follows: $pH = 7.47$; $PCO_2 = 3.3$; $PO_2 = 15.3$; bicarbonate $= 17.53$. The most likely diagnosis is:

    A. Respiratory acidosis with metabolic compensation
    B. Acute metabolic acidosis
    C. Respiratory alkalosis with metabolic compensation
    D. Metabolic acidosis with respiratory compensation
    E. Acute respiratory alkalosis

10. Nocturia

A 21-year-old woman complains of urinary frequency, nocturia, constipation and polydipsia. Her symptoms started 2 weeks ago and prior to this she would urinate twice a day and never at night. She has also noticed general malaise and some pain in her left flank. A urine dipstick is normal. The most appropriate investigation is:

    A. Serum phosphate
    B. Serum calcium
    C. Parathyroid hormone (PTH)
    D. Plasma glucose
    E. Serum potassium

11. Breathlessness

A 58-year-old man presents with breathlessness, he reports feeling unwell over the last three months with nausea, vomiting and difficulty breathing. You notice his ankles are swollen and he has bruises on his arms. The patient mentions he has not been urinating as often as normal. The most appropriate investigation is:

    A. Urine microscopy
    B. Renal ultrasound
    C. Serum electrolytes, urea and creatinine
    D. Renal biopsy
    E. Chest x-ray

12. Abdominal pain

A 24-year-old man presents with a four-month history of abdominal pain which has been getting worse. The patient describes the pain as generalized, dull in character and does not radiate but often occurs alongside loin pain. An irregular mass is palpable in both flanks and a mid-systolic click can be auscultated. The most appropriate investigation is:

A. MRI scan
B. Abdominal US scan
C. Excretion urography
D. CT scan
E. Abdominal x-ray

13. Proteinuria

A 55-year-old woman is seen in clinic, she has a ten-year history of type 2 diabetes treated with glibenclamide. Her blood pressure is 148/93 with new onset proteinuria, her serum results show elevated lipid levels, glycated haemoglobin of 5.5 per cent and fasting glucose of 6.0 mmol/L. A renal biopsy shows the presence of Kimmelstiel–Wilson lesions. The most appropriate management is:

A. Increase oral hypoglycaemic dosage
B. Angiotensin II receptor agonist (or blocker)
C. Start cholesterol lowering therapy
D. Start ACE inhibitors
E. Start renal dialysis

14. Weight loss

A 52-year-old man complains of a 3-week history of malaise and shortness of breath. He has lost weight in the last few months but attributes this to a loss of appetite possibly due to stress at work. On examination, he has a palpable mass in the right lumbar region. He has no urinary symptoms. However, the urine dipstick detected blood. The most likely diagnosis is:

A. Renal abscess
B. Renal cyst
C. Renal carcinoma
D. Adrenal tumour
E. Pyelonephritis

15. Hypercalciuria

A 37-year-old man presents with a 5-day history of haematuria. Abdominal examination is unremarkable. Urine analysis reveals hypercalciuria and excretion urography reveals small calculi within the papilla of the patient's right kidney. The patient has presented several times in the past with UTIs and renal stones, but is otherwise healthy. The most likely diagnosis is:

    A.   Medullary sponge kidney
    B.   Renal cell carcinoma
    C.   Medullary cystic disease
    D.   Horse-shoe kidney
    E.   Tertiary hyperparathyroidism

16. Long-term ibuprofen use

A 38-year-old woman presents to her GP with a 2-week history of dysuria, haematuria and shortness of breath. She suffers from chronic headaches and has been taking ibuprofen in order to treat them. She has a history of cardiovascular disease in the family and a friend recommended she use aspirin to keep healthy. The most appropriate investigation is:

    A.   Retrograde pyelography
    B.   Renal biopsy
    C.   Abdominal x-ray
    D.   Antegrade pyelography
    E.   CT scan of the kidney

17. Oliguria

A 64-year-old man is undergoing treatment for polycythaemia vera with chemotherapy, he has no other medical problems. Shortly after starting treatment, the patient becomes lethargic, feels unwell and suffers weight loss. He attributes this is to the chemotherapy. After 2 weeks, the patient becomes oliguric, complains of bilateral flank pain and becomes oedematous. The most likely diagnosis is:

    A.   Analgesic nephropathy
    B.   Renal infarction
    C.   Hyperuricaemic nephropathy
    D.   Acute tubulointerstitial nephritis
    E.   Chronic renal failure

18. Collapse

A 67-year-old diabetic female is brought into accident and emergency following a collapse at her home. She was found by her daughter who said she saw the patient going to the toilet and then hearing her collapse. The patient did not lose consciousness and appears well. Her supine blood pressure is 100/70 and standing 115/79. Urine dipstick is positive for glucose, nitrates, leukocytes and haematuria. The most likely diagnosis is:

A. Diabetic ketoacidosis
B. UTI
C. Orthostatic hypotension
D. Diabetic nephropathy
E. Hypoglycaemia

19. Sacral oedema

An 18-year-old man presents with general malaise and lethargy for the last 2 weeks, he denies any weight loss and has maintained a good appetite. On examination, there are no abnormalities except for sacral oedema and a polyphonic wheeze. Urine dipstick is positive for protein only and blood pressure is 140/90. The most likely diagnosis is:

A. Nephritic syndrome
B. Nephrotic syndrome
C. Goodpasture's disease
D. Thin-basement membrane nephropathy
E. Minimal change glomerulonephritis

20. Haematuria (2)

A 6-year-old has a sore throat and has been given antibiotics. Three weeks later, he represents feeling feverish with nausea, vomiting and tea-coloured urine. Urine dipstick confirms haematuria and protein. Blood pressure is 100/60 mmHg. The most likely diagnosis is:

A. Nephritic syndrome
B. UTI
C. Acute tubulointerstitial nephritis
D. Minimal change glomerulonephritis
E. Post streptococcal glomerulonephritis

21. Haematuria (3)

A 21-year-old man complains his urine has turned a faint red in the last week. He denies any significant changes in his diet or lifestyle and has no other medical problems except for sensorineural deafness diagnosed when he was young. On examination, you notice retinal flecks and urine dipstick confirms protein and blood. The most likely diagnosis is:

A. Alport's syndrome
B. Benign familial haematuria
C. Wolfram syndrome
D. IgA nephropathy
E. Down's syndrome

22. Chronic cigarette smoking

A 65-year-old overweight man presents with a 2-week history of haematuria. The patient denies any other symptoms and his blood pressure is 128/83 mmHg. He suffers from no other medical problems but admits to being a chronic smoker since the age of 16. He has tried to lose weight using herbal remedies for three years, but he has only noticed significant weight loss in the last week despite stopping the remedies months ago. The most likely diagnosis is:

A. Chinese herb nephropathy
B. Bladder cancer
C. Schistosomiasis
D. Acute tubulointerstitial nephritis
E. Renal cancer

23. Abdominal aortic aneurysm rupture

A 53-year-old man with HIV suffers a ruptured aortic aneurysm and is rushed into theatre, he undergoes a successful operation and is recovering on the wards in a stable condition. One day after the operation, he becomes oliguric with mildly elevated urea and creatinine. After 1 week, he becomes polyuric with a GFR of 30. The most likely diagnosis is:

A. Haemolytic–uraemic syndrome
B. Acute tubular necrosis
C. SIADH
D. HIV nephropathy
E. Acute renal failure

24. C-ANCA positive assay

A 64-year-old woman with type 1 diabetes presents to clinic with several months of sinus problem and a 4-day history of oliguria. Her blood pressure is 137/80, serum results show mildly elevated urea and creatinine, absence of anti-GBM antibodies, while a C-ANCA assay is positive. Red blood cell (RBC) casts are present in the urine and her renal biopsy reveals glomerular crescents. The most likely diagnosis is:

A. Post-streptococcal glomerulonephritis
B. Goodpasture's syndrome
C. Minimal change glomerulonephritis
D. Rapidly progressive glomerulonephritis
E. Wegener's granulomatosis

25. Abdominal bruits

A 68-year-old obese Asian man is seen in the hypertension clinic. His blood pressure is 151/93 and he suffers from poorly controlled type 2 diabetes. Blood results demonstrate elevated serum urea and creatinine. An ultrasound scan shows asymmetry between the two kidneys and on examination audible abdominal bruits are auscultated. Urine dipstick did not detect any blood or protein. The best investigation is:

A. CT angiography
B. Doppler ultrasonography
C. Abdominal x-ray
D. Renal arteriography
E. Renal biopsy

26. Suprapubic pain

A 63-year-old woman presents in accident and emergency with a 3-day history of worsening abdominal pain and mild flank pain. Examination reveals pain in the suprapubic region, but otherwise the abdomen is soft with no masses. The patient denies any other symptoms, such as dysuria, but mentions she has had difficulty passing urine in the last week and is only able to provide a small urine sample which is odorous and bloody. She has no other medical problems, but admits to being a long-term smoker. An ultrasound scan of renal system is most likely to show:

A. Bladder dilation
B. Ureteral stricture
C. Bilateral hydronephrosis
D. Renal cysts
E. Renal cancer

27. Type 1 diabetes

A 19-year-old man is recently diagnosed with type 1 diabetes and attends your clinic to ask about possible complications in the future. He mentions an uncle who has end-stage renal disease due to poorly controlled diabetes and specifically enquires about testing for early signs of renal impairment. The most appropriate investigation is:

    A. Blood pressure
    B. Microalbuminuria
    C. Serum creatinine
    D. Serum electrolytes
    E. Urine dipstick for glucose

28. Periorbital oedema

A 21-year-old man presents with lethargy over the last week, he has periorbital oedema and proteinuria. The patient mentions he has been to hospital a number of times in the past due to the same symptoms as well as mild eczema. Light microscopy of a renal biopsy showed normal morphology. Electron microscopy of the renal biopsy reveals the diffuse effacement of the epithelial podocytes. The most appropriate treatment is:

    A. Cyclosporin
    B. No treatment
    C. Probenecid
    D. Renal transplant
    E. Oral prednisone

29. Hyperphosphataemia

A 49-year-old woman attends your clinic suffering from chronic renal failure due to progressive glomerular disease. She appears well and her blood pressure is 141/92 mmHg. Blood tests reveal elevated phosphate, serum creatinine and urea, while calcium levels are low. Her estimated glomerular filtration rate is 35 mL/min/1.73 m^2. You also notice the patient's cholesterol levels are moderately raised. The most appropriate management is:

    A. Sevelamer
    B. Parathyroidectomy
    C. Oral vitamin D
    D. Cinacalcet
    E. Renal dialysis

30. Rigors

A 66-year-old woman with poorly controlled type 2 diabetes presents to accident and emergency with a 2-day history of severe pain in the right flank, nausea and fevers that come and go. On examination, the patient appears unwell, sweaty and has visible rigors with a temperature of 38°C. The patient denies any recent travel. Urine dipstick is positive for protein, blood, leukocytes and nitrites. A CT scan of the abdomen reveals gas in the renal parenchyma area. The most likely diagnosis is:

A. Renal stones
B. Renal infarction
C. Diabetic nephropathy
D. Renal TB
E. Pyelonephritis

ANSWERS

Haematuria

1 C   Haematuria may be macroscopic with blood evident in the urine or microscopic requiring urine dipstick testing. The anatomical origin of macroscopic haematuria can often be deduced from its presentation in the urine, although this should not be relied upon. Bleeding from the bladder or above usually presents throughout voiding, terminal bladder or prostatic bleeding occurs at the end of voiding, while urethral sites present at the beginning. Microscopic haematuria identified by urine dipstick requires microscopic analysis to confirm red blood cell presence. Red cell casts are red blood cells that have leaked into renal tubules and clump together forming a cast-like structure which is excreted into the urine. The presence of red cell casts are therefore strongly suggestive of glomerular pathology. False-positive results may arise from haemoglobin or myoglobin in the urine. IgA nephropathy or Berger's disease (C) is the most common cause of glomerulonephritis and may present at any age. Haematuria is usually macroscopic and occurs in intervals corresponding with glomerular attacks, infections such as pharyngitis can exacerbate the condition. Henoch–Schonlein purpura (A) differs from Berger's disease through more systemic involvement, often presenting with arthritis of the large joints, abdominal pain and a characteristic purpuric rash of the extensor skin surfaces. The absence of pain and genital symptoms excludes a UTI (E). Diabetic nephropathy (D) typically presents with proteinuria and not haematuria. Benign prostatic hypertrophy (B) occurs in much older patients often alongside poor urine flow.

Hyponatraemia

2 E   This patient has a significant hyponatraemia with a mildly low potassium level and low osmolality. Sodium homeostasis involves insensible and obligatory loss followed by the dominant influence of the kidney. Factors controlling sodium reabsorption include the renin-angiotensin-aldosterone system, natriuretic peptides and indirectly anti-diuretic hormone (ADH). Hyponatraemia arising from water overload (E) often occurs in patients following surgical procedures with inappropriate fluid management. In this case, excess dextrose solution causes dilutional hyponatraemia resulting in acute delirium. Addison's disease (A) results in a deficiency of mineralocorticoid activity causing an accumulation of potassium and reduced sodium reabsorption which is not reflected in the patient's biochemistry results. The SIADH (B) is due to inappropriately elevated levels of ADH which leads to increased retention of water causing hyponatraemia and reduced serum osmolality. The syndrome does not typically cause hypokalaemia and the urine would be more concentrated

due to water reabsorption. Diabetic nephropathy (C) is a progressive disease that arises in diabetic patients, pathology is characterized by an initial increase in glomerular filtration rate and glomerular basement membrane hypertrophy. As the disease progresses, glomerulosclerosis occurs as a result of accumulation of extracellular matrix and destroying the filtering ability of the glomerular membrane. This allows protein leakage. Severe diabetic nephropathy may present with symptoms of the nephrotic syndrome and acute derangement of biochemistry does not occur. Excess insulin injection (D) would cause hypoglycaemia and a reduction in potassium due to a shift of potassium to the intracellular compartment. Patients become irritable, sweat and eventually can fall into a coma.

Fever

3 A   The majority of tubulointerstitial nephritis (A) is due to drug hypersensitivity reactions, most commonly penicillin or non-steroidal anti-inflammatory drugs which are commonly given. Patients typically present with fever, skin rashes and may also have painful joints. Blood results will often have raised eosinophils. Eosinophils are involved in allergic responses, such as asthma and drugs, parasitic infection and also tissue inflammation. Renal failure (B) is the sudden loss of renal function which in the acute phase is reversible, plasma urea and creatinine typically increase due to the loss of filtering function of the kidney and patients tend to be oliguric rather than polyuric. In diabetes (C), although patients would tend to visit the toilet more due to hyperglycaemia causing an osmotic diuresis, other important features would include weight loss, polydipsia and the presence of glucose and possibly ketones on urine dipstick. A UTI (D) is characterized by features that include dysuria, elevated white cell count and raised leukocytes and nitrites in the urine. Reiter's disease (E) is a sterile synovitis that typically follows an infection and involves the classical triad of urethritis, arthritis and conjunctivitis.

Pitting oedema

4 B   This patient has the classic triad of proteinuria, low serum albumin and oedema that occurs in the nephrotic syndrome. This can occur due to a number of disease processes such as diabetes and SLE, as well as those specific to the kidney, including minimal-change nephropathy and focal-segmental glomerulosclerosis. First-line management should include dietary measures to restrict sodium intake and a diuretic (B). Potental diuretics include furosemide which is often required to control any associated severe oedema. High protein diets (A) do not have any benefit to the management of nephrotic syndrome, a normal low salt diet should be encouraged. Albumin infusion can be used as adjuncts in patients who are resistant to diuretic therapy but never in isolation as they have transient beneficial effects. Bed rest (E) should also be discouraged in patients since coagulation factors, for example antithrombin, are also lost as part of the proteinuria creating a hypercoagulable state, patients are therefore at risk of thromboembolism, including renal vein thrombosis. Therefore, prophylactic anticoagulation (C) is desirable to protect against hypercoagulation and should always be considered, Angiotensin-converting enzyme (ACE) inhibitors (D) protect against proteinuria by reducing the filtration pressure upon the glomerular capillaries.

Flank pain

5 E   This patient has a suspected renal stone, the most useful investigation would be an abdominal ultrasound scan (E) specifically of the kidneys, ureters and bladder (KUB). The differential diagnosis should include other causes of abdominal pain, such as acute appendicitis. The most common stone consists of calcium oxalate and up to 80 per cent of renal stones are visible on ultrasound. The KUB US scan is poor at differentiating different stones and can often miss smaller stones. Intravenous urography (IVU) (C) is more useful for detecting obstructions in the renal tract and US scans should always be done before IVU as smaller stones often become non-visible. IVU is also more invasive than US scanning with particular risk from contrast-induced damage and radiation. A CT scan (D) is superior to IVU and US scans as it is able to differentiate up to 99 per cent of renal stones and it is also useful for exploring other causes of an acute abdomen. However, the radiation risk to the patient makes this investigation much more invasive and it is not as readily available as an US scan. An MRI scan (B) has only a few advantages over a CT scan, these include the ability to assess renal arteries and there is no risk from radiation. However, MRI has poor differentiation ability and stones can often appear similar to tumours or blood clots. Where it is particularly important to avoid radiation, i.e. a pregnant woman, an MRI scan should be considered. An abdominal x-ray (A) is reasonable in detecting renal stones (up to 80 per cent) since the majority consist of calcium which shows up well on radiograph films, however, there is again a radiation risk to the patient which is avoidable in US scans.

Dysuria

6 A   Tuberculosis (A) affecting the renal system is often insidious and easily overlooked. Symptoms usually include pain affecting the back, flanks and suprapubic region. Non-specific symptoms including haematuria, increased frequency and nocturia should always be considered when urine examination reveals a pyuria in the absence of a positive culture, otherwise called a 'sterile pyuria'. A diabetic nephropathy (C) usually presents with increased proteinuria, initially as microalbuminuria which gradually progresses. Other signs can include a normocytic anaemia and raised erythrocyte sedimentation rate (ESR), patients do not typically have haematuria. The classic presentation in bladder cancer (D) is painless, gross haematuria, although any patient with unexplained haematuria should be investigated for bladder cancer. Important causative factors include smoking and exposure to aromatic amines present in dyes and paints. A sterile pyuria is not a feature in bladder cancer unless the patient had been recovering from a UTI infection that was partially treated. Renal cell carcinoma (B) usually involves the triad of haematuria, flank pain and an abdominal or flank mass with or without non-specific symptoms, such as weight loss, fever and malaise. Nephritic syndrome (E) does involve haematuria (micro- or macroscopic) but presents with hypertension and proteinuria which causes oedema. Dysuria and neutrophils are not usually associated.

Periorbital oedema

7 D   This patient is suffering from post-streptococcal glomerulonephritis (D), which forms part of the nephritic syndrome consisting of haematuria (micro- or macroscopic), hypertension, proteinuria and oedema. In severe cases, oliguria and uraemia can also occur. Patients usually suffer from a streptococcal infection 1–3 weeks prior to presenting with the above symptoms or signs of the nephritic syndrome. During this time, immune complexes are formed and deposited in the glomeruli causing damage. The nephrotic syndrome (A) involves albuminuria usually in the order of ≥3.5 g/d in adults causing oedema and is also associated with hyperlipidaemia (increased LDL/HDL ratio). Nephritic syndrome (B) involves haematuria (micro- or macroscopic) alongside hypertension and proteinuria. Renal failure (C) is an abrupt reduction in kidney function, usually ≤48 hours, with an increase in serum creatinine of ≥26.4 μmol/L or reduction in urine output. A Von Grawitz tumour (E), otherwise known as renal cell cancer, typically occur in males (2:1 male to female ratio) originating from the proximal tubular epithelium. The average age of presentation is 50 years with symptoms including pain, haematuria and usually a mass in the flank alongside other symptoms of malignancy such as weight loss.

Urinary tract infection in pregnancy

8 D   The treatment of symptomatic and asymptomatic bacteriuria is important to prevent complications in pregnancy. Empiric treatment for common organisms such as *Escherichia coli* and *Proteus* should be administered while maintaining safety. Penicillins and cephalosporins, such as cephalexin (D), are safe for use during pregnancy. Ampicillin (E) is no longer recommended due to increasing resistance. Nitrofurantoins are also effective. Trimethoprim (A) is a folic acid antagonist and therefore should be avoided in pregnancy, especially in the first trimester of pregnancy as in this patient. Fluoroquinolones (B) and tetracyclines (C) are also known teratogens and must also be avoided in pregnancy.

Distress

9 E   The history in this case suggests the patient's chest pain is due to muscular injury rather than anything more sinister. The patient's anxiety about cardiovascular morbidity has ultimately resulted in hyperventilation causing an acute respiratory alkalosis (E). Acid base abnormalities can be solved by either considering the Henderson–Hasselbach equation ($CO_2 + H_2O \leftrightarrow H_2CO_3 \leftrightarrow H^+ + HCO_3^-$), whereby change in the product(s) on one side of the equation is balanced by a shift in equilibrium. For example, in this case the patient's hyperventilation causes a reduction in CO_2, in order to increase the CO_2 the equilibrium shifts towards $CO_2 + H_2O$ which causes a reduction in H^+ (alkalosis) and HCO_3^-. This process occurs in respiratory alkalosis with metabolic compensation (C). If the patient had a true cardiac arrest it would cause a surge in lactic acidosis hence H^+ concentration increases causing a metabolic acidosis (B). In order to balance this change, the equilibrium shifts away from H^+ and causes increased CO_2 production which can manifest as an increased respiratory rate, otherwise called 'metabolic acidosis with respiratory compensation' (D). In a respiratory acidosis with metabolic compensation (A) scenario, a patient may have a respiratory abnormality such as chronic hypoventilation. The accumulation of CO_2 which leads to increased H^+ is compensated for by bicarbonate which is subsequently reduced. In more chronic conditions, the bicarbonate becomes elevated.

Nocturia

10 B   This patient has symptoms of hypercalcaemia, the major causes of which can be divided into primary, secondary and tertiary disorders. Primary usually includes malignancies such as adenomas producing PTH, secondary conditions are due to a compensatory increase in parathyroid hormone due to low serum calcium, such as in vitamin D deficiency. Secondary conditions can eventually become tertiary disorders with autonomous PTH production, such as in renal failure. The symptoms of hypercalcaemia can vary depending on severity, patients may be asymptomatic or suffer a number of features affecting different organ symptoms. General symptoms include malaise, abdominal pain and depression. Renal tubule impairment can lead to polyuria, polydipsia and nocturia. Bone pain occurs due to the effect of PTH upon bone metabolism, renal stones can also form due to increased serum calcium and dehydration. Serum calcium (B) must be measured first as this will be able to confirm an abnormal level of calcium in the body. Measuring PTH (C) may or may not provide useful diagnostic information, for example in a tumour producing excess calcium the PTH would be low. Serum phosphate (A) is useful to measure in patients with anorexia, weight loss and osteoporosis as this suggests deficiency, although this is very rare due to an abundance in natural foods. Plasma glucose (D) would be useful in a patient with suspected diabetes, however flank pain and constipation are not typical presentations and urine dipstick would reveal the presence of glucose and ketones. Derangement of serum potassium (E) does not produce the symptoms described in this patient. Hyperkalaemia predisposes to cardiac arrhythmias (loss of p-waves, widened QRS complex and tented T-waves) and muscle weakness, while in severe hypokalaemia there is muscle weakness, atrial and ventricular ectopics.

Breathlessness

11   C   This patient is suffering from symptoms of renal failure which is defined as an abrupt, reversible deterioration in renal function causing uraemia and often associated with oliguria. The uraemia can result in non-specific symptoms such as nausea and vomiting, failure to excrete H^+ results in acidosis causing hyperventilation. Oedema can also result as the kidney loses its diuretic ability, erythropoietin is also produced by the kidney. With increasing impairment there is also reduced haemostatic function causing easy bruising. Serum electrolytes, urea and creatinine (C) is the first-line investigation in this case in order to determine the current level of renal function. Biochemical impairment is reflected by sodium, potassium (increased in renal failure), urea (increased in renal failure) and creatinine (increased in renal failure). The RIFLE criteria (risk, injury, failure, loss, end-stage renal disease) is useful in determining the difference between an acute, chronic or acute-on-chronic presentation of renal failure which can otherwise be difficult in clinical practice. The patient does not have typical features of a UTI, therefore a urine microscopy (A) is not appropriate although it may show evidence of red cell casts to support the blood investigations. Oliguria and easy bruising deviates away from respiratory pathology which would be revealed using a chest x-ray (E). A renal ultrasound scan (B) would reveal the degree of gross damage to the kidneys and structure problems, such as dilatation of the urinary tract due to obstruction, while a biopsy would show histological changes (D). However, these tests are more useful for determining the cause of renal failure and are not appropriate as first-line investigations until the diagnosis of renal failure has been established.

Abdominal pain

12   B   This patient is most likely suffering from polycystic kidney disease which involves the presence of multiple cysts within the renal parenchyma. Patients commonly present with loin or abdominal pain as the kidneys hypertrophy, bleeding or infection of the renal cysts and symptoms of renal failure as renal function becomes increasing impaired. Polycystic kidney disease is most commonly due to PKD1 situated on chromosome 16. Other associations include mitral valve prolapse and berry aneurysms. In this case scenario, an abdominal ultrasound scan (B) is the least invasive investigation to conduct while providing good differentiating ability. Although an MRI scan (A) is better for differentiating soft tissues it is far more expensive and often less readily available. Similarly, a CT scan (D) is more invasive with regards to radiation risk and does not match the US scan in soft tissue identification. Excretion urography (C) has been largely replaced by US scan and can be damaging to the kidneys due to the use of contrast. An abdominal x-ray (E) would not be helpful in determining the cause of loin pain in this case.

Proteinuria

13 D The mainstay of treatment in diabetic patients with new onset proteinuria is to aggressively control blood pressure, ideally below 130/80 mmHg. ACE inhibitors (D) are therefore first-line therapy, angiotensin receptor blockers can also be used. Oral hypoglycaemic (A) agents should be avoided since they are excreted by the renal system. ACE II antagonists (B) are second-line treatment if there are contraindications to ACE inhibitor use. In patients with persistent proteinuria due to diabetic nephropathy, ACE and ARB may be combined together provided the patient is monitored regularly under specialist care. Renal dialysis (E) is only needed if the patient has progressive end stage renal failure. Cholesterol-lowering therapy (C) would be useful in lowering patient's cardiovascular risk factor but does not help in improving impaired renal function.

Weight loss

14 C Renal cell carcinoma (C) is often characterized by the triad of haematuria, flank pain and an abdominal or flank mass alongside symptoms of malignancy, such as weight loss and malaise. Patients may also have peripheral signs of anaemia due to erythropoietin deficiency and this can include pallor and shortness of breath, but anaemia is not an essential feature. A renal abscess (A) often presents insidiously and can be difficult to diagnose with non-specific symptoms, such as abdominal pain, weight loss and malaise. Patients tend to have spiking fevers and pain which may or may not be localized to the flank. A CT scan or ultrasound can be used to localize a suspected renal abscess. Renal cysts (B) can be solitary or present in multiples and are usually asymptomatic, often being found incidentally on ultrasound scans. Occasionally, they may present with pain or haematuria if they grow too large in size. Unless part of a larger pathology, such as polycystic kidneys, renal cysts do not impair renal function and would not cause shortness of breath, pallor or fever as in this patient. Pyelonephritis (E) is easier to diagnose than renal abscesses. They usually manifest as local symptoms of UTI, such as dysuria, haematuria and loin pain, as well as systemic symptoms that suggest infection into the upper urinary tract, such as fever and rigors. An adrenal tumour (D) manifests differently dependent on the location of the malignancy, a medullary tumour produces adrenaline and noradrenaline and is otherwise called a 'phaeochromocytoma'. A tumour in the cortex may produce excess aldosterone (Conn's syndrome), cortisol (Cushing's syndrome) or sex hormones.

Hypercalciuria

15 A Medullary sponge kidney (A) is a congenital disorder of the kidneys that is characterized by the formation of cystic sacs within the papillary zone of the kidney creating a sponge-like appearance. The cysts create an obstruction that prevents the optimal flow of urine through the renal tubules, predisposing to UTIs, haematuria and renal calculi. Although a congenital abnormality, patients rarely present with symptoms before the age of 30. Other associations with medullary sponge kidney include hemihypertrophy, hypercalciuria and renal tubular acidosis. Diagnosis is confirmed by excretion urography revealing cysts and calculi within the renal papilla. Renal cell cancer (B) is unlikely in the absence of abdominal pain, flank mass and weight loss. Renal stone formation and urinary tract infection are also not often associated with renal cell carcinoma. Medullary cystic disease (C) occurs in childhood and is characterized by interstitial inflammation and atrophy of the tubules. Despite its name, cystic formation is not a common early feature and is usually situated within the medulla. Growth retardation, polyuria and polydipsia are the most common presenting symptoms. Horse-shoe kidney (D) describes the fusion of the lower renal poles and patients are usually asymptomatic but may have an increased incidence of UTIs and renal stones. Tertiary hyperparathyroidism (E) is the autonomous production of parathyroid hormone after a long period of untreated secondary hyperparathyroidism in patients with severe chronic kidney disease. Features of elevated calcium include constipation, loin pain, renal stone formation and abdominal pain.

Long-term ibuprofen use

16 E This patient is most likely suffering from analgesic nephropathy in view of the chronic history of NSAID consumption. Chronic intake can result in papillary necrosis and tubulointerstitial nephritis leading to anaemia, UTIs and haematuria. Diagnosis is made by ultrasound or CT scan (E) alongside this clinical picture. An ultrasound is particularly useful if patients complain of sudden flank pain which can result from sloughed papillae causing urinary obstructions. Antegrade pyelography (D) is used to investigate a potential area of obstruction within the kidney which is not indicated in this case. Retrograde pyelography (A) is conducted to investigate obstructions via a catheter. A renal biopsy (B) would be useful to assess the degree of damage to the kidney but this is not essential as stopping analgesics or replacing them with alternatives, such as paracetamol, can reduce or even improve the condition. An abdominal x-ray alone would not be a useful modality for revealing renal damage in this case (C).

Oliguria

17 C   Acute hyperuricaemic nephropathy (C) is a common finding in patients suffering from hyperuricaemia. This is a common occurrence in patients with increased cell turnover, such as myeloproliferative disorders or following chemotherapy. Uric acid crystallizes within the renal system causing obstructions which can manifest as flank pain, oliguria, hypertension, oedema and uraemic symptoms. Analgesic nephropathy (A) is usually due to chronic NSAID intake causing papillary necrosis and tubulointerstitial nephritis. Presentation can include anaemia, urinary tract infections and haematuria. Acute tubulointerstitial nephritis (D) is a drug hypersensitivity reaction, usually due to penicillin or NSAID medication. Patients typically present with fever, skin rashes and joint pain alongside an eosinophilia. Renal infarction (B) can be a difficult diagnosis to make due to the broad clinical presentation that can result, dependent on the degree of ischaemia and necrosis that may occur. In moderate to severe arterial occlusion, patients may present with pain affecting the back, abdomen or flanks. Patients will often have several cardiovascular risk factors that predispose them to thromboembolism, such as atrial fibrillation, clotting abnormalities, etc. In this patient, polycythaemia alone is unlikely to have caused a severe acute renal infarction in both kidneys and, given the recent commencement of chemotherapy, an acute hyperuricaemic nephropathy is more likely. Another potential differential is renal vein thrombosis. Chronic renal failure (E) occurs as a long-standing illness causing significant reduction in renal function, usually in an insidious manner rather than the abrupt situation in this case.

Collapse

18 B   The prevalence of UTIs (B) is increased in elderly female patients, especially those suffering diabetes. Most bacteria convert nitrates to nitrites which, alongside leukocytes, are detected on urine dipstick. Severe infections can result in sepsis, hypovolaemia and collapse. The absence of ketones negates diabetic ketoacidosis (A), the presence of glucose can be due to poor glycaemic control and this also makes hypoglycaemia (E) less likely. The symptoms of hypoglycaemia normally manifest as sweating, tachycardia, palpitations and tremor. Although hypoglycaemia can cause collapse with the risk of patients going into a hypoglycaemic coma, preceding symptoms such as irritability and sweating tend to be present. Postural/orthostatic hypotension (C) is defined as a drop of 20 mmHg in systolic blood pressure when changing from a standing to sitting position. Diabetic nephropathy (D) typically presents with proteinuria and not haematuria which is suggested by this patient's urine dipstick results.

Sacral oedema

19 E   Minimal change nephropathy (E) is the most common cause of nephrotic syndrome in children and young adults. The nephrotic syndrome (B) is likely in this patient with proteinuria resulting in oedema, however, the cause of these symptoms is minimal change glomerulonephritis, hence this is the best answer. The nephritic syndrome (A) consists of haematuria (micro- or macroscopic) which differs from the nephrotic syndrome since in the latter the damaged pores are large enough to allow passage of proteins, but not RBCs. Also, part of the nephritic syndrome is hypertension and proteinuria which causes oedema. Thin basement membrane nephropathy (D) is one of the most common causes of asymptomatic haematuria alongside IgA nephropathy, it is a benign condition characterized by thinning of the glomerular basement membrane which does not impact renal function, hence signs such as sacral oedema would not be present. Goodpasture's disease (C) is the triad of glomerulonephritis, pulmonary damage causing haemorrhage and the presence of anti-glomerular basement membrane antibodies. This is due to a type II autoimmune reaction whereby the anti-GBM antibodies attack type IV collagen of the lungs and the renal glomerulus.

Haematuria

20 E   This patient has the typical findings that manifest in a case of post-streptococcal glomerulonephritis (E). The group A streptococcus infection causes deposition of immune complex in the glomeruli. Within this period, the streptococcal organisms themselves are destroyed, hence a UTI (B) coinciding this presentation is not likely. Also, other symptoms suggestive of a UTI are absent, such as dysuria. This patient does not fulfil the triad required for nephritic syndrome (A) since there is no hypertension despite the presence of haematuria and proteinuria. An acute tubulointerstitial nephritis (C) is usually accompanied by fever, skin rashes and painful joints. Minimal change nephropathy (D) is the most common cause of the nephrotic syndrome in children. In this case, haematuria is not a feature of minimal change glomerulonephritis, although proteinuria are present but there is no oedema, which does not fulfil the criteria present in the nephrotic syndrome.

Haematuria

21 A   Alport syndrome (A) is caused by a genetic defect in type IV collagen synthesis causing the triad of hereditary nephritis, sensorineural deafness and ocular abnormalities which can include cataracts and macular retinal flecks. Renal abnormalities are progressive in such patients and include proteinuria, haematuria and eventually renal failure. Thin basement membrane nephropathy or benign familial haematuria (B) is a common cause of asymptomatic haematuria. Apart from glomerular basement membrane thinning, there are no other associated abnormalities and patients have an excellent prognosis. IgA nephropathy (D) is the most common cause of glomerulonephritis and one of the most common causes for asymptomatic haemauria. Glomerular attacks occur episodically and, during these, haematuria presents. Features such as retinal flecks are not present. Wolfram syndrome (C) is a rare genetic disease that causes diabetes insipidus, diabetes mellitus, optic atrophy and deafness. This is not likely given the absence of glucose on urine dipstick. Patients suffering from Down's syndrome (E) have a range of abnormalities and are often recognized from their characteristic facial appearance. The kidney, however, tends to be spared in such patients. Brushfield spots may be mistaken for retinal flecks in such patients and while sensorineural deafness can occur in Down's syndrome, this is not congenital as occurs in Alport's syndrome.

Chronic cigarette smoking

22 B The renal system from the kidneys to the urethra is lined by transitional cell epithelium which is vulnerable to a number of predisposing factors of cancers, in particular bladder cancer (B). Such factors include cigarette smoke, chemicals used in the rubber and dye industry and medications such as aristolochic acid present in many herbal remedies for weight loss. The most common symptom of bladder cancer is painless haematuria alongside significant weight loss. Chinese herb nephropathy (A) results from the same offending chemical aristolochic acid, as a mistaken chosen component in the herbal preparation. However, the nephropathy is characterized by an aggressive progression to end-stage renal failure with hypertension, proteinuria and haematuria. In the absence of flank pain and an abdominal or flank mass renal cell carcinoma (E), the patient does have the worrying sign of significant unintended weight loss (remedies for weight loss having been stopped a considerable time before weight loss was noticed). Acute tubulointerstitial nephritis (D) is a drug hypersensitivity reaction most commonly to penicillin or NSAIDs and painless haematuria is suggestive of a more sinister pathology. Schistosomiasis (C) can cause bladder cancer through chronic inflammation, however, other symptoms include a local dermatitis at the area of penetration while more systemic features include fevers, muscle pain and allergic rashes.

Abdominal aortic aneurysm rupture

23 B Acute tubular necrosis (B) is most commonly due to renal ischaemia, as in this case, though direct pharmacological toxicity can also be the cause among many others including haemorrhage, diuretics, contrast during radiological procedures and heart failure. The clinical course is dependent on the offending factor and degree of damage but most commonly early oliguria followed by recovery of renal function with an increase in renal output. GFR, however, may remain low due to tubular damage. Full renal capacity is usually regained within 6 weeks of the initial stressor. Haemolytic uraemic syndrome (HUS) (A) defines the acute injury to the kidney from RBC fragmentation which usually originates from thrombosis within arteries. HUS is therefore the triad of microangiopathic haemolysis, thrombocytopenia and acute renal injury. The syndrome of inappropriate anti-diuretic hormone (C) (SIADH) is the result of inappropriately elevated levels of ADH causing the acute retention of water. As a result, there is hyponatraemia and reduced serum osmolality which is not present in this patient. In severe cases, patients can become very agitated and at risk of seizures. HIV nephropathy (D) is a common occurrence in HIV sufferers and can be due to direct HIV infection. Features include nephritic range proteinuria, large kidneys on ultrasound scan and typically collapsing focal segmental glomerulosclerosis on renal biopsy. In this acute case, the impact of renal hypoperfusion is the likely cause of the patient's presentation. Although this is an example of acute renal failure (E), the specific cause is the most appropriate answer.

C-ANCA positive assay

24 E Wegener's granulomatosis (E) is part of the small vasculitides that also includes other diseases such as Churg–Strauss syndrome. Wegener's typically affects the lungs and kidneys although other body systems can be involved. The pathology of Wegener's is autoimmune in nature. Antineutrophil cytoplasmic antibodies (ANCAs) attack small to medium-sized blood vessels resulting in necrotizing granulomatous inflammation. There is a broad spectrum of symptoms but specific to the renal system patients can be asymptomatic to presenting with renal failure on presentation. Patients characteristically have a crescentic necrotizing glomerulonephritis with the presence of RBC casts. Minimal change nephropathy (C) most commonly occurs in young children causing the nephrotic syndrome. There is also a high association with asthma and eczema. Rapidly progressive glomerulonephritis (D) is characterized by the presence of RBC casts (dysmorphic RBCs damaged as they pass into the renal tubules) which are present in the haematuria. Patients rapidly develop renal failure over weeks and may have glomerular crescents on histology. There are several common causes of rapidly progressive glomerulonephritis, such as ANCA-associated glomerulonephritis, including Wegener's granulomatosis, Goodpasture's disease and a severe form of lupus nephritis. Goodpasture's disease (B) is due to a type 2 autoimmune reaction with antibodies attacking the glomerular basement membrane and lung membrane. Patients often present with upper respiratory tract complaints such as haemoptysis with renal manifestations, such as anaemia and glomerulonephritis, occuring later. ANCA may be positive but are not a dominant feature. Post-streptococcal glomerulonephritis (A) is usually associated with haematuria and hypertension following a streptococcal infection which leads to an acute nephritis due to deposition of immune complex.

Abdominal bruits

25 D This patient is mostly likely suffering from a renovascular disease which causes progressive narrowing of the renal vessels which, if not treated, can cause renal necrosis. This is further supported by the patient's cardiovascular risk factors alongside the presence of abdominal bruits which is strongly suggestive of renovascular compromise. Renal arteriography (D) shows the exact location of an occlusion within the renal vasculature and remains the gold standard. The procedure involves radiological dyes injected into the vasculature which are then detected using x-rays. CT angiography (A) produces high resolution pictures but involves the exposure of radiation and is still not as sensitive as renal arteriography. An abdominal x-ray (C) would not be able to reliably identify the position of the kidneys and is not appropriate to demonstrate abnormalities in the vasculature without more sophisticated methods such as contrast. An MRI arteriography (B) of the kidney is useful in identifying the vascular stenosis. The sensitivity and specificity is dependent on the experience of individual centres. Although Doppler ultrasonography is the least invasive of the investigations listed, the sensitivity is less than MRI or CT scanning and direct visualization of a renal artery stenosis is difficult to achieve. A renal biopsy (E) is suitable for histological diagnosis and could be used to demonstrate any renal impairment that may have resulted from poor perfusion of the kidneys. It would not be helpful in identifying obstructions in the renal vasculature.

Suprapubic pain

26 C This patient is suffering from acute urinary retention most likely due to bladder malignancy. The obstruction to urine outflow causes urine to accumulate within the bladder and then create a back-pressure upon the kidneys resulting in bilateral hydronephrosis (C). In comparison, the bladder is a strong muscular organ which requires a significant build up of pressure before it becomes dilated (A). A ureteral stricture (B) is more likely to be painful and cause asymmetrical dilation of kidney. Renal cancer (E) presents characteristically with a palpable mass with pain normally localized to the flanks. Renal cysts (D) are usually asymptomatic and also do not normally cause suprapubic pain.

Type 1 diabetes

27 B Diabetic nephropathy is an insidious complication of diabetes which is often missed since renal compensation can cause patients to present only when they are close to end-stage renal failure. Detection of microalbumin (B) in the urine has been shown to be a good marker for identifying patients most likely at risk of further renal damage. Urine dipsticks are not sensitive enough to detect microalbumin which normally should not be present in the urine. Measurement of blood pressure (A) is a broad marker of cardiovascular integrity. It can both cause and be the product of renal impairment and is not appropriately specific to monitor loss of renal function. Similarly, serum electrolytes (D) such as sodium and potassium can be abnormal due to a number of causes not necessarily related to loss of renal function due to diabetes, for example SIADH. Elevation in serum creatinine (C), which is usually excreted by the kidney, is a late marker of function renal impairment and not appropriate for early risk identification. Urine dipstick for glucose (E) is a screening test for glycaemic control, however, it does not predict specific increased risk for nephropathology but simply increases the likelihood of all diabetic complications.

Periorbital oedema

28 E This patient is suffering from minimal change disease which is the most common cause of nephrotic syndrome in children but can also present in young adults. Only electron microscopy is able to detect any abnormalities of the glomerulus which typically demonstrates fusion of the podocyte foot processes. Although this finding is not pathognomonic, it is highly predictive in children or young adults with nephrotic syndrome with associated eczema or asthma and its positive response to steroids (E). Since this patient has presented a number of times with the nephrotic syndrome, not providing treatment (B) is not helpful given the good response minimal change disease patients demonstrate to steroids or immunosuppressants. Probenecid (C) is primarily used in the prophylaxis against gout as it acts to increase urinary excretion of uric acid. Renal transplant (D) is the treatment for several chronic kidney diseases or end stage renal function. Cyclosporin (A) is an alternative second-line therapy for patients who are steroid-resistant or continually relapse. Cyclosporin therapy requires longer-term therapy compared to steroids but must be continually monitored as accumulation is nephrotoxic, hence it is not appropriate as first-line therapy when compared to oral steroids.

Hyperphosphataemia

29 A This patient is suffering from secondary hyperparathyroidism due to renal failure which explains the abnormal calcium and phosphate levels. Hyperphosphataemia can cause vascular calcification and should be treated as soon as possible. Gut phosphate binders such as sevelamer (A) binds to ingested phosphate within the gut, thereby lowering serum phosphate levels. It also lowers calcium and lowers cholesterol. Parathyroidectomy (B) is reserved for patients refractive to medical therapy and should not be used as first-line therapy. Oral vitamin D therapy (C) is useful in early renal disease as it lowers PTH levels, however it is not appropriate as first-line therapy since it increases calcium and phosphate reabsorption and so can inadvertently exacerbate the patient's symptoms. Once phosphate levels have been lowered, vitamin D therapy is then beneficial. Calcimimetics such as cinacalcet (D) are successful in treating secondary hyperparathyroidism through PTH suppression which then lowers calcium and phosphate levels. The first stage of management is with correction calcium, phosphate by appropriate use of oral phosphate binder and then vitamin D therapy. Renal dialysis (E) is not necessary in this case since adequate medical treatments are available to treat hyperphosphataemia.

Rigors

30 E Pyelonephritis (E) is a potentially life-threatening disease that most commonly occurs due to gram-negative infection. Patients with poorly controlled diabetes have increased risk of infection. Parenchymal infection results in gas accumulation which is identifiable on CT scan, patients may otherwise present similarly to a case of pyelonephritis, however rapid treatment is required to prevent a more fulminating clinical course. Gas in the renal parenchyma is not ever seen in answers A–D. Renal stones (A) can cause exquisite pain, often in a loin to groin pattern, they are rarely coincident with renal infection as suggested by the urine dipstick and such stones are also very well identified by CT scanning. Renal infarction (B) commonly presents with flank pain or chronic abdominal pain. Patients usually have cardiovascular risk factors which can precipitate thromboembolism such as atrial fibrillation. CT scan is usually successful in identifying areas of infarct. Diabetic nephropathy (C) causes progressive damage to the filtering capacity of the kidney due to poor diabetes control. There is an initial increase in GFR that eventually causes glomerulosclerosis typically called 'Kimmelstiel–Wilson lesions'. This allows the passage of protein into the urine but not blood, which is detected in this patient. Renal TB (D) can often be vague in presentation, symptoms tend to be long term and include urinary frequency, dysuria and blood or pus in the urine. Patients are often treated unsuccessfully for UTI before TB is considered.

SECTION 5: ENDOCRINOLOGY

Questions

QUESTIONS

1. Balanitis

A 60-year-old man visits his GP complaining of tiredness. He has noticed weight loss over the last six months and irritation of the tip of his penis which appears inflamed on examination. He mentions he has been visiting the toilet more often than usual and feeling thirsty. The most appropriate investigation would be:

    A. Oral glucose tolerance test
    B. Measurement of glycated haemoglobin
    C. Random plasma glucose test
    D. Water deprivation test
    E. Measurement of triglyceride levels

2. Tiredness

A 33-year-old obese woman complains of tiredness. She has recently given birth to a healthy baby boy and is enjoying being a mother. However, she is becoming more reliant on her partner for support as she always feels exhausted and often becomes depressed. The patient has a poor appetite and often does not finish her meals, despite this she has gained 5 kg in the last 2 weeks. The most likely diagnosis is:

    A. Postpartum depression
    B. Eating disorder
    C. Hyperthyroidism
    D. Hypothyroidism
    E. Occult malignancy

3. Weight gain

A 28-year-old woman has noticed a change in her appearance; most notably her clothes do not fit properly and are especially tight around the waist. Her face appears flushed and more rounded than usual, despite exercising regularly and eating healthily her weight has steadily increased over the last 3 weeks. On visiting her GP, he notices her blood pressure has increased since her last visit and she has bruises on her arm. She is especially worried about a brain tumour. The most appropriate investigation would be:

    A. Low-dose dexamethasone test
    B. High-dose dexamethasone test
    C. Urinary catecholamines
    D. Computed tomography (CT) scan
    E. Urinary free cortisol measurement

4. Sleep apnoea

A 49-year-old man presents with a history of difficulty sleeping. He reports feeling increasingly tired and general weakness which he attributes to his poor sleep pattern. Additionally, the patient has noticed he has gained weight and sweats very easily. On examination, the patient has coarse facial features. The most likely diagnosis is:

    A. Hyperthyroidism
    B. Cushing's disease
    C. Acromegaly
    D. Hypothyroidism
    E. Diabetes

5. Visual disturbance

A 42-year-old woman presents with visual disturbances. She reports having double vision which was intermittent initially but has now become much more frequent. In addition, she becomes breathless very easily and experiences palpitations. On examination, raised, painless lesions are observed on the front of her shins and finger clubbing. The most likely diagnosis is:

    A. De Quervain's thyroiditis
    B. Thyroid storm
    C. Phaeochromocytoma
    D. Graves' disease
    E. Plummer's disease

6. Goitre

A 16-year-old girl presents to her GP complaining of a swelling in her neck which she has noticed in the last 2 weeks. She has felt more irritable although this is often transient. On examination, a diffuse swelling is palpated with no bruit on auscultation. The most likely diagnosis is:

    A. Hyperthyroidism
    B. Simple goitre
    C. Riedel's thyroiditis
    D. Thyroid carcinoma
    E. Thyroid cyst

7. Dizziness

A 22-year-old woman complains of dizziness and feeling light-headed. She works in an office and most frequently experiences this when standing up to visit the toilet. She has never fainted. The patient has lost 5 kg, but attributes this to eating more healthily. She has noticed a recent scar on the back of her hand which has started to turn very dark. The most appropriate investigation is:

   A. Synacthen test
   B. Low-dose dexamethasone test
   C. Cortisol measurement
   D. Urinary free cortisol measurement
   E. Abdominal ultrasound (US) scan

8. Polyuria

A 29-year-old man presents with a 4-week history of polyuria and extreme thirst. The patient denies difficulty voiding, hesitancy or haematuria, although the urine is very dilute. The patient does not believe he has lost any weight and maintains a good diet. No findings are found on urine dipstick. The most appropriate investigation is:

   A. Serum osmolality
   B. Fasting plasma glucose
   C. Urinary electrolytes
   D. Magnetic resonance imaging (MRI) scan of the head
   E. Water deprivation test

9. Confusion (1)

A 69-year-old man presents with confusion. His carers state that over the last month he has become increasingly lethargic, irritable and confused. Despite maintaining a good appetite, he has lost 10 kg in the last month. Blood results are as follows:

Sodium	125 mmol/L
Potassium	4 mmol/L
Urea	3
Glucose (fasting)	6 mmol/L
Urine osmolality	343 mmol/L

The most likely diagnosis is:

   A. Hypothyroidism
   B. Dilutional hyponatraemia
   C. Addison's disease
   D. Acute tubulointerstitial nephritis
   E. Syndrome of inappropriate anti-diuretic hormone (SIADH)

10. Stridor

A 54-year-old woman presents to her GP complaining of a change in her breathing sound. She first noticed numbness, particularly in her fingers and toes, three months ago but attributed this to the cold weather. Her partner now reports hearing a high pitched, harsh sound while she is sleeping. Her BMI is 27. While measuring blood pressure, you notice the patient's wrist flexing. The most likely diagnosis is:

    A. Obstructive sleep apnoea
    B. Hypocalcaemia
    C. DiGeorge syndrome
    D. Guillain–Barré syndrome
    E. Raynaud's syndrome

11. Depression

A 39-year-old man presents with a three-month history of depression. The patient recently lost a family member and around the same period began to feel unwell with constipation and a depressed mood. He has started taking analgesia for a sharp pain in his right lower back that often radiates towards his front. The most appropriate investigation is:

    A. Serum parathyroid hormone
    B. Serum thyroid stimulating hormone
    C. Colonoscopy
    D. Fasting serum calcium
    E. MRI scan

12. High blood pressure

A 47-year-old woman presents to clinic after being referred from her GP for consistently elevated blood pressure. Her last reading was 147/93. The female does not report any symptoms but recently lost her job and attributes the elevated reading to stress. Her blood tests are as follows:

Sodium	146
Potassium	3.4
Glucose (random)	7.7
Urea	4

The most appropriate investigation is:

    A. CT scan
    B. 24-hour ambulatory blood pressure
    C. Abdominal ultrasound scan
    D. Aldosterone–renin ratio
    E. Glucose tolerance test

13. Panic attack

A 65-year-old woman complains of panic attacks. She has recently retired as a school teacher, but 2–3 times a week she suffers extreme anxiety, becomes short of breath and sweats excessively. Elevated catecholamines are detected in the urine. The most appropriate medical treatment is:

A. Phenoxybenzamine alone
B. Prolopanolol alone
C. Phenoxybenzamine followed by propanolol
D. Sodium nitroprusside
E. Propanolol followed by phenoxybenzamine

14. Weight loss

A 47-year-old woman complains of weight loss. She has a family history of type 1 and type 2 diabetes but has never been diagnosed herself despite the finding of islet cell antibodies. In the last few months, however, she has noticed progressively increasing polyuria and poydipsia and 5 kg of weight loss. Her fasting plasma glucose is 8 mmol/L and urine dipstick shows the presence of ketones. The most likely diagnosis is:

A. Type 1 diabetes
B. Non-ketotic hyperosmolar state
C. Type 2 diabetes
D. Occult malignancy
E. Latent autoimmune diabetes of adults (LADA)

15. Diabetes management (1)

A 50-year-old Asian man is referred to the diabetes clinic after presenting with polyuria and polydipsia. He has a BMI of 30, a blood pressure measurement of 137/88 and a fasting plasma glucose of 7.7 mmol/L. The most appropriate first-line treatment is:

A. Dietary advice and exercise
B. Sulphonylurea
C. Exenatide
D. Thiazolidinediones
E. Metformin

16. Neuropathy

A 55-year-old diabetic woman presents with altered sensations in her hands and feet. She finds it difficult to turn pages of books and discriminating between different coins. When walking, the floor feels different and she likens the sensation to walking on cotton wool. The most likely diagnosis is:

   A. Autonomic neuropathy
   B. Diabetic amyotrophy
   C. Acute painful neuropathy
   D. Symmetrical sensory neuropathy
   E. Diabetic mononeuropathy

17. Abdominal lump

A 29-year-old woman is referred to a diabetic clinic for poor diabetes management. She was diagnosed with type 1 diabetes at the age of 12 and prescribed actrapid insulin injections. Recently, the patient has been suffering fluctuations in her plasma glucose levels and her previously well-controlled glycated haemoglobin has risen to 8.1 per cent. The patient admits she has recently been avoiding using her injections. On examination, the patient has a raised, smooth lump that is firm on palpation at the lower abdomen. The most likely diagnosis is:

   A. Worsening of diabetes
   B. Lipohypertrophy
   C. Injection scarring
   D. Lipoma
   E. Injection abscess

18. Headache

A 15-year-old girl complains of headaches which started 6 weeks ago. The headaches initially occurred 1–2 times a week but now occur up to five times a week, they are not associated with any neurological problems, visual disturbances, nausea or vomiting. The girl also reports a white discharge from both of her nipples. She has not started menstruating. The most appropriate investigation is:

   A. Lateral skull x-ray
   B. CT scan
   C. MRI scan
   D. Thyroid function tests
   E. Serum prolactin measurement

19. Striae

A 7-year-old girl presents with red striae which her mother noticed around her abdomen. The girl also has plethoric cheeks and, on her back, several faint, irregular brown macules are observed. The mother is particularly concerned about the early breast development that seems apparent on her daughter. Serum phosphate is decreased. The most likely diagnosis is:

A. Paget's disease of the bone
B. McCune–Albright syndrome
C. Cushing's disease
D. Hypopituitarism
E. Neurofibromatosis

20. Delayed puberty

An 18-year-old man presents to clinic worried about his scant pubic hair development. Examination reveals undescended testes and plasma testosterone, luteinizing hormone and follicle stimulating hormone were found to be low. A karytotype test was 46, XY. The patient was otherwise well, but during neurological examination struggled during the olfactory test. The most likely diagnosis is:

A. Hypogonadotropic hypogonadism
B. Klinefelter's disease
C. Androgen insensitivity syndrome
D. 5-alpha reductase deficiency
E. Kallman's syndrome

21. Room temperature intolerance

A 47-year-old woman is referred to the endocrine clinic complaining of a two-month history of tiredness. Despite wearing several items of clothing, the patient appears intolerant to the room temperature. She has noticed an increase in weight, particularly around her waist. The most appropriate investigation is:

A. Radioiodine scan
B. Thyroid stimulating hormone (TSH)
C. Total tetraiodothyronine level (T_4)
D. Tri-iodothyronine level (T_3)
E. Ultrasound scan of the neck

22. Painful neck

A 58-year-old woman presents with an acutely painful neck, the patient has a fever, blood pressure is 135/85 mmHg and heart rate 102 bpm. The patient explains the pain started 2 weeks ago and has gradually become worse. She also notes palpitations particularly and believes she has lost weight. The symptoms subside and the patient presents again complaining of intolerance to the cold temperatures. The most likely diagnosis is:

    A. Thyroid papillary carcinoma
    B. Plummer's disease
    C. De Quervain's thyroiditis
    D. Hyperthyroidism
    E. Thyroid follicular carcinoma

23. Abdominal pain

A 6-year-old girl presents to accident and emergency with severe abdominal pain, nausea and vomiting. On examination, the patient is tachypnoeic, capillary refill is 3 seconds and she has a dry tongue. While listening to the patient's lungs, you detect a sweet odour from her breath. The most likely diagnosis is:

    A. Diabetic ketoacidosis
    B. Non-ketotic hyperosmolar state
    C. Gastroenteritis
    D. Pancreatitis
    E. Adrenal crisis

24. Bilateral adrenalectomy complication

A 45-year-old Asian man is diagnosed with Cushing's disease in India. He undergoes a bilateral adrenalectomy and recovers well from the operation. On his return to the UK one year later, he complains of a constant dull headache, peripheral visual disturbances and increasing pigmentation of the skin creases of both hands. The most likely diagnosis is:

    A. Ectopic ACTH secreting tumour
    B. Prolactinoma
    C. Nelson syndrome
    D. Addison's disease
    E. Side effects from iatrogenic steroid intake

25. Loss of consciousness

A 29-year-old woman is found unconscious by her partner and rushed to accident and emergency. She is a type 1 diabetic and has maintained excellent glucose control using insulin injections. Blood biochemistry results demonstrate a moderately raised level of insulin, no detectable C-peptide and very low blood glucose. Her partner mentions she is a lawyer and has been working particularly hard in the last week, eating quick meals and occasionally missing meals. The most likely diagnosis is:

A. Hyperosmolar coma
B. Diabetic ketoacidosis
C. Insulin overdose
D. Hypoglycaemic coma
E. Autonomic neuropathy

26. Diabetes management (2)

A 49-year-old man has recently been diagnosed with type 2 diabetes and is being carefully monitored. He has been advised to maintain a healthier diet and lifestyle, he attends a follow-up clinic and claims to have been following the diet stringently since his last appointment three months ago. The most appropriate investigation is:

A. Random plasma glucose
B. Fasting plasma glucose
C. Urine dipstick
D. Glycated haemoglobin
E. Weight measurement

27. Diabetes treatment

A 41-year-old man has been recently diagnosed with type 2 diabetes and has been following a plan of lifestyle measures to improve his diet and increase his level of exercise. On returning to clinic, his BMI is 23, fasting plasma glucose 9.0 mmol/L, blood pressure 133/84 mmHg and HbA1$_c$ of 7.1 per cent. The most appropriate treatment option is:

A. Metformin
B. Sulphonylurea
C. Insulin
D. Exenatide
E. Further diet and exercise

28. Parasthesia

A 33-year-old man complains of a tingling sensation in his hands for several months which occasionally awakens him during sleep. The patient has noticed he has gained weight and no longer wears his wedding ring as it has become too tight. You notice the patient is sweating while speaking to you and has quite a large jaw, furrowed tongue and large hands. His blood pressure reading is 142/91 mmHg. The most appropriate investigation would be:

    A.   MRI scan of the pituitary
    B.   Glucose tolerance test
    C.   Growth hormone levels
    D.   Thyroid function tests
    E.   Serum prolactin levels

29. Prognathism

A 19-year-old woman presents with concerns about changes to her facial appearance, in particular her nose and jaw seem quite large, she is also quite sweaty and despite using antiperspirants is finding it difficult to control and is afraid of embarrassment at university. A glucose tolerance test is performed and found to be raised. The most appropriate management would be:

    A.   Trans-sphenoidal surgery
    B.   Octreotide
    C.   Bromocriptine
    D.   Pituitary radiotherapy
    E.   Pegvisomant

30. Impaired fasting glucose

A 29-year-old man presents to his GP complaining of being constantly thirsty, tired and visiting the toilet more often than usual during the last 4 days. He has noticed his clothes have become more baggy and he now needs to tighten his belt. His parents both have diabetes requiring insulin therapy. A fasting plasma glucose result is most likely to be:

    A.   9.0 mmol/L
    B.   6.0 mmol/L
    C.   16.3 mmol/L
    D.   5.0 mmol/L
    E.   3.0 mmol/L

31. Ketonuria

A 22-year-old woman is found unconscious in her room by her boyfriend and brought into accident and emergency. A urine dipstick is positive for glucose and ketones and blood analysis shows the following results:

pH	6.9
PCO_2	3.0 kPa
PO_2	13 kPa
Sodium	144 mmol/L
Potassium	5.0 mmol/L
Urea	11
Glucose	20
Chloride	100
Bicarbonate	2.9

The most likely anion gap is:

A.   180
B.   118
C.   139.2
D.   46.1
E.   28

32. Quadrantanopia

A 37-year-old man presents with symptoms of an acute headache, vomiting, malaise and visual disturbance. A neurological examination reveals a bitemporal superior quadrantanopia. A CT scan shows a hyperdense area within the pituitary gland. The most likely diagnosis is:

A.   Kallman syndrome
B.   Septo-optic dysplasia
C.   Sheehan's syndrome
D.   Empty sella syndrome
E.   Pituitary apoplexy

33. Facial plethora

A 38-year-old woman presents to clinic complaining of changes in her appearance and weight gain. She has recently been through a divorce and attributed her weight gain to this. However, despite going to the gym her clothes are still tight, especially around her waist, her face seems puffy and flushed. The most likely diagnosis is:

A.   Hyperthyroidism
B.   Cushing's disease
C.   Acromegaly
D.   Hypothyroidism
E.   Diabetes

34. Collapse

A 60-year-old diabetic man recovering from sepsis after collapsing at home was treated with appropriate antibiotics after blood culture and aggressive fluid management with 0.9 per cent saline for 2 days for hypotension. Although blood pressure returned to normal, the patient had the following abnormal biochemical blood results:

pH	7.32
PCO_2	5.2
PO_2	11.1
Sodium	147 mmol/L
Potassium	3.5 mmol/L
Chloride	119 mmol/L
Bicarbonate	19.5

The most likely diagnosis is:

    A. Diabetic ketoacidosis
    B. Lactic acidosis
    C. Conn's syndrome
    D. Renal tubular acidosis type 1
    E. Hyperchloremic acidosis

35. Confusion

A 57-year-old woman, who has recently returned from a holiday in America, presents with dull grey-brown patches in her mouth and the palms of her hand which she has noticed in the last week. She has also noticed she gets very dizzy when rising from a seated position and is continually afraid of fainting. The most likely diagnosis is:

    A. Addison's disease
    B. SIADH
    C. Conn's syndrome
    D. Waterhouse–Friderichsen syndrome
    E. 17-hydroxylase deficiency

ANSWERS

Balanitis

1 C   Type 2 diabetes symptoms are usually well recognized, as in this patient, with polyuria and weight loss occurring due to the osmotic diuresis that results from elevated blood glucose. In subacute presentations, more subtle signs include lethargy and opportunistic infections, such as Candida, causing pruritus vulvae in females or penile inflammation (balantis) in males. The criteria for diabetes diagnosis depends on the clinical presentation. In symptomatic patients, a single abnormal glucose reading is adequate and this may be a fasting plasma glucose $\geq$7.0 mmol/L or as in this case a random plasma glucose (C) of $\geq$11.1 mmol/L. In asymptomatic presentations, two abnormal readings are required, e.g. two fasting plasma glucose $\geq$7.0 mmol/L or two random plasma values $\geq$11.1 mmol/L. Water deprivation (D) is useful in investigating polydipsia for conditions such as diabetes insipidus. An oral glucose tolerance test (A) is only used for borderline cases or diagnosis of gestational diabetes. Other investigations, such as triglyceride (E), cholesterol and glycated haemoglobin (B), can be conducted after diagnosis to monitor the progress of the condition and used as potential risk factors for other conditions.

Tiredness

2 D   Hypothyroidism (D) is a common disease with a higher prevalence in females and is usually a primary disorder affecting the thyroid gland itself. Thyroid hormones control the metabolic rate in many tissues, underactivity produces symptoms which are often insidious. These include tiredness, depression, cold intolerance, constipation and weight gain. The main causes include iodine deficiency, autoimmune pathology such as Hashimoto's thyroiditis and, in females who have recently given birth, postpartum thyroiditis. Hyperthryoidism (C) results in an excess of thyroid hormones which inappropriately increases metabolic rate with symptoms such as weight loss, increased sweating, restlessness and palpitations. A goitre can occur in both hypo- and hyperthyroidism. Postpartum depression (A) is often accompanied by confusion and is characterized by low mood, anhedonia and anergia. Severely affected patients can have delusional thoughts about their newborn child, such as it being evil, and even progress to thoughts of harming the child or suicidal ideation. Eating disorders (B), such as bulimia or anorexia nervosa, often result in drastic changes in body weight resulting from psychological problems with self-image and include behaviours such as self-induced vomiting to avoid weight gain or binge eating. Most malignancies (E) result in considerable weight loss though this is dependent on the type of cancer and often symptoms provide clues as to the location, e.g. neurological problems.

Weight gain

3 E   The patient appears to be suffering from cushingoid symptoms. After a history to exclude causes such as high-dose steroid intake, the main differential diagnoses include an adrenal tumour, an ectopic tumour producing ACTH (Cushing's syndrome) or a pituitary tumour (Cushing's disease). Although a 24-hour urinary free cortisol level measurement (E) does not confirm the exact diagnosis, it does indicate if there is a pathological excess of cortisol (levels can vary up to 700 nmol/L in the morning to 280 nmol/L at midnight). A low dose (0.5 mg) dexamethasone test (A) involves measuring ACTH after dexamethasone administration. In Cushing's disease and syndrome, there is no suppression of ACTH. A high-dose dexamethasone test (B) will differentiate between Cushing's disease and Cushing's syndrome since only in the former is there suppressed ACTH production after high-dose dexamethasone administration. A CT scan (D) can be used to identify a pituitary tumour if requiring surgical management. Urinary catecholamine (C) measurement is used in the diagnosis of a phaeochromocytoma, an adrenal tumour producing excess catecholamines measurable in the urine. Differentiating an adrenal tumour producing excess cortisol can be done by administering metyrapone, an 11-β hydroxysteroid dehydrogenase inhibitor, which effectively ceases adrenal cortisol production. If cortisol is still high it is due to an ectopic source, e.g. lung tumour.

Sleep apnoea

4 C   Acromegaly (C) is most commonly due to a pituitary tumour usually identified on MRI scan, patients most frequently present with changes in appearance followed by visual defects and headaches. Sleep apnoea is often a common complaint among patients due to weight gain. Other manifestations include large hands and feet, hirsutism, prominent and coarse facial features, carpal tunnel syndrome, hypertension, diabetes and heart failure among others. The glucose tolerance test is diagnostic for suspected acromegaly, GH levels can be measured directly, although elevated findings are not sufficient for diagnosis. Hyperthryoidism (A) produces symptoms that are usually secondary to an elevation in metabolic rate, such symptoms include diarrhoea, goitre, sweating and intolerance to the temperature whereby the patient consistently feels hot irrespective of the true environmental temperature. Sleep apnoea is not usually a complaint among patients since they often lose weight despite an increased appetite. Cushing's disease (B) results from a pituitary tumour producing excess ACTH, the excess cortisol levels result in symptoms such as striae, bruising, thin skin, weight gain (particularly in the abdominal region) and often a dorsocervical fat pad (buffalo hump). Hypothyroidism (D) features include tiredness, depression, cold intolerance, constipation and weight gain. Patients do not tend to sweat more and the disease does not coarsen facial features. In diabetes (E), patients' symptoms often result in weight loss though in type 2 diabetes they may suffer from sleep apnoea due to their high BMI.

Visual disturbance

5 D   Graves' disease (D) is the most common cause of hyperthyroidism. The condition is due to IgG antibodies binding to the TSH receptor, this in turn causes excess production of thyroid hormone. The antibodies also bind to other areas of the body such as the extraocular muscles leading to gaze abnormalities, the shins causing raised lesions known as 'pretibial myxoedema' and rarely the fingers causing clubbing known as 'thyroid acropachy'. These collective signs are only seen in Graves' disease, hence it is the only correct answer. De Quervain's thyroiditis (A) is a transient thyroid state most likely due to a viral infection. The patient usually complains of a fever and painful neck with some signs of hyperthyroidism, such as tachycardia, as well as raised ESR levels. A few weeks later, the patient suffers from transient hypothyroid symptoms before returning to a euthyroid state. Phaeochromocytomas (C) are malignancies of the sympathetic nervous system, 90 per cent arise in the adrenal medulla and produce excess catecholamines. The symptoms of a phaeochromocytoma are often similar to hyperthyroidism and include anxiety, palpitations and headache. However, these symptoms are usually intermittent and the main risk to patients is from cardiovascular compromise. Plummer's disease (E) is a solitary nodule in the thyroid gland producing excess thyroid hormones. It is usually refractory to antithyroid treatment. A thyroid storm or crisis (B) is a rapid deterioration in patients suffering from hyperthyroidism, often stimulated by a stressor such as infection. Patients present with acute-onset, severe tachycardia, distress and hyperpyrexia.

Goitre

6 B   A simple goitre (B) is an idiopathic enlargement of the thyroid. Often the condition is associated with thyroid antibodies, but these do not cause any symptoms. Riedel's thyroiditis (C) is a rare inflammatory disease of the thyroid gland that is characterized by fibrosis of the thyroid gland and other structures in the neck. It is often stony or woody on palpation and patients are usually asymptomatic. The patient does not have any features of hyperthyroidism (A) in which a thyroid bruit can be present. A thyroid cyst or nodule (E) is usually harmless and is a fluid-filled swelling often presenting as a single compressible small lump rather than a diffuse swelling. A full history and examination should always be conducted with ultrasound and fine needle examination to exclude malignancy. Thyroid cancer (D) is a rare but important diagnosis, they often present as irregular thyroid nodules but can metastasize to the lung, brain, liver and bone. Papillary and follicular cancers usually have good prognoses compared to medullary and anaplastic cancers.

Dizziness

7 A   This patient has Addison's disease whereby the adrenal gland is destroyed, usually due to infection (TB) or autoimmunity. The reduced cortisol, aldosterone and sex steroids produce a myriad of signs and symptoms, most importantly postural hypotension due to reduced aldosterone and increased pigmentation often in palmar creases and newly formed scars. This latter sign is due to elevated melanocyte-stimulating hormone (MSH) which is derived from the POMC molecule which breaks down into MSH and ACTH. Other symptoms include weight loss, malaise and vitiligo. The synachten test (A) involves giving an infusion of ACTH which would be expected to cause an increase in measured cortisol. A short synacthen test confirms primary Addison's disease, whereas ACTH deficiency or suppression by steroids can be confirmed by doing a long synacthen test. Urinary free cortisol (D) and the low-dose dexamethasone test (B) is appropriate for investigating Cushing's syndrome and is not correct for this patient. A single cortisol measurement (C) is not very valuable for confirming diagnosis due to poor sensitivity and specificity, as well as the diurnal nature of cortisol. A random measurement below 100 nmol/L during the day is more suggestive of Addison's disease, while a value of >550 nmol/L makes the diagnosis less likely. An abdominal US scan (E) would not be appropriate until less invasive blood tests which can confirm Addison's had been conducted.

Polyuria

8 E   This patient is likely to be suffering from psychogenic polydipsia. The water deprivation test (E) is the most appropriate investigation to confirm this diagnosis. In a normal patient, the serum osmolality remains within the normal range (275–295 mOsm/kg), while the urine osmolality rises to >600 mOsm/kg as water is reabsorbed. In diabetes insipidus, the serum osmolality is elevated with no compensatory concentration of urine osmolality. If the patient responds to desmopressin, this confirms cranial DI rather than nephrogenic DI, hence a water deprivation test is the most appropriate answer. An MRI scan (D) is most appropriate for investigating a pituitary tumour. This commonly presents with visual field impairment and symptoms of elevated prolactin not seen in this patient. The fasting plasma glucose (B) would be appropriate for investigating a patient with suspected diabetes mellitus, however this is often accompanied by weight loss. Serum osmolality (A) would be useful in gauging how serious the patient's degree of dehydration is, but would not be diagnostic. Urinary electrolytes (C) and fasting plasma glucose would be useful in gauging the severity of the patient's clinical state, but would not confirm the diagnosis.

Confusion

9 E   The syndrome of inappropriate anti-diuretic hormone (E) (SIADH) is due to inappropriately elevated levels of ADH which leads to the retention of water. The syndrome is therefore characterized by reduced serum sodium levels (hyponatraemia) and reduced serum osmolality, while urine osmolality and urine sodium levels are elevated. Patients are also euvolaemic without signs of oedema. In patients suffering from heart failure, liver failure or the nephrotic syndrome, the reduced circulatory volume acts as a stimulus for the ADH secretion. Despite the patient being in a hypo-osmolar state, ADH secretion is increased causing hyponatraemia, however such patients will be hypervolaemic as in dilutional hyponatraemia (B) due to fluid overload. The SIADH can arise from an inappropriate source of ADH such as tumours both in and out of the pituitary or failure in the feedback mechanism. Hypothyroidism (A) and Addison's disease (C) can also cause the SIADH, however the above patient does not exhibit any of the other signs of these diseases such as weight gain and hypotension, respectively. Acute tubulointerstitial nephritis (D) affects the tubules or interstitium of the kidney and most commonly arises due to hypersensitivity reactions from medications such as non-steroidal anti-inflammatory drugs (NSAIDs). Patients usually present with fever, arthralgia and renal failure.

Stridor

10 B   This patient exhibits many of the signs present in hypocalcaemia (B) including tingling in the fingers and toes and carpopedal spasm. In the latter, occlusion of the brachial artery, which occurs when measuring blood pressure, causes muscle spasming of the hand and forearm (Trosseau's sign). Other signs include facial muscle twitching when the facial nerve is tapped on the same side (Chvostek's sign), prolonged QT interval, hyperreflexia and stridor. Hypocalcaemia most commonly arises due to renal failure. DiGeorge syndrome (C) is a congenital condition that arises due to an abnormality at chromosome 22q11 causing malformation of the third and fourth pharyngeal arches. Patients present at a young age with cardiac abnormalities, abnormal facies, cleft palate and hypocalcaemia. Raynaud's syndrome (E) is characterized by triphasic changes in the peripheral digits, usually the fingers, stressors such as cold temperature causes arterial spasming which reduces the blood flow to the end arteries. Patients will notice their fingers turn white, blue and then red as the blood flow returns. In mild disease, this can be associated with mild tingling while severe disease can cause severe pain and even necrosis. Obstructive sleep apnoea (A) is a disorder of sleep that is characterized by loss of airway patency causing a significant reduction in airflow despite constant breathing effort. This can occur for a number of reasons such as obesity, asthma and hypothyroidism. However, there are not usually any underlying neurological signs. Guillain–Barré syndrome (D) is an immune-mediated disease which usually results following an infection such as cytomegalovirus (CMV) and campylobacter causing a polyneuropathy. The demyelination typically occurs in a symmetrical ascending pattern starting with the distal limbs. Paralysis of the respiratory muscles can occur, requiring emergency treatment, but there are no signs of hypocalcaemia as in the above patient.

Depression

11 D This patient appears to be suffering from symptoms of elevated calcium levels, these can include depression, constipation and renal stone formation causing abdominal pain. The normal calcium homeostatic pathway is controlled by parathyroid hormone (PTH). When calcium levels fall, as in malnutrition, PTH levels increase causing calcium reabsorption by the kidneys and the gastrointestinal system, while calcium stored in the bones is released. PTH malignancies are the most common cause of elevated calcium, however the diagnosis of hypercalcaemia itself is only confirmed by measuring the serum calcium itself (D). PTH (A) levels would then reveal whether the hypercalcaemia is due to hyperparathyroidism but are not appropriate before serum calcium measurements. Primary hyperparathyroidism occurs due to parathyroid adenomas producing excess PTH. Secondary hyperparathyroidism is a compensatory increase in PTH in renal failure or vitamin D deficiency. Tertiary hyperparathyroidism is autonomous PTH production after long-standing secondary hyperparathyroidism. An MRI scan (E) would not be appropriate without first measuring blood levels of PTH if a PTH tumour were suspected. Although hyperthyroidism can cause hypercalcaemia, TSH (B) is not measured before serum calcium or PTH. A colonoscopy (C) would be appropriate to investigate unexplained constipation, especially if a gastrointestinal (GI) malignancy were suspected alongside worrying symptoms such as significant weight loss. Less invasive investigations such as blood tests should always be considered before more invasive investigations.

High blood pressure

12 B The main differential in this patient is hyperaldosteronism arising from an adrenal tumour (Conn's syndrome). The excess aldosterone causes hypertension, elevated sodium reabsorption and potassium excretion. However, given the patient history, the elevated blood pressure could easily be due to the stress of having blood pressure measured or the patient's personal situation. A 24-hour ambulatory blood pressure measurement (B) is therefore the most appropriate investigation to eliminate essential hypertension. Since the blood results are only mildly deranged and essential hypertension has not been eliminated, an aldosterone–renin ratio (D), CT scan (A) or abdominal ultrasound (C) would not be the first-line investigations to consider. They would be useful to investigate Conn's syndrome if essential hypertension was excluded as a differential. A glucose tolerance test (E) is inappropriate in this case since the random glucose reading is not abnormal and the patient is not suffering from symptoms suggestive of diabetes.

Panic attack

13 C Phaeochromocytomas are malignancies of the sympathetic tract, most commonly arising as tumours of the adrenal medulla. The excess catecholamines put the patient at considerable risk of cardiovascular compromise, initial treatment must therefore protect against this with complete alpha and beta blockade (C). Phenoxybenzamine (A) is a non-reversible alpha antagonist which acts to protect against the effects of hypertension. Propanolol (B) is a non-selective beta-blocker which negates the increased heart contractility (inotropic effects) and heart rate (chronotropic effect). Alpha and beta blockade alone is not sufficient to protect the patient. The alpha blockade by phenoxybenzamine must be started first before propanolol to prevent exacerbating the hypertension (E). Sodium nitroprusside (D) is a potent vasodilator and is used during surgery when removing the adrenal tumour. Since severe hypertension can occur, sodium nitroprusside is used in this instance only.

Weight loss

14 E This patient is suffering from an atypical presentation of a rare type of diabetes. In type 1 diabetes (A) patients suffer symptoms due to insulin deficiency. The elevated blood glucose causes polyuria and polydipsia due to osmotic diuresis, patients tend to present in childhood and puberty although this is not an essential aspect for diagnosis. In type 2 diabetes (C) patients tends to have a stronger family history and present later in life with obesity and insulin resistance. Autoimmune sequelae, such as antibodies, are less well established. A more insidious disease progress towards insulin deficiency occurs in latent autoimmune diabetes of adults (E) whereby patient's begin to show symptoms and signs such as weight loss, hyperglycaemia and ketonuria in adulthood. Despite diet and medication, these symptoms tend to persist and islet cell antibodies are strongly predictive of disease. Although an occult malignancy (D) is possible, the association of polyuria, polydipsia, family history, antibodies and late presentation make LADA much more likely to be correct. Non-ketotic hyperosmolar states (B) usually occur in type 2 diabetics suffering from insulin deficiency, the condition increases thrombotic risk, mental function dysfunction, coma and serum glucose levels usually ≥ 33 mmol/L.

Diabetes management

15 A The initial management of type 2 diabetes (T2DM) should begin with lifestyle changes (A) which involve obtaining a dietary history, physical exercise per week and other factors such as a smoking history. Expert clinical advice may then be offered with the help of a registered dietician, regular exercise encouraged and smoking cessation encouraged. The aim should be to normalize blood glucose, blood pressure and lipid levels. Unfortunately, T2DM becomes progressively worse with time until eventually exogenous insulin replacement is required. Metformin (E) is particularly proficient in lowering serum glucose and should be used in overweight/obese patients with particular difficulty in controlling glucose levels. Insulin secretagogues (B) (sulphonylureas and rapid-acting insulin secretagogues, such as nateglinide and repaglinide) are particularly effective in controlling HbA1$_c$ levels and improving cardiovascular outcomes. They should be used as first-line treatment if patients are not overweight and require rapid glucose control due to hyperglycaemic symptoms. Patients unable to maintain or achieve adequate glucose control may use sulphonylureas as second-line therapy. Exenatide (C) and thiazolidinediones (D) tend to be considered following lifestyle, metformin and sulphonylurea action to control HbA1$_c$ levels.

Neuropathy

16 D Diabetic neuropathy is likely to occur through various pathways, occlusion of the vasa nervorum may explain mononeuropathies (E) that occur in isolation and not symmetrically as in this patient. Diffuse symmetrical neuropathies produce more variable presentations and are likely to be due to metabolic damage. The build up of sorbitol and fructose in Schwann cells due to hyperglycaemia is a popular theory. Symmetrical sensory neuropathy (D) is characterized by early loss of vibration, pain and temperature sense in a glove and stocking pattern. In advanced disease, patients often lose their balance and complain of altered sensations. Painful neuropathies (C) are less common and patients typically present with burning sensations or painful parasthesia of their feet, shins or thighs. Diabetic amyotrophy (B) is characterized by painful wasting of the patients' quadriceps muscles and is usually asymmetrical. Control of glucose levels over time usually resolves the condition. Autonomic neuropathy (A) is rarely symptomatic, but can present with a number of different problems of the sympathetic and parasympathetic system. This includes vagal neuropathy causing tachycardia at rest, gastroparesis which rarely can lead to vomiting, erectile dysfunction and atonic bladder.

Abdominal lump

17 B Management of diabetes care should always involve explaining the risks of treatment, especially in young children who are using insulin injections. Shallow injections should be avoided as they are painful and can lead to scarring (C). Allergic responses may occasionally occur, but are usually mild and resolve spontaneously. Importantly, patients should be encouraged to alternate injection sites between the thighs, abdomen and shoulder to prevent build up of adipose tissue creating smooth, firm lumps known as lipohypertrophy (B). This is not dissimilar to a lipoma (D) which are benign masses consisting of fatty tissue enclosed by a fibrous capsule. They are usually mobile, painless and soft on palpation. Worsening diabetes (A) does not cause lipohypertrophy, but would likely worsen symptoms of diabetes such as weight loss and osmotic diuresis. Patients also increase their risk of diabetic complications such as retinopathy, neuropathy and nephropathy. An injection abscess (E) can occur in any situation where needles are being used in poor sanitary conditions; the presentation, however, is usually of a pus-filled cavity that is painful and erythematous.

Headache

18 E This patient is most likely suffering from hyperprolactinaemia, which is most commonly caused by a prolactinoma which is a pituitary adenoma causing stalk compression or hypothyroidism. Prolactin levels (E) must first be measured in order to confirm the diagnosis before more invasive tests are used to determine the cause. An MRI scan (C) is the most definitive investigation in this patient as the patient's complaint of headaches alongside the rest of the history point towards a pituitary tumour. Prolactin levels above 1000 mU/L also strongly suggest this. A CT scan (B) is not able to reveal pituitary masses as readily as MRI scans can and also involve considerable radiation levels which are especially important in sensitive areas such as the brain. In large lesions, a lateral skull x-ray (A) can reveal fossa enlargement, lesions are often also discovered incidentally, however lateral skull x-rays are rarely used as definitive investigation. Thyroid function tests (D) are important to conduct as they can also cause hyperprolactinaemia; however, as the patient does not have features of thyroid disease they are not first line.

Striae

19 B McCune–Albright syndrome (B) is a genetic disorder that causes the uncontrolled secretion of a number of endocrine glands causing abnormalities of the skin, bones and hormonal disturbances. It is usually suspected when the following pathologies occur: precocious puberty, cushingoid features, hyperpituitarism (acromegaly, gigantism), café-au-lait spots and hypophasphataemia. Cushing's disease (C) is due to a pituitary tumour producing excess ACTH which results in excess cortisol levels. Symptoms such as striae, bruising, thin skin, weight gain, particularly abdominally, and often a dorsocervical fat pad (buffalo hump) are observed which are not features in this case. Paget's disease of the bone (A) most commonly presents with bone pain, hearing loss and deformation of bones. The pathogenesis has yet to be elucidated though viral cause is theorized, initially a marked increased in bone resorption occurs followed by fibrous replacement leading to the aforementioned symptoms. Café-au-lait spots and sphenoid dysplasia do not occur. Hypopituitarism (D) can present with a spectrum of symptoms which include malaise, weight gain, temperature intolerance, loss of libido and hair loss. Neurofibromatosis (E) is another genetic disorder that causes tumour growth from nerve tissue. Patients can present with learning difficulty, absence seizures and features secondary to impingement by neurofibromas, such as headaches and deafness. Café-au-lait spots can also occur but usually in association with axillary freckling.

Delayed puberty

20 E Kallman syndrome is a rare genetic condition which results from deficient hypothalamic gonadotropin-releasing hormone which results in hypogonadism, infertility and variable pubertal maturation. Kallman syndrome (E) is differentiated from idiopathic hypogonadotropic hypogonadism (A) by the additional abnormality of hypo-anosmia. Klinefelter syndrome (B) is a chromosomal disorder defined most commonly by a 47,XXY karyotype. It is normally the most common chromosomal abnormality associated with hypogonadism. Androgen insensitivity syndrome (C) causes a female phenotype in male genotypes due to an X-linked recessive abnormality of the androgen receptor. Individuals fail to develop their external genitalia due to poor sensitivity to androgens. 5-alpha reductase deficiency (D) leads to a deficiency of dihydrotestesterone so that genetically male patients only are affected. Such patients usually appear female although they are born with male gonads. The sense of smell is not affected.

Room temperature intolerance

21 B This patient is suffering from hypothyroidism. The most appropriate first-line investigation is measurement of TSH (B) as this indicates if a primary disease affecting the thyroid is present. In a patient with symptoms of hypothyroidism due to a primary disorder of the thyroid, the TSH would be elevated. Similarly, in symptoms of hyperthyroidism due to a primary abnormality of the thyroid, the TSH would be depressed. The total tetraiodothyronine level (T_4) (C) would be decreased hypothyroidism and elevated in hyperthyroidism, but this could be due to abnormalities of TSH secretion or a primary disorder of the thyroid. Hyperthyroidism due to elevated levels of tri-iodothyronine level (T_3) (D) occurs much less commonly than T4 and hence is measured less often. A radioiodine scan (A) is useful for studying causes of hyperthyroidism, such as Plummer's disease. The patient in this question is suffering from symptoms of hypothyroidism. Ultrasound scan of the neck (E) is most useful for differentiating between solid and cystic nodules; these usually do not alter thyroid function.

Painful neck

22 C This patient is suffering from symptoms of hyperthyroidism (D) but with some atypical features that provide clues to the most accurate diagnosis. De Quervain's thyroiditis (C) causes a transient change in thyroid state usually due to a viral infection. The patient usually complains of a fever and painful neck with some signs of hyperthyroidism, such as tachycardia, as well as raised ESR levels. This is due to thyroid hormone release as viral organisms infect the thyroid cells. Patients will suffer hypothyroidism as thyroid hormone is depleted before becoming euthyroid again. Plummer's disease (B) usually presents with a solitary nodule in the thyroid gland producing excess thyroid hormones. Thyroid papillary (A) and follicular carcinoma (E) can present with all the features described in this case but are usually painless and less often associated with fever. Apart from De Quervain's thyroiditis, no other pathology swings from hyperthyroidism to hypothyroidism before returning to a euthyroid state.

Abdominal pain

23 A In diabetic ketoacidosis (A), the body enters a catabolic state as it perceives a lack of energy stores. Ketones are produced from the breakdown of fat which causes an acidotic state in the body. Patients commonly present with nausea, vomiting, dehydration and abdominal pain. The acidosis is partially compensated by hyperventilation (Kussmaul respiration) and the sweet breath is acetone as the body tries to equilibrate the serum pH. A non-ketotic hyperosmolar state (B) usually occurs in type 2 diabetes whereby the hyperglycaemic state causes a hyperosmolar state causing polyuria and dehydration which exacerbate the elevated glucose concentration. Ketones are not responsible as there is a small presence of insulin inhibiting lipolysis. In an adrenal crisis (E), the adrenal gland is destroyed, usually due to infection (TB) or autoimmunity. The reduced cortisol, aldosterone and sex steroids produce a myriad of signs and symptoms, most importantly postural hypotension due to reduced aldosterone and increased pigmentation often in palmar creases and newly formed scars. This latter sign is due to elevated melanocyte-stimulating hormone (MSH) which is derived from the POMC molecule which breaks down into MSH and ACTH. Other symptoms include weight loss, malaise and vitiligo. Gastroenteritis (C) and pancreatitis (D) have more prominent symptoms of abdominal pain and do not usually feature acetone breath.

Bilateral adrenelectomy complication

24 C Nelson syndrome (C) occurs in patients who undergo bilateral adrenalectomies, the loss of negative feedback over time causes a macroadenoma to form in the pituitary which secretes adrenocorticotropin (ACTH). A spectrum of symptoms may arise due to the effects of serum

ACTH, as well as the deficiency in other pituitary hormones. An ectopic tumour secreting ACTH (A) can produce similar symptoms, however they usually originate from oat cell of small cell lung carcinomas which are associated with weight loss rather than headaches and visual disturbances. Iatrogenic steroid side effects (E) would cause symptoms imitating cortisol excess such as striae, bruising, thin skin and weight gain. A prolactinoma (B) can cause some of the symptoms the patient complains of, such as headache and visual disturbances, due to impingement upon surrounding structures. However, symptoms in males does not involve hyperpigmentation and usually include loss of libido, impotence and gynaecomastia. Addison's disease (D) causes similar symptoms described in the question stem, however the cause of adrenal function loss is due to autoimmune action or infection.

Loss of consciousness

25 D In this case, the most likely answer is a hypoglycaemic coma (D). The history indicates that the patient has been missing meals but adheres to her insulin regime. The raised insulin level and absent C-peptide indicates no endogenous insulin production (which would produce insulin and C-peptide) but exogenous insulin. The patient has therefore not eaten sufficiently to maintain an adequate glucose level despite taking a recommended dose of insulin. This differs from an insulin overdose (C) where an excess level of insulin is injected causing an abnormally low glucose level. A diabetic ketoacidosis (B) occurs due to the body's attempt to compensate for the perceived lack of glycogen stores due to insulin deficiency. Therefore, by definition, serum insulin levels would be low or absent. A hyperosmolar coma (A) affects type 2 diabetics whereby the hyperglycaemic state causes hyperosmolarity causing polyuria and dehydration. The glucose, however, is low in this case. Diabetic neuropathy can cause a myriad of symptoms due to autonomic dysfunction (E) including urinary incontinence, constipation and postural hypotension. However, there is usually a collection of such symptoms rather than an isolated event. Patients affected also tend to have poor diabetic control.

Diabetes management

26 D Glycated haemoglobin (D) reflects the level of blood glucose due to glucose attachment to red blood cells non-enzymatically. Since red blood cells have a half-life of 120 days, they will reflect the glucose level of the patient for approximately three months. Measuring the random plasma glucose (A) and fasting glucose (B) will show the state of glucose control at the instant of measurement, but provides no information about the degree of control the patient has over a longer period of time. Patients may therefore fast closer to the date of their appointments despite poor compliance. Similarly, urine dipstick (C) can only reflect the control of glucose homeostasis at the instance of measurement, it is also only appropriate as a screening measurement and must be quantified with blood tests. Weight measurement (E) would be useful to measure to record the change in BMI over time; however, it provides no information to the state of diabetes control.

Diabetes treatment

27 B If after a trial of lifestyle measures aimed at improving diet content and increasing exercise fails to control blood glucose levels and HbA1$_c$, patients may be started on medical therapy. Diet and exercise (E) should continue to be employed alongside medical therapy, but since adequate control has not been achieved following this measure it is not appropriate to continue without medical adjuncts. Sulphonylureas (B) can be considered as first-line medical treatment if the patient is not overweight or if their blood glucose levels are particularly elevated, as in this patient. If neither of these factors exist, as in most patients, metformin (A) is used as first-line treatment. HbA1$_c$ values are used to monitor patient progress and, in the case of improvement, patients are monitored for side effects. If patients on metformin fail to improve their HbA1$_c$ (this can be taken as <6.5 per cent, but patients and clinicians usually agree on a target value) sulphonylureas can be used together to augment therapy. Insulin therapy (C) is usually started after a trial of lifestyle measures, metformin and sulphonylurea has failed to control blood glucose and HbA1$_c$ values (>7.5 per cent or on a target value agreed upon by patient and clinician). Exenatide (D) may also be considered at this juncture instead of insulin if body weight is a particular issue in the patient's management.

Parasthesia

28 B The glucose tolerance test (B) is diagnostic in patients with suspected acromegaly, many of whom will appear diabetic. Growth hormone (GH) levels (C) can be raised during periods of stress and for most of the time remain <1 mU/L. A raised GH level is therefore not sufficient to diagnose acromegaly though low or undetectable levels can exclude this diagnosis. An MRI scan (A) is the best modality to reveal a pituitary adenoma secreting GH, however this investigation should always follow an abnormal glucose tolerance test reading. Hyperprolactinaemia (E) is commonly associated in acromegaly patients as the pituitary adenoma often co-secretes GH and prolactin and is useful to measure in a confirmed diagnosis of acromegaly and especially if a patient presents with symptoms of elevated prolactin. Thyroid function tests (D) would not be correct in this case. Although the patient does show some symptoms of hypothyroidism, such as weight gain and carpal tunnel syndrome, patients tend not to have elevated blood pressure and increased sweating which would be a feature in hyperthyroidism.

Prognathism

29 A Left untreated, acromegaly patients succumb to cardiovascular related morbidities, such as hypertension and heart failure, as well as an increased incidence of colon cancer. Trans-sphenoidal surgery (A) is first line therapy and is particularly effective against microadenomas. Pituitary radiotherapy (D) usually follows unsuccessful surgery, it is also more useful as an adjunct to other medical treatments as response to radiotherapy alone is often slow. Octreotide (B) is a somatostatin receptor agonist which is effective in reducing growth hormone levels and are often used for short-term treatment, but are not definitively used as first-line therapy. Bromocriptine (C) is a dopamine agonist and is primarily used to reduce the size of tumours before more definitive treatment such as surgery. This is useful since high GH levels are a poor prognostic markers prior to surgery. Pegvisomant (E) is a GH antagonist and is effective in lowering IGF-1 levels rather than GH or tumour size. They are used in patients refractory to surgical, radiotherapy and somatostatin therapy.

Impaired fasting glucose

30 A Diabetes symptoms with polyuria, polydipsia and weight loss occur due to the osmotic diuresis that results from elevated blood glucose. In symptomatic patients, a single abnormal glucose reading is adequate and this may be a fasting plasma glucose ≥7.0 mmol/L or a random plasma glucose of ≥11.1 mmol/L, hence the most appropriate answer is (A) while answer (C) is most likely to occur in a patient with significant symptoms with a random plasma glucose measurement. Asymptomatic patients require two abnormal readings, such as two fasting or two random plasma glucose measurements ≥7.0 mmol/L. Answer (D) is within the normal fasting plasma glucose range (3.9–5.5 mmol/L), while answer (E) is hypoglycaemia. Answer (B) is mildly impaired fasting plasma glucose which is unlikely in a patient who is symptomatic.

Ketonuria

31 D This patient is suffering from an episode of diabetic ketoacidosis; the accumulation of ketones causes a metabolic acid. Calculating the anion gap is useful, narrowing the number of differentials that can cause a metabolic acidosis by showing whether it is due to the retention of H^+ and Cl^- or due to other acids which can help support the suspected diagnosis. The pH balance in the body is maintained by cations such as Na^+, K^+ and anions such as Cl^-, HCO_3^- (there are other cations and anions, but these are the main ones used in anion gap calculations). The anion gap is therefore calculated by $([Na^+] + [K^+]) - ([HCO_3^-] + [Cl^-])$. The anion gap calculation in this case is $([144]) + ([5]) - ([2.9]) - ([100])$ giving 46.1 mmol/L (D). A normal anion gap is 10–18 mmol/L. A normal anion gap in an acidotic patient suggests the retention of H^+/Cl^- or the loss of Na^+/HCO_3^-. This can be due to diarrhoea, renal tubular acidosis or hyperparathyroidism, among other causes. In a metabolic acidosis with an elevated anion gap, as in this case, an unmeasured anion is present in increased quantities, such as lactate or ketones. Causes include lactic acidosis, ketoacidosis and excess salicylates.

Quadrantanopia

32 E Pituitary apoplexy (E) is characterized by a sudden headache, vomiting, visual disturbances and hormonal dysfunction. The cause is most commonly due to the abrupt growth of a pituitary adenoma or pituitary infarction. The headache in apoplexy is usually very abrupt and can be mistaken for a subarachnoid haemorrhage, although usually not as severe. The presentation can be unilateral or generalized. Visual defects are most commonly of the superior quadrant bitemporally. Visual disturbances, such as loss of vision and opthalmoplegia affecting cranial nerves III, IV and VI, help differentiate apoplexy from other intracranial pathology. Hypopituitarism can also follow an apoplexy although this is dependent on degree of damage and often patients present feeling very tired or nauseous. Kallman syndrome (A) is characterized by gonadotrophin deficiency and congenital anosmia. Septo-optic dysplasia (B) is a congenital disorder characterized by the triad of optic nerve hypoplasia, hypopituitarism and forebrain abnormalities. The empty sella syndrome (D) is the observation of absent pituitary tissue within the sella turcica observed on imaging, however pituitary function is normal due to ectopic or unusual position of pituitary tissue within the sella fossa. Sheehan syndrome (C) is also called postpartum hypopituitarism and is most commonly a rare complication of pregnancy. Patient's present with agalactorrhoea, amenorrhoea and hypothyroidism after pregnancy.

Facial plethora

33 C Acromegaly (C) is most commonly due to a pituitary tumour, usually identified on MRI scan. Patients most frequently present with changes in appearance followed by visual defects and headaches. Sleep apnoea, due to weight gain, is often a common complaint among patients. Other manifestations include large hands and feet, hirsutism, prominent and coarse facial features, carpal tunnel syndrome, hypertension, diabetes and heart failure, among others. The glucose tolerance test is diagnostic for suspected acromegaly, GH levels can be measured directly, although elevated findings are not sufficient for diagnosis. Hyperthyroidism (A) produces symptoms that are usually secondary to an elevation in metabolic rate, such symptoms include diarrhoea, goitre, sweating and intolerance to the temperature, whereby the patient consistently feels hot irrespective of the true environmental temperature. Sleep apnoea is not usually a complaint among patients since they often lose weight despite an increased appetite. Cushing's disease (B) results from a pituitary tumour producing excess ACTH, excess cortisol levels result in symptoms such as striae, bruising, thin skin, weight gain, particularly abdominally, and often a dorsocervical fat pad (buffalo hump). Hypothyroidism (D) features include tiredness, depression, cold intolerance, constipation and weight gain. Patients do not tend to sweat more and the disease does not coarsen facial features. In diabetes (E) patients, symptoms often result in weight loss although in type 2 diabetes they may suffer from sleep apnoea due to their high BMI.

Collapse

34 E The patient is mildly acidotic with slightly deranged sodium and borderline normal potassium values. The low bicarbonate and raised chloride, however, are the most strikingly abnormal values. An anion gap calculation $[(Na^+ + K^+) - (Cl^- + HCO_3^-)]$ produces 11.8 which is normal (8–16). An elevated anion gap would suggest excess anions as in lactic acidosis. The differentials for acidosis with a normal anion gap include loss of bicarbonate via the gastrointestinal system, e.g. diarrhoea. Hyperchloraemic metabolic acidosis (E) can also occur resulting from elevated chloride anion levels present in normal saline solution, the acid–base balance shifts to produce excess HCl causing a metabolic acidosis, as in the above patient. Although the sodium and potassium are slightly deranged, Conn's syndrome (C) causes a significantly elevated level of aldosterone from an adrenal tumour which results in significantly deranged sodium and potassium values. Patients also tend to be fluid overloaded resulting in elevated blood pressure. Renal tubular acidosis type 1 (D) results from an inability of the kidney to excrete H^+, resulting in a significant metabolic acidosis. The disease is usually associated with rickets or osteomalacia as Ca^{2+} buffers the excess H^+, the increased Ca^{2+} can also result in increased nephrocalcinosis and recurrent infections. A diabetic ketoacidosis (A) and lactic acidosis (B) result in significant H^+ excess alongside hypokalaemia, usually resulting in an increased anion gap value.

Confusion (2)

35 A This patient is suffering from Addison's disease (A) whereby the adrenal gland is destroyed, usually due to infection (TB) or autoimmunity. The reduced cortisol, aldosterone and sex steroids produce a myriad of signs and symptoms: most importantly, postural hypotension due to reduced aldosterone and increased pigmentation often in palmar creases and newly formed scars. This latter sign is due to elevated MSH which is derived from the POMC molecule which breaks down into MSH and ACTH. Other symptoms include weight loss, malaise, postural hypotension and vitiligo. The SIADH is due to inappropriately elevated levels of ADH (B) which leads to the retention of water. The syndrome is therefore characterized by reduced serum sodium levels (hyponatraemia) and reduced serum osmolality, while urine osmolality and urine sodium levels are elevated. Patients are also euvolaemic without signs of oedema. In patients suffering from heart failure, liver failure or the nephrotic syndrome, the reduced circulatory volume acts as a stimulus for the ADH secretion. Conn's syndrome (C) causes a significantly elevated level of aldosterone secondary to an adrenal tumour. The Waterhouse–Friderichsen syndrome (D) is adrenal haemorrhage that most commonly occurs due to meningococcal infiltration. Patients tend to present with abdominal pain, although symptoms of hypoadrenalism do occur and include fatigue, weakness, dizziness and vomiting. Symptoms of the underlying disease process are also often present, such as fever. This condition tends to occur in younger patients and rarely affects adults. Patients therefore tend to be fluid overloaded resulting in elevated blood pressure. 17-hydroxylase deficiency (E) is usually recognized around puberty, patients present with hypertension, hypokalaemia and hypogonadism. The aldosterone synthesis pathway is overstimulated, while cortisol and sex steroid synthesis is reduced.

SECTION 6:
RHEUMATOLOGY

QUESTIONS

1. Stiff hands (1)

A 36-year-old woman presents to the rheumatology outpatient clinic with a two-month history of stiff hands and wrists. She mentions that the pain is particularly bad for the first few hours after waking up and is affecting her work as a dentist. On examination, the wrists, metacarpophalangeal joints and proximal interphalangeal joints are swollen and warm. What is the most likely diagnosis?

    A. Rheumatoid arthritis
    B. Osteoarthritis
    C. Septic arthritis
    D. Polymyalgia rheumatica
    E. Reactive arthritis

2. Stiff hands (2)

A 45-year-old woman presents to the rheumatology outpatient clinic with a three-month history of stiff hands and wrists. She mentions that the pain is particularly bad first thing in the morning. On examination, the wrists, metacarpophalangeal joints and proximal interphalyngeal joints are swollen and warm. A diagnosis of rheumatoid arthritis is suspected. Which of the following investigations is most specific for confirming the diagnosis?

    A. X-rays
    B. Rheumatoid factor levels
    C. Anti-citrullinated peptide antibody (anti-CCP) levels
    D. C-reactive protein
    E. Erythrocyte sedimentation rate

3. Stiff hands (3)

A 40-year-old woman presents to the rheumatology outpatient clinic with a three-month history of stiff hands and wrists. She mentions that the pain is particularly bad first thing in the morning. On examination, the wrists, metacarpophalangeal joints and proximal interphalangeal joints are swollen and warm. A diagnosis of rheumatoid arthritis is suspected. Blood tests for rheumatoid factor return as positive. What is the most appropriate management?

    A. Non-steroidal anti-inflammatory drugs (NSAIDs)
    B. Intramuscular depot injection of methylprednisolone plus NSAIDs
    C. Anti-TNF therapy
    D. Intramuscular depot injection of methylprednisolone plus NSAIDs and methotrexate and sulfasalazine
    E. Physiotherapy

4. Stiff hands (4)

A 50-year-old woman, who has received a recent diagnosis of rheumatoid arthritis, presents to her GP with ongoing pain and stiffness in her hands and feet. Which joints are usually spared at onset of rheumatoid arthritis?

    A. Proximal interphalangeal joints
    B. Distal interphalangeal joints
    C. Metacarpophalangeal joints
    D. Wrists
    E. Metatarsophalangeal joints

5. Stiff hands (5)

A 55-year-old man presents to his GP with a 2-week history of pain in his hands. The pain is particularly bad in his right hand. On examination, brown discoloration of the nails with onycholysis is noted and the distal interphalangeal joints are tender on palpation. What is the most likely diagnosis?

    A. Rheumatoid arthritis
    B. Dermatomyositis
    C. Reactive arthritis
    D. Osteoarthritis
    E. Psoriatic arthritis

6. Painful knees (1)

A 75-year-old woman presents to accident and emergency complaining of pain in her knees. She mentions that this has been troubling her for several months. Pain is generally worse in the evenings and after walking. On examination, there are palpable bony swellings on the distal interphalangeal joints of the fingers on both hands. In addition, there is reduced range of movement and crepitus in the knees. What is the most likely diagnosis?

    A. Rheumatoid arthritis
    B. Osteoarthritis
    C. Reactive arthritis
    D. Polymyalgia rheumatica
    E. Gout

7. Painful knees (2)

A 79-year-old woman presents to her GP with pain in the left knee. This is particularly bad in the evenings and is stopping her from sleeping. The GP explains that her discomfort is most likely due to osteoarthritis and arranges for her to have an x-ray of the knee. Which of the following descriptions are most likely to describe the x-ray?

    A. Reduced joint space, subchondral sclerosis, bone cysts and osteophytes
    B. Increased joint space, subchondral sclerosis, bone cysts and osteophytes
    C. Reduced joint space, soft tissue swelling and peri-articular osteopenia
    D. Increased joint space, soft tissue swelling and peri-articular osteopenia
    E. Normal x-ray

8. Painful knees (3)

A 76-year-old man presents to accident and emergency with pain in his knees. It is worse in the right knee. He describes the pain as being worse in the evening and after exertion. On examination, bony nodules are palpable on the distal interphalangeal joints of both his hands. The right knee is swollen and there is a reduced range of active movement. X-rays show reduction in the joint space, subchondral sclerosis and osteophyte formation. What is the most appropriate treatment?

    A. Anti-TNF therapy
    B. NSAIDs and urgent orthopaedic follow up
    C. NSAIDs and GP follow up
    D. NSAID and intramuscular depot injection of methylprednisolone with GP follow up
    E. Admit the patient for orthopaedic assessment

9. Painful knees (4)

A 32-year-old man presents to accident and emergency with a 1-day history of pain in the right knee. He also mentions that he has had a fever and is feeling generally unwell. On examination, the right knee is swollen, warm and extremely painful to move. What is the most appropriate next step?

    A. Empirical intravenous antibiotic treatment
    B. X-rays of the right knee
    C. Aspiration of the joint and blood cultures
    D. Referral for physiotherapy
    E. Immobilize the joint

10. Painful knees (5)

A 30-year-old man presents to his GP with a 1-week history of painful, swollen knees and a painful right heel. Further history reveals that he has been experiencing burning pains while urinating for the past 2 weeks and that his eyes have become red and itchy. What is the most likely diagnosis?

    A. Septic arthritis
    B. Gout
    C. Ankylosing spondylitis
    D. Enteropathic arthritis
    E. Reactive arthritis

11. Painful knees (6)

A 70-year-old woman presents to accident and emergency with sudden onset pain and swelling in the right knee. Her past medical history includes hypertension and hypercholesterolaemia. She is currently taking aspirin, ramipril and simvastatin. On examination, she is apyrexial and the right knee is swollen. There is reduced range of movement in the knee due to swelling and pain. X-ray of the right knee shows chondrocalcinosis. What is the most likely diagnosis?

    A. Gout
    B. Pseudo-gout
    C. Septic arthritis
    D. Reactive arthritis
    E. Osteoarthritis

12. Painful knees (7)

A 74-year-old woman presents to accident and emergency with sudden onset pain and swelling in the left knee. On examination, she is apyrexial and the left knee is swollen. There is reduced range of movement in the knee due to swelling and pain. X-ray of the right knee shows chondrocalcinosis. Microscopy of the fluid aspirated from the joint is most likely to show:

    A. Rhomboidal, weakly positively birefringent crystals under polarized light microscopy
    B. Needle-shaped negatively birefringent crystals under polarized light microscopy
    C. Atypical mononuclear cells
    D. Reed Sternberg cells
    E. Tophi

13. Back pain (1)

A 23-year-old man presents to the rheumatology clinic with lower back and hip pain. These have been occurring every day for the past two months. Pain and stiffness are worse in the mornings. He also mentions that his right heel has been hurting. He is previously fit and well, but had occasions of lower back pain when he was a teenager. His symptoms have stopped him from playing tennis. Recent blood tests organized by his GP have shown a raised C-reactive protein (CRP) and erythrocyte sedimentation rate (ESR). What is the most appropriate treatment?

  A. NSAID and spinal exercises
  B. NSAID and bed rest
  C. Oral prednisolone
  D. Methotrexate plus sulfasalazine
  E. Bed rest

14. Back pain (2)

A 32-year-old man presents to the minor injuries walk-in clinic, complaining of back pain. This had started suddenly that morning after he had lifted a heavy box at home. He mentions that the pain has been shooting down his left leg and he cannot walk without the support of his friend. He has not passed urine since the onset of pain. On neurological examination of the lower limbs, tone and power cannot be assessed due to pain but there are decreased ankle reflexes and a sacral anaesthesia. What is the most appropriate next step?

  A. Give NSAID analgesia and complete neurological examination
  B. Send the patient home with NSAID analgesia and bed rest advice
  C. Arrange urgent MRI of spine
  D. Give NSAID analgesia and catheterize the patient
  E. Send the patient home with NSAID analgesia and advice to avoid heavy lifting

15. Back pain (3)

A 70-year-old woman with a history of vertebral crush fractures presents to the osteoporosis outpatient clinic. Which of the following investigations is most useful to assess the extent of her osteoporosis?

  A. Spinal x-rays
  B. MRI scan
  C. Full blood count, bone and liver biochemistry blood tests
  D. Vitamin D levels
  E. DEXA scan

16. Blurred vision

A 20-year-old man presents to accident and emergency with sudden onset pain in the right eye, with associated blurred vision and discomfort when gazing at the lights. He has a history of back pain and has recently been diagnosed with ankylosing spondylosis. What is the most likely cause of his eye pain?

    A. Conjunctivitis
    B. Retinal detachment
    C. Anterior uveitis
    D. Corneal ulceration
    E. Acute glaucoma

17. Shoulder pain (1)

A 70-year-old woman presents to her GP complaining of severe unilateral headache over the left side of her head. On further questioning, she mentions that she has been having bilateral shoulder and neck pains over the past few weeks. She has also been feeling lethargic. On examination, the left side of her scalp is painful to touch. What is the most likely diagnosis?

    A. Polyarteritis nodosa
    B. Polymyositis
    C. Hypothyroidism
    D. Migraine
    E. Giant cell arteritis

18. Shoulder pain (2)

A 77-year-old woman presents to accident and emergency complaining of severe unilateral headache over the left side of her head. On examination, the left side of her scalp is painful to touch. Blood tests reveal a raised ESR and CRP. What is the most appropriate management?

    A. Steroid therapy and arrange urgent temporal artery biopsy
    B. NSAID analgesia and arrange urgent temporal artery biopsy
    C. Paracetamol analgesia and discharge with advice to bed rest
    D. Arrange urgent MRI head
    E. NSAID analgesia and arrange urgent electromyography

19. Shoulder pain (3)

A 60-year-old woman presents to her GP with a two-month history of lethargy and weakness. She mentions that she is finding it increasingly difficult to climb the stairs and do the housework. On examination, there is wasting and weakness of the proximal muscles in the upper and lower limbs. What is the most likely diagnosis?

    A. Dermatomyositis
    B. Polymyositis
    C. Polymyalgia rheumatica
    D. Kawasaki's disease
    E. Polyarteritis nodosa

20. Shortness of breath (1)

A 30-year-old Afro-Carribean woman presents to accident and emergency with a 1-week history of progressive shortness of breath and fever. On further questioning, she mentions that her hands have been painful and stiff over the past few months and she has been having recurrent mouth ulcers. Chest x-ray confirms bilateral pleural effusions and blood tests reveal a raised ESR and a normal CRP. What is the most likely diagnosis?

    A. Systemic lupus erythematosus
    B. Systemic sclerosis
    C. Sjögren's syndrome
    D. Discoid lupus
    E. Beçhet's disease

21. Shortness of breath (2)

A 34-year-old Afro-Carribean woman has been admitted for management and investigation of increasing shortness of breath. On further questioning, she mentions that her hands have been painful and stiff over the past few months and she has been having recurrent mouth ulcers. Chest x-ray confirms bilateral pleural effusions and blood tests reveal a raised ESR and a normal CRP. A diagnosis of systemic lupus erythematosus (SLE) is suspected and a full autoantibody screen is sent to the laboratory. Which of the following auto-antibodies is most specific to the suspected diagnosis?

    A. Anti-nuclear antibody
    B. Rheumatoid factor
    C. Anti-double stranded DNA antibody
    D. Anti-centromere antibody
    E. Anti-mitochondrial antibody

22. Shortness of breath (3)

A 55-year-old woman presents to her GP with shortness of breath and dry cough. The symptoms began a few months ago and have progressed. She has a past medical history of rheumatoid arthritis, diagnosed ten years earlier. On respiratory examination, there are bibasal fine inspiratory crackles on auscultation. What is the most likely cause of her symptoms?

  A. Pulmonary oedema
  B. Consolidation
  C. Pleural effusions
  D. Pulmonary fibrosis
  E. Intrapulmonary nodules

23. Shortness of breath (4)

A 27-year-old woman presents to accident and emergency complaining of sudden onset shortness of breath and right-sided pleuritic chest pain. She has a past medical history of three miscarriages and a deep venous thrombosis in the right leg. On examination, pulse is 110 bpm, respiratory rate is 24 bpm, oxygen saturation is 88 per cent on room air. An arterial blood gas shows pH 7.40, PO_2 8.0, PCO_2 3.1. What is the diagnostic investigation of choice?

  A. Full blood count
  B. Chest x-ray
  C. D-dimer
  D. CT pulmonary angiogram (CTPA)
  E. ECG

24. Shortness of breath (5)

A 27-year-old woman presents to accident and emergency complaining of sudden onset shortness of breath, right-sided pleuritic chest pain and haemoptysis. She has a past medical history of three miscarriages and a deep venous thrombosis in the right leg. CTPA confirms a large pulmonary embolism. What is the most likely underlying diagnosis?

  A. SLE
  B. Primary anti-phospholipid syndrome
  C. Raynaud's disease
  D. Systemic sclerosis
  E. Beçhet's disease

25. Shortness of breath (6)

A 27-year-old woman presents to accident and emergency complaining of sudden onset shortness of breath, right-sided pleuritic chest pain and haemoptysis. She has a past medical history of three miscarriages and a deep venous thrombosis in the right leg. CTPA confirms a large pulmonary embolism. A diagnosis of anti-phospholipid syndrome is suspected and a full autoantibody screen is sent. Which of the following auto-antibodies would confirm the diagnosis if detected?

A. Anti-cardiolipin antibody
B. Anti-centromere antibody
C. Anti-nuclear antibody
D. Anti-mitochondrial antibody
E. Anti-histone antibody

26. Dry eyes

A 45-year-old woman presents to the rheumatology clinic with a three-month history of itchy, dry eyes and a persistently dry mouth. She also mentions that her fingers have been extremely cold, occasionally turning blue after going outside in the morning. Schirmer's test is positive. What is the most likely diagnosis?

A. Systemic sclerosis
B. Raynaud's disease
C. SLE
D. Primary Sjögren's syndrome
E. Secondary Sjögren's syndrome

27. Cold hands

A 24-year-old woman presents to her GP complaining of cold hands and feet. This has been ongoing for the past three months and is especially bad when she goes out in the mornings and may last for hours. On further questioning, she mentions that her hands sometimes turn blue or red and that gloves are unhelpful. She has otherwise been feeling well and has no past medical history. What is the most appropriate treatment?

A. Propanolol
B. Aspirin
C. Nifedipine
D. Subcutaneous injection of low molecular weight heparin
E. Prednisolone

28. Chest discomfort

A 42-year-old woman presents to accident and emergency with retrosternal discomfort. She was diagnosed with systemic sclerosis a year ago. Which of the following statements is true about systemic sclerosis?

A. Microstomia is only seen in diffuse cutaneous systemic sclerosis
B. Skin involvement is limited to face, hands and feet in limited cutaneous systemic sclerosis
C. Oesophageal dysmotility is only seen in limited cutaneous systemic sclerosis
D. Anti-double stranded DNA antibodies are normally detected in patients with systemic sclerosis
E. Raynaud's phenomenon occurs as a result of skin fibrosis (scleroderma)

29. Painful joints

A 30-year-old woman presents to accident and emergency with worsening stiffness in the hands, wrists and feet. She mentions that the pain has been particularly bad in the mornings. On examination, there is a palpable spleen. Initial blood tests reveal a low neutrophil count and a raised C-reactive protein. The most likely diagnosis is:

A. Felty's syndrome
B. Reactive arthritis
C. Still's disease
D. Infectious mononucleosis
E. Serum sickness

30. Joint pain (1)

A 53-year-old man, who works as a chef, presents to accident and emergency with sudden onset severe pain, tenderness and swelling of the first metatarsophalangeal joint. The pain is making it difficult for him to mobilize. He has had two previous similar episodes. Blood tests reveal a raised serum urate level. The most likely diagnosis is:

A. Gout
B. Pseudo-gout
C. Septic arthritis
D. Reactive arthritis
E. Osteoarthritis

31. Joint pain (2)

A 59-year-old man presents to his GP with sudden onset severe pain, tenderness and swelling of the first metatarsophalangeal joint. He is known to suffer from acute gout and has had several previous similar episodes. What is the most appropriate treatment?

    A.   Allopurinol
    B.   NSAIDs
    C.   Conservative measures including reduced alcohol intake and weight loss
    D.   Intra-articular steroid injection
    E.   Methotrexate

32. Skin reaction (1)

A 30-year-old Turkish man presents to accident and emergency with oral ulcers, genital ulcers and painful legs. On examination, there are apthous ulcers in the mouth, genital ulceration, erythema nodosum over the shins. He is admitted under the medical team on call and a skin pathergy test is positive. What is the most likely diagnosis?

    A.   Henoch–Schönlein purpura
    B.   Lyme disease
    C.   Berger's disease
    D.   Caplan's syndrome
    E.   Behçet's disease

33. Skin reaction (2)

A 23-year-old woman presents to accident and emergency with a purpuric rash over the buttocks and lower limbs and haematuria. She is finding it difficult to mobilize due to pain in her ankles and knees. What is the most likely diagnosis?

    A.   Henoch–Schönlein purpura
    B.   Perthes' disease
    C.   Behçet's disease
    D.   Still's disease
    E.   Ehlers–Danlos syndrome

34. Bone pain (1)

A 67-year-old man presents to his GP with pain in his pelvis. During the consultation, he mentions that his friends have been commenting that his head appears larger than before. In addition, he has noticed deterioration in hearing in his left ear. On neurological examination, a left-sided sensorineural deafness in detected. Closer inspection of the legs reveals bowing of the tibia. What is the most likely diagnosis?

    A. Osteomalacia
    B. Osteoporosis
    C. Acromegaly
    D. Rickets
    E. Paget's disease

35. Bone pain (2)

In a patient with Paget's disease of the bone, which of the following blood test results are most likely to be seen?

    A. Normal serum calcium, normal serum phosphate, raised serum alkaline phosphatase
    B. Normal serum calcium, normal serum phosphate, normal serum alkaline phosphatase
    C. Raised serum calcium, low serum phosphate, normal serum alkaline phosphatase
    D. Normal serum calcium, low serum phosphate, raised serum alkaline phosphatase
    E. Low serum calcium, low serum phosphate, low serum alkaline phosphatase

ANSWERS

Stiff hands (1)

1 A   Rheumatoid arthritis (A) is a chronic, systemic inflammatory disease, which produces a symmetrical, deforming polyarthritis. The typical presentation of rheumatoid arthritis is with symmetrical pain and stiffness of the small joints of the hands and feet. Pain is characteristically worse in the morning and improves with exercise. As the disease progresses, it may cause deformity of the affected joints. Less commonly, rheumatoid arthritis may present with a monoarthritis. Diagnosis is made from the presence of articular and extra-articular features characteristic of the disease. The most recent criteria for diagnosis is the 2010 American College of Rheumatology and the European League Against Rheumatism criteria:

	Score
A. Joint involvement	
1 large joint	0
2–10 large joints	1
1–3 small joints (with or without involvement of large joints)	2
4–10 small joints (with or without involvement of large joints)	3
>10 joints (including at least one small joint)	5
B. Serology	
Negative RF[a] and negative anti-citrullinated protein antibody	0
Low-positive RF[a] or low-positive anti-citrullinated protein antibody	2
High-positive RF or high-positive anti-citrullinated protein antibody	3
C. Acute phase reactants	
Normal CRP and normal ESR	0
Abnormal CRP or abnormal ESR	1
D. Duration of symptoms	
<6 weeks	0
≥6 weeks	1

[a]Rheumatoid factor

This criteria set can be applied to patients that have synovitis in at least one joint and the absence of an alternative diagnosis. A total score of 6 or greater is diagnostic.

Primary nodal osteoarthritis (B) affects the hands. However, this answer is incorrect as the distal interphalangeal joints (DIPs) are usually more involved than the proximal interphalangeal joints (PIPs). In addition, pain is characteristically worse at the end of the day. Septic arthritis (C) usually presents as a monoarthritis, making this answer incorrect. Polymyalgia rheumatica (D) is incorrect as this disorder is rare in those under the age of 60 and is characterized by pain and stiffness in the shoulders, neck, hips and lumbar spine, which is worse in the morning. Reactive arthritis (E) is usually an asymmetrical, lower-limb arthritis. Therefore this answer is also wrong.

Stiff hands (2)

2 C   Anti-citrullinated peptide (anti-CCP) antibodies (C) levels are the most specific investigation for rheumatoid arthritis. X-rays (A) early in the disease course will demonstrate soft tissue swelling but are unlikely to show much else. However, x-rays of the hands, feet and any other affected joint should be performed early in the disease to establish a baseline. Rheumatoid factor (B) is positive in approximately 70 per cent of patients with rheumatoid arthritis. However, it is not specific to rheumatoid arthritis and may be raised in a number of other conditions. Rheumatoid factor should be tested for in patients with suspected rheumatoid arthritis. Anti-CCP antibodies can be subsequently sent if rheumatoid factor is negative or to inform decision making about starting therapy. It is important to note that anti-CCP antibodies are not presently a routine test for all patients with suspected rheumatoid arthritis. C-reactive protein (D) is raised in many infective and inflammatory conditions. It is therefore not the most specific test for rheumatoid arthritis. However, it is raised in rheumatoid arthritis and can be used to monitor the disease and guide treatment decisions. Erythrocyte sedimentation rate (E) is raised in rheumatoid arthritis and a range of other conditions. It is, therefore, not the correct answer.

Stiff hands (3)

3 A   Most patients will be offered NSAIDs (A) first by their GP, or over the counter, but if these fail, referral to hospital rheumatology is required. If NSAIDs do not resolve symptoms, therapy would be escalated to include methotrexate and one other disease-modifying anti-rheumatic drug (DMARD), such as sulfasalazine plus a steroid (D). DMARDs should be offered early within the treatment of the disease to limit joint destruction. Short-term steroid therapy is useful for controlling disease flares and can be given by oral, intramuscular and intra-articular routes. Intramuscular depot injection of methylprednisolone plus NSAIDs (B) will be very useful in managing symptoms of the flare, but will not alter the disease course. Anti-TNF therapy (C) is reserved for patients who have active disease despite DMARDs (usually two trials of DMARDs should be tried before considering anti-TNF). Physiotherapy (E) is very useful and should be encouraged, but alone cannot control symptoms or disease course, making this answer incorrect.

Stiff hands (4)

4 B   The hand changes associated with rheumatoid arthritis are frequently tested in clinical and written exams. The most common presenting features are pain and stiffness of the small joints of the hands and feet, which is worse in the mornings. The most common joints at onset of disease are proximal interphalangeal joints (A), metacarpophalangeal joints (C), wrists (D) and metatarsophalangeal joints (E). The distal interphalangeal joints (B) are usually spared at onset, making this the correct answer here. It is important to note, however, that this is a variable disease and some patients may present with other joint involvement including elbows, shoulders, knees or ankles. As the disease progresses and joint damage occurs in the hands, a variety of deformities may be seen. These include ulnar deviation and palmar subluxation of the metacarpophalangeal joints, Boutonniere deformity (flexion of PIPs, hyperextension of DIPs), swan-neck deformity (hyperextension of PIP, flexion of DIPs) or dorsal subluxation of the ulnar styloid. Inflammation of the flexor tendon sheath may result in carpal tunnel syndrome and inflammation of the extensor tendon sheath can cause tendon rupture. Therefore, it is worth looking out for scars of carpal tunnel decompression and tendon repair during clinical examination.

Stiff hands (5)

5 E   Approximately 5 per cent of patients with psoriasis develop arthritis. The pattern of arthritis is variable but most commonly affects the distal interphalangeal joints and is asymmetrical. Nail or skin changes of psoriasis are usually present, but may develop after the arthritis. It is also important to note that psoriatic arthritis may present as a symmetrical polyarthritis, resembling rheumatoid arthritis. A small number of patients with psoriatic arthritis may develop arthritis mutilans, where peri-articular osteolysis and bone shortening occur, producing marked deformity. The pattern of asymmetrical arthritis affecting the distal interphalangeal joints with nail changes should indicate that psoriatic arthritis (E) is the correct answer. The distal interphalangeal joints are usually spared at onset of rheumatoid arthritis (A) and the asymmetrical pattern described with nail changes mean that this is the incorrect answer. Dermatomyositis (B) presents with symmetrical proximal muscle weakness with characteristic skin changes. It does not cause a polyarthritis of the hands, thus making this answer incorrect. Reactive arthritis (C) is an asymmetrical lower limb arthritis, making this answer wrong. Osteoarthritis (D) may affect the distal interphalangeal joints, but does not cause nail changes, making this answer incorrect as well.

Painful knees (1)

6 B   Osteoarthritis (B) is the most common type of arthritis. It is increasingly common with age and most people over the age of 60 will have some evidence of the disease on x-rays. It is important to note that osteoarthritis occurs as a result of a complex pathological process. Osteoarthritis may be localized or generalized, with pain characterisitically worse in the evenings. Localized osteoarthritis includes nodal osteoarthritis, which usually involves the distal interphalangeal joints. However, the proximal interphalangeal joints are also affected. With time, the hands become stiff and painful and painless bony swellings develop – Heberden's nodes on the DIPs and Bouchard's nodes on the PIPs. Bony swelling of the first carpometacarpal joint may result in a squared hand appearance in nodal osteoarthritis. Localized osteoarthritis may also affect the weight-bearing joints of the hips and knees. Generalized osteoarthritis may include features of nodal disease plus widespread joint involvement including DIPs, first metatarsophalangeal joints, knees and hips. Increased pain in the evenings, nodal disease and knee involvement point to osteoarthritis being the correct answer here. Rheumatoid arthritis (A) is worse in the mornings and the DIPs are usually spared at disease onset, making this answer wrong. Reactive arthritis (C) does not involve the hands or cause nodal disease, making this answer incorrect. Polymyalgia rheumatica (D) is wrong as this does not usually involve the hands or knees and is worse in the mornings. Gout (E) normally presents as an acute monoarthritis, making this answer incorrect.

Painful knees (2)

7 A   The main radiographical features of osteoarthritis are reduced joint space, subchondral sclerosis, bone cysts and osteophytes (A). Knowledge of the radiograhical features of osteoarthritis is commonly examined in both written and clinical exams. Joint space is reduced radiographically in osteoarthritis, making answers (B) and (D) incorrect. Reduced joint space, soft tissue swelling and peri-articular osteopenia (C) are radiographical features of rheumatoid arthritis. Additional features include bony erosions and joint subluxation. X-ray findings are likely to be present in this patient, making normal x-ray (E) the incorrect option. However, it is important to note that the extent of radiographical abnormality may not correlate well with the extent of symptoms, and treatment options should be based on the patient and the level of disability rather than the extent of joint damage seen on the x-ray.

Painful knees (3)

8 C   The case in this question is describing a patient with osteoarthritis. Appropriate analgesia and GP follow up (C) is the most appropriate treatment plan in this question. Analgesia should follow the WHO analgesic ladder with simple analgesia as first-line therapy. NSAID analgesia is likely to be effective for pain relief. Given that the patient has had ongoing symptoms for some months and is able to mobilize, follow up from the GP is the best option. Anti-TNF therapy (A) and steroid therapy (D) are not used in the treatment of osteoarthritis. Orthopaedic follow up (B) to consider surgical options would be appropriate if the pain is uncontrollable and particularly if the patient is getting pain at rest or during the night. Admission (E) should be considered in some patients where the pain is too severe for discharge or social circumstances or co-morbidities mean that management of symptoms at home will not be possible.

Painful knees (4)

9 C The case presented in this question should raise the suspicion of septic arthritis. This is a medical emergency and if left untreated can result in rapid destruction of the joint. *Staphlococcus aureus* is the most common organism that causes septic arthritis, although gonococcus is also common in young people. Septic arthritis presents as a hot, red, swollen joint that is extremely painful. The systemic features and fever in the case should also point to septic arthritis, but patients may also have no systemic features. The management of patients with suspected septic arthritis should be swift. Aspiration of the joint and blood cultures (C) should be taken first and sent to the microbiology laboratory for culture. Empirical intravenous antibiotic treatment (A) must then be commenced without delay. An example of an empirical regime for septic arthritis would include flucloxacillin, benzylpenicillin and gentamicin. These can then be altered when sensitivites are known. X-rays of the right knee (B) should be performed but are unlikely to aid the diagnosis. Other blood tests including full blood count and CRP should also be sent. The joint should be initially immobilized (E), but this is not the most appropriate next step. Physiotherapy (D) should be started early, but after an initial period of immobilization, making this the wrong answer.

Painful knees (5)

10 E Reactive arthritis (E) is a sterile arthritis, which follows an attack of dysentery (caused by *Campylobacter*, *Salmonella*, *Shigella* or *Yersinia* spp.) or urethritis (caused by *Chlamydia* or *Ureaplasma* spp.). Clinical features of reactive arthritis are an acute, asymmetrical lower limb arthritis occurring 1–4 weeks following an infection. Other features of reactive arthritis include conjunctivitis (as described by this case), enthesitis (which may result in plantar fasciitis or Archilles tendonitis), circinate balanitis (painless superficial ulceration of glans penis), keratoderma blenorrhagica (painless, red plaques on the soles and palmes), nail dystrophy, mouth ulcers and, rarely, aortic incompetence. The triad of urethritis, arthritis and conjunctivitis is known as Reiter's disease. Treatment of reactive arthritis is with NSAIDs and local steroid injection for symptomatic control. Any underlying infection should be treated but is unlikely to influence the course of the arthritis. Individuals who develop recurrent attacks of arthritis can be considered for therapy with sulfasalazine or methotrexate. Septic arthritis (A) is a monoarthritis, presenting as a hot, swollen, tender joint. Therefore this is the incorrect answer. Gout (B) also usually presents as an acute monoarthritis and does not cause conjunctivitis or urethritis, making this answer incorrect. Ankylosing spondylosis (C) does not affect the knees or cause urethritis, although it can cause conjunctivitis. Enteropathic arthritis (D) is an asymmetrical lower limb arthritis, associated with inflammatory bowel disease. The absence of bowel symptoms in this patient means this is the incorrect answer.

Painful knees (6)

11 B   Pseudo-gout (B) is caused by the presence of calcium pyrophosphate crystals in the joint, causing an acute synovitis. Pseudo-gout most commonly affects elderly women and usually involves the knee or wrists. It may also be seen in younger patients with underlying conditions causing the deposition of calcium pyrophosphate crystals such as hypothyroidism, hyperparathyroidism, acromegaly Wilson's disease or haemochromatosis. X-ray of the affected joint may show chondrocalcinosis (calcification of the hyaline cartilage). Treatment of pseudo-gout is with aspiration of the joint and NSAIDs. Intra-articular steroid injection can be used if pain is not controlled. The acute synovitis of pseudogout resembles gout (A). While acute gout most commonly affects the first metatarsophalangeal joint, other joints may be affected. However, the finding of chondrocalcinosis makes pseudo-gout more likely than gout. Septic arthritis is a differential diagnosis of pseudo-gout and should be considered, despite the apyrexia. Therefore, the joint aspirate should be sent for culture. The chondrocalcinosis on x-ray makes the diagnosis of pseudo-gout more likely than septic arthritis (C) in this question. Reactive arthritis (D) presents as an asymmetrical polyarthritis of the lower limbs, making this answer incorrect. Osteoarthritis (E) may affect the knee. However, the chondrocalcinosis again makes pseudo-gout the more likely answer. In addition, a history of pain in the knee would be expected.

Painful knees (7)

12 A   The presence of rhomboidal, weakly positively birefringent crystals (A) under polarized light microscopy in joint fluid is diagnostic of pseudo-gout. Needle-shaped negatively birefringent crystals (B) are seen in gout. Atypical mononuclear cells (C) are found on microscopy of blood samples in patients with infectious mononucleosis. Microscopic analysis of lymph node biopsy specimens in patients with Hodgkin's lymphoma may show Reed–Sternberg cells (D). Tophi (E) are the white deposits seen in skin and soft tissue in some patients with gout. They are composed of sodium urate and the presence of tophi in a patient with long-standing gout is called 'chronic tophaceous gout'.

Back pain (1)

13 A This is a difficult question as it requires knowledge of the diagnosis and then knowledge of the treatment. The case presented is of a patient with ankylosing spondylosis. The diagnosis is clinical, with involvement of the sacroiliac joint as the earliest manifestation. The disease course is variable and may progress to a marked kyphosis of the spine. Other features include enthesitis (such as the Archilles tendon enthesitis in this case), costochondritis, peripheral joint involvement (usually asymmetrical and involving the large joints), aortic regurgitation, apical pulmonary fibrosis and amyloidosis. The ESR and CRP are usually raised. Initial x-rays may be unremarkable. However, later in the disease, syndesmophytes (bony spurs due to inflammatory enthesitis) may be seen between vertebrae resulting in the characteristic bamboo spine appearance. Ankylosing spondylosis is managed with exercises, not bed rest. NSAIDs are given, unless there are contraindications, for the management of pain. Therefore, NSAID and spinal exercises (A) is the correct answer and NSAID and bed rest (B) and bed rest (E) are incorrect. Local steroid injections may be used for pain relief, particularly for peripheral arthritis and enthesitis. However, oral prednisolone (C) is not normally used. Methotrexate and sulfasalazine (D) may be given to patients with peripheral arthritis, but do not help the back pain, making this answer incorrect.

Back pain (2)

14 C The history and examination should raise the suspicion of cauda equina syndrome. This is a medical emergency and permanent neurological deficit may occur without urgent intervention. The shooting pain down the left leg, absence of ankle jerk reflex and urinary retention suggest that the L5/S1 disk has prolapsed into the cauda equina and nerve root. The patient must be sent to accident and emergency (C) without delay for assessment, MRI of the spine and subsequent neurosurgical referral. Therefore, sending the patient home, as described by options (B) and (E) is inappropriate. A complete neurological examination (A) is desirable, but should not delay transfer to accident and emergency for MRI. Similarly, the patient will require a catheter (D), but this should not delay transfer to accident and emergency. It is important to note that while intramuscular NSAID analgesia can be used for patients with cauda equina syndrome, stronger opiate analgesia may be required.

Back pain (3)

15 E Osteoporosis is a loss of the bone mass. It is important to note that the mineralization of the bone is normal. This loss of bone mass means there is an increasing likelihood of fracture with increasing age. Due to the accelerated loss of bone mass following the menopause, elderly women are at a higher risk of osteoporosis than men. There are numerous risk factors for the development of osteoporosis. Among them are Caucasian and Asian ethnic groups, female sex, increasing age, early menopause, smoking, excess alcohol, corticosteroid use, hypogonadism and rheumatoid arthritis. The reduced bone mass of osteoporosis may result in vertebral crush fractures, the majority of which are asymptomatic. The extent of osteoporosis is best investigated with a dual energy x-ray absorptiometry (DEXA) scan (E). This gives a T score, which is the number of standard deviations the patient's bone mineral density differs from the population average for a young healthy adult. The World Health Organization defines osteoporosis as a T score of −2.5 or greater (i.e. the bone mineral density of more than 2.5 standard deviations below that of the average for a young healthy adult). A T score of between −1.5 and −2.5 is defined as osteopenia. Spinal x-rays (A) are useful to assess vertebral crush fractures but cannot assess extent of osteoporosis. MRI scans (B) are not used to assess osteoporosis, so this answer is incorrect. Full blood count, bone and liver biochemistry tests (C) are not affected by osteoporosis, making this answer incorrect. Vitamin D deficiency may contribute towards the development of osteoporosis but levels (D) cannot assess extent of disease. Treatment options in osteoporosis include use of bisphosphonates, hormone replacement therapy and raloxifene (a selective oestrogen receptor modulator).

Blurred vision

16 C Anterior uveitis (C) is associated with ankylosing spondylosis and may occur in up to one-third of patients. The symptoms described in this patient with ankylosing spondylosis means anterior uveitis is the correct answer. Conjunctivitis (A) is associated with ankylosing spondylosis but would present with red, itchy eyes without blurred vision or photophobia, making this answer incorrect. Retinal detachment (B) is not associated with ankylosing spndylosis and usually presents with flashes of light in the affected eye and increase in the number of floaters followed by visual loss. Therefore, this answer is incorrect. Corneal ulceration (D) is not associated with ankylosing spondylosis and presents with redness and eye pain without visual loss, making it the wrong answer. Acute glaucoma (E) may present with eye pain but is not associated with ankylosing spondylosis, making this answer incorrect. Patients would present with a red eye, sudden onset eye pain, decreased visual acuity and nausea or vomiting.

Shoulder pain (1)

17 E   This is a relatively straightforward question. Giant cell arteritis (E) is a large vessel vasulitis, which occurs in association with polymyalgia rheumatica. Features of giant cell arteritis include severe headaches, which are usually unilateral and involve the temporal region with associated scalp tenderness. There may also be jaw claudication on eating. Involvement of the ophthalmic arteries may result in visual loss, which may be permanent if the condition is untreated. Polyarteritis nodosa (A) is a medium-sized vessel vasculitis, which may affect a number of organs. However, headache is not a feature, making this the incorrect answer. Polymyositis (B) presents with proximal muscle weakness, resembling polymyalgia rheumatica. Again, headache is not a feature making this answer wrong. Hypothyroidism (C) can result in proximal muscle weakness but does not cause unilateral headache, making this answer incorrect. The presentation of migraine (D) is variable and includes unilateral headache, with or without aura. However, the presence of scalp tenderness and features of polymyalgia rheumatica make giant cell arteritis a more likely option.

Shoulder pain (2)

18 A   The ESR and CRP are usually raised in patients with giant cell arteritis. Due to the risk of irreversible visual loss, patients with giant cell arteritis must be started on high-dose steroids (usually 60 mg of prednisolone/day) immediately. The response to steroids is usually rapid (within 48 h). A temporal artery biopsy should be arranged within the next 3–4 days to confirm the diagnosis. It is important to note that the arteritis may be patchy and thus absent in the section of vessel biopsied. Therefore, if the temporal artery biopsy is negative, it does not exclude the diagnosis. Therefore, steroid therapy and arrange an urgent temporal artery biopsy (A) is the correct option here. NSAID analgesia (B) may help with symptoms but does not treat the underlying arteritis and the risk of visual loss remains. Therefore, these options are incorrect. Paracetamol analgesia and discharge (C) with advice to bed rest does not address the underlying artertitis or confirm the diagnosis, making this answer wrong. MRI head and electromyography are not diagnostic investigations in temporal arteritis (E), making these options incorrect.

Shoulder pain (3)

19 B   Polymyositis (B) occurs due to inflammation of striated muscle, resulting in proximal muscle weakness. It affects women more than men. The onset usually occurs over a period of months and may include systemic features such as lethargy and weight loss. The proximal muscles of the shoulder and pelvis girdle become weak and wasted. The disease may then progress to involve the pharyngeal, laryngeal or respiratory muscles. When features of polymyositis are accompanied with overlying skin changes, it is termed 'dermatomyositis' (A). These include a heliotrope (lilac) rash over the eyelids, scaly red papules over the knuckles, elbows or knees (Gottron's papules), a macular rash over the back and shoulders (shawl sign) or painful cracking over the tips of the fingers (mechanic's hands). The absence of these features makes dermatomyositis the incorrect answer. Polymyalgia rheumatica (C) may affect the proximal muscles. However, it is associated with pain, which is an uncommon feature of polymyositis. Although investigations have not been mentioned in this question, it is worth noting that polymyalgia rheumatica is associated with a raised ESR while in polymyositis, the ESR is usually not raised. Kawasaki's disease (D) is a medium-vessel vasculitis that affects mainly children and does not cause proximal muscle weakness, making this answer incorrect. Polyarteritis nodosa (E) is also a medium vessel vasculitis, which affects multiple organs. Proximal muscle weakness is not a feature, making this answer incorrect.

Shortness of breath (1)

20 A SLE is a multisystem, inflammatory disorder which is nine times more common in women than men. It is also more common in people of Afro-Carribean origin and peak age of onset is usually 20–40 years of age. Multiple genetic and aetiological factors have been associated with the development of this disease. SLE has an extremely variable presentation, with clinical features usually caused by underlying vasculitis. These include polyarthritis (the most common clinical feature, often a symmetrical small joint polyarthritis similar to that seen in early RA), photosensitive rashes (characteristic erythematous rash over malar eminences, sparing the nasolabial folds), mouth ulcers, serositis (affecting pleura or pericardium) or renal disease (usually nephrotic syndrome of renal failure due to underlying glomerulonephritis). The features presented in this case are, therefore, most suggestive of SLE (A) as the diagnosis. The raised ESR and CRP should also identify SLE as the correct answer. Systemic sclerosis (B) can be localized or diffuse and does not characteristically cause mouth ulcers, pleural effusions or a raised ESR. Sjögren's (C) is a syndrome of dry eyes and dry mouth. It can be a primary syndrome or occur secondary to other autoimmune diseases. While it is associated with arthralgia, the pleural effusion, mouth ulcers and blood results make this diagnosis unikely. Discoid lupus (D) is a variant of SLE where skin involvement is the only feature. Therefore, this is the incorrect answer. Behçet's disease (E) usually manifests with oral ulceration. However, the peripheral polyarthritis, pleural effusuions and blood results (in Behçet's both ESR and CRP may be elevated) make this the incorrect answer in this case.

Shortness of breath (2)

21 C Anti-double stranded DNA antibody (C) is the most specific antibody for SLE and is raised in 60 per cent of cases. Levels of other autoantibodies may also be raised in SLE but these are less specific. They include anti-nuclear antibody (A) and rheumatoid factor (B). Anti-centromere antibody (D) levels may be raised in patients with limited systemic sclerosis but not in patients with SLE. Raised anti-mitochondrial antibody (E) levels are associated with primary biliary cirrhosis.

Shortness of breath (3)

22 D The collection of shortness of breath, dry cough and bibasal fine inspiratory crackles should point to pulmonary fibrosis (D) as the answer in this question. In patients with rheumatoid arthritis, this may occur as a result of extra-articular manifestation of the disease. Pulmonary fibrosis is also a side effect of methotrexate, a disease-modifiying anti-rheumatic drug, which is commonly used in rheumatoid arthritis. Pulmonary oedema (A) will cause shortness of breath and be heard as fine inspiratory crackles during respiratory examination. However, it would characteristically produce a productive cough of frothy sputum. In addition, pulmonary oedema is not an extra-articular manifestation of rheumatoid arthritis or a side effect of the drugs used to treat it, making this answer incorrect. Consolidation (B) occurs as a result of an infective process and can present in a number of ways including shortness of breath, productive cough or pleurisy. On respiratory examination, there is likely to be bronchial breathing and end expiratory crackles. Pleural effusions (C) are an extra-articular manifestation in rheumatoid arthritis. Clinical features would include shortness of breath and, on examination, there would be reduced air entry, stony dullness to percussion and reduced vocal resonance. Therefore, this is the incorrect answer. Intrapulmonary nodules (E) are also an extra-articular manifestation of rheumatoid arthritis, but do not cause the clinical features outlined in this question, making this answer wrong.

Shortness of breath (4)

23 D The clinical features outlined in this question of sudden onset shortness of breath and pleuritic chest pain with tachycardia and tachypnoea with a low oxygen saturation on room air, should raise the suspicion of pulmonary embolism. The blood gas demonstrates a low PO_2 and PCO_2. This indicates that the patient is hypoxic despite hyperventilation. The diagnostic investigation of choice in patients with pulmonary embolism is CTPA (D). Full blood count (A) is not useful in the diagnosis of pulmonary embolism. Chest x-ray (B) is often normal in patients with pulmonary embolism but may show a wedge-shaped infarct. D-dimer (C) is a fibrin degradation product that is commonly used in the diagnosis of deep venous thrombosis or pulmonary oedema. When negative, it indicates that venous thrombosis is unlikely. D-dimer may be positive for a number of reasons. Therefore, it is often used in patients where the clinical picture is unclear. In the case outlined in the question, there should be a high degree of suspicion for pulmonary embolism and a CTPA should be arranged without delay, making D-dimer the incorrect answer. ECG (E) may be useful and may commonly demonstrate sinus tachycardia. In addition, ECG might show signs of right heart strain, such as right bundle branch block or right axis deviation. Rarely, the S1Q3T3 pattern is seen (large S wave in lead I, Q wave in lead III and inverted T wave in lead III). While ECG is useful, it is not the diagnostic investigation of choice, making this the incorrect answer.

Shortness of breath (5)

24 B Recurrent venous or arterial thromosis with a history of miscarriages should point to primary anti-phospholipid syndrome (B) as the correct answer in this question. Anti-phospholipid syndrome is associated with SLE (A) and a proportion of patients with SLE may develop secondary anti-phospholipid syndrome. The absence of any clinical features of SLE in this case means that this answer is the incorrect option. Raynaud's disease (C) is digital ischaemia due to vasospasm, often precipitated by the cold in the absence of an underlying cause. When an underlying cause, for example SLE, is present, it is termed Raynaud's phenomenon. Recurrent venous thrombosis and miscarriage are not features of systemic sclerosis (D) or Beçhet's disease (E), making these answers incorrect.

Shortness of breath (6)

25 A The presence of anti-cardiolipin antibodies (A) would confirm the diagnosis. Both anti-cardiolipin antibody and lupus anticoagulant antibodies should be sent. Raised levels of anti-centromere (B) antibodies are associated with limited systemic sclerosis, not anti-phospholipid syndrome, making this answer incorrect. Anti-nuclear antibody (C) levels may be raised in a number of conditions including SLE, systemic sclerosis and rheumatoid arthritis, but are usually negative in anti-phospholipid syndrome. Raised anti-mitochondrial antibody (D) levels are associated with primary biliary cirrhosis, but not anti-phospholipid syndrome, making this answer incorrect. Similarly, raised anti-histone (E) antibody levels are associated with drug-induced SLE, but not anti-phospholipid syndrome.

Dry eyes

26 D Primary Sjögren's syndrome (D) occurs due to underlying fibrosis of exocrine glands. Clinical features include decreased tear production, decreased salivation and parotid gland swelling. There may be systemic disease, including arthritis, vasulitis or organ involvement (including pulmonary disease, renal tubular involvement, thyroid disease, myaesthenia gravis, primary biliary cirrhosis). Schirmer's test uses filter paper under the lower eyelid to measure tear production. Reduced tear production and salivation are not features of systemic sclerosis (A), making this answer incorrect. While Raynaud's phenomenon is a systemic manifestation of Sjögren's syndrome, primary Raynaud's disease (B) just affects the hands and is thus the incorrect answer. Secondary Sjögren's syndrome may occur in patients with other connective tissue disorders including SLE or systemic sclerosis. The absence of features suggestive of these other connective tissue disorders means SLE (C) and secondary Sjögren's syndrome (E) are the incorrect answers.

Cold hands

27 C The case in this question is describing Raynaud's syndrome. Vasospasm results in peripheral digital ischaemia. Precipitating factors include exposure to cold. Patients may describe their hands becoming pale, then blue and then red. Raynaud's disease is when Raynaud's syndrome occurs without an underlying cause, as in this case. However, Raynaud's syndrome is associated with a wide range of underlying connective tissue diseases. In these cases, it is termed Raynaud's phenomenon. Treatment of Raynaud's disease is with conservative measures such as warm gloves. In addition, nifedipine (C) can be used, making this the correct answer. Propanolol (A) is contraindicated in patients with Raynaud's syndrome as it may worsen the digital ischaemia. Aspirin (B), subcutaneous injection (D) and prednisolone (E) are not treatments for Raynaud's syndrome.

Chest discomfort

28 B Systemic sclerosis is a multisystem disease of unknown cause. It may be limited to skin and soft tissue in limited cutaneous systemic sclerosis or also involve the organs in diffuse cutaneous systemic sclerosis. Skin involvement of the face may be seen in both forms and may produce the characteristic beak-like nose and small mouth, termed microstomia (A). In limited cutaneous systemic sclerosis, skin involvement is limited to the hands, face and feet, making this the correct answer (B). In diffuse cutaneous systemic sclerosis, skin across most of the body can be affected in the worst cases. Oesophageal dysmotility (C) may occur in both forms of the disease, making this option incorrect. Raised levels of anti-nuclear antibody, anti-centromere antibody (limited cutaneous systemic sclerosis), anti-Ro and anti-topoisomerase antibodies are associated with systemic sclerosis. Anti-double stranded DNA antibodies (D) are normally associated with SLE not systemic sclerosis, making this answer wrong. Raynaud's phenomenon (E) results from digital ischaemia, not skin fibrosis as mentioned here.

Painful joints

29 A Felty's syndrome (A) is splenomegaly and neutropenia in a patient with
rheumatoid arthritis. Reactive arthritis (B) is an asymmetrical lower limb
arthritis occurring 1–4 weeks following an infection. A range of other
clinical features may also be present (see question 8). Still's disease (C) is
systemic juvenile idiopathic arthritis and is characterized by swinging
pyrexia, rash and arthritis. Juvenile idiopathic arthritis is the most common
form of persistent arthritis in those under 16 years of age. There is a
variable pattern of arthritis including oligoarthritis, polyarthritis and
systemic arthritis. Infection mononucleosis (D) may cause splenomegaly.
However, arthritis and neutropenia are not features of infectious
mononucleosis, making this answer incorrect. Serum sickness (E) is caused
by a hypersensitivity reaction to antibodies derived from animals. The
clinical features include fever, rashes, arthralgia, malaise, splenomegaly
and lymphadenopathy. Arthritis affecting and hands and feet and
neutropenia are not common features, making this option incorrect.

Joint pain (1)

30 A This case describes a typical presentation of acute gout (A). It is caused
by a raised plasma urate level and most commonly affects the first
metatarsophalangeal joint. Occassionally it is polyarticular. Acute
manifestations may be precipitated by a range of causes such as trauma,
surgery or the use of diuretics. Pseudo-gout (B) may present as a monoarthritis but usually affects other joints such as the knee, wrist or hip. In
addition, the raised urate levels are not seen. Septic arthritis (C) should be
considered in any acutely inflamed joint. The raised urate levels mean that
this diagnosis is less likely. Reactive arthritis (D) presents as an asymmetrical
polyarthritis of the lower limbs, making this answer incorrect. Osteoarthritis
(E) is unlikely to present as an acute arthritis affecting just the first
metatarsophalangeal joint. The raised urate levels and the clinical
presentation mean that a diagnosis of osteoarthritis is unlikely.

Joint pain (2)

31 B The most appropriate treatment of acute episodes is with a strong NSAID
(B) such as indomethacin. If NSAIDs are contraindicated, for example in
peptic ulcer disease, colchicine can be used. For patients with recurrent
attacks of gout, such as this case, serum urate should be reduced with
conservative measures and long-term allopurinol (A). Conservative
measures (C) include weight loss and avoiding excess alcohol, purine-rich
food and low-dose aspirin. However, the treatment of the acute episode is
the immediate priority here. Allopurinol may exacerbate an acute episode
and must only be started after the attack has resolved. Steroids (D) by oral,
intramuscular, intra-articular routes can be given in an acute episode

when NSAIDs and colchicine are contraindicated, for example in renal failure. Methotrexate (E) is a DMARD that is not used in the management of gout.

Skin reaction (1)

32 E Behçet's disease (E) is a systemic vasculitis of unknown cause. Clinical features of the disease include oral ulceration, genital ulceration, ocular involvement (including anterior uveitis, posterior uveitis or retinal vascular lesions), cutaneous lesions (including erythema nodosum or papulopustular lesions), arthritis (mono- or oligo-arthritis), gastrointestinal features (including diarrhoea and anorexia) and neurological features (including encephalitis, confusion or cranial nerve palsies). A skin pathergy test is when a needle prick leads to papule formation within 48 hours and is specific to Behçet's disease. Ulceration of the mouth, genitals and erythema nodosum are not features of Henoch–Schönlein purpura (A), making this answer incorrect. Clinical features of Lyme disease (B) are a skin rash called 'erythema chronicum migans', headache, fever, myalgia, arthralgia and lymphadenopathy. Berger's disease (C) or IgA nephropathy is the most common glomerulonephritis and usually presents with haematuria. Caplan's syndrome (D) is a combination of rheumatoid arthritis and pneumoconiosis, resulting in intrapulmonary nodules which can be seen on chest x-ray.

Skin reaction (2)

33 A Henoch–Schönlein purpura (A) is small vessel vasculitis, which usually occurs in children after an upper respiratory tract infection. Clinical manifestations include a lower limb purpuric rash, arthritis (most commonly involving the ankles, knees or elbows) and abdominal pain. Haematuria may occur due to underlying glomerulonephritis. Perthes disease (B) is characterized by avascular necrosis of the proximal femoral epiphysis. A purpuric rash and haematuria are not features, making this answer incorrect. Similarly, while oral and genital ulceration are features in Beçhet's disease, (C) purpuric rash and haematuria are not seen. Similarly, purpuric rash and haematuria are not features of Still's disease (D), making this answer incorrect. Ehlers–Danlos syndrome (E) is a hypermobility syndrome caused by a defect in collagen. The features outlined in this case are not seen in Ehlers–Danlos, making this the incorrect answer.

Bone pain (1)

34 E Paget's disease (E) is a disorder of bone remodelling, in which the constant resorption and formation of bone can lead to deformity. Sites that are typically affected include the skull, spine, pelvis, femur and tibia. Typical deformities include skull changes and bowed tibia. The remodelling of bone can lead to nerve compression. Nerves affected may include cranial nerve VIII, resulting in sensorineural deafness. This is a frequently examined point! It is important to note that other cranial nerves may be affected. In addition, Paget's disease may often be asymptomatic or present with bone pain (typically of the spine or pelvis) or joint pain. X-rays of the bones involved in Paget's disease may show lytic lesions. Osteomalacia (A) and ricketts are caused by deficiency of vitamin D, causing inadequate mineralization of bone. Osteomalacia occurs in adults and deformity is uncommon, nerve compression is not a feature. Rickets (D) occurs in children and can cause bone deformity, typically bow legging. However, skull changes and nerve compression do not occur, making this answer incorrect. Patients with osteoporosis (B) have loss of bone mass. They usually present with fractures. The clinical features described in this question with bony deformity are not features. Acromegaly (C) is unlikely in this question as typical features include prognathism, coarsening of facial features, deepening of the voice, hypertension and diabetes. Bowing of the tibia would not be a feature.

Bone pain (2)

35 A The increased bone turnover in Paget's disease is reflected by a normal serum calcium and phosphate and a raised alkaline phosphatase (A). The alkaline phosphatase in Paget's may be markedly raised at over 1000 U/L. Normal serum calcium, phosphate and alkaline phosphatase (B) may be seen in the absence of disease. It is important to note that normal blood tests are also seen in osteoporosis. Raised serum calcium, low serum phosphate and normal serum alkaline phosphatase (C) are seen in patients with primary hyperparathyroidism. Normal serum calcium, low serum phosphate and raised serum alkaline phosphatase (D) may be seen in hyperparathyroidism secondary to osteomalacia. The raised alkaline phosphatase is indicative of osteoblast activity causing bone resorption. Meanwhile, the raised levels of parathyroid hormone may increase serum calcium levels to normal and leave a low serum phosphate level. A low serum calcium, low serum phosphate and low serum alkaline phosphatase (E) is not characteristic of Paget's.

SECTION 7:
HAEMATOLOGY

QUESTIONS

1. Blood group

A woman with BO positive blood and her partner with AB positive blood have a child together. Which of the following cannot be the child's blood type?

A. AB positive
B. BB positive
C. AO positive
D. AA positive
E. BB negative

2. Blood transfusion

A 24-year-old man is involved in a road traffic accident and rushed to accident and emergency accompanied by his mother who was unharmed. An examination shows severe abdominal injuries, peripheral cyanosis and cold extremities. The doctor on call decides a blood transfusion is necessary. The mother thinks the patient is blood group B negative but is unsure. The most appropriate blood group to give the patient is?

A. Group O positive blood
B. Group B positive blood
C. Group B negative blood
D. Group O negative blood
E. Group A negative blood

3. Epistaxis

A 16-year-old boy presents to his GP complaining of nosebleeds and bleeding after brushing his teeth. He is unsure of how long this has been occurring but decided to seek advice after having to continually excuse himself from lessons. On examination you notice he has some skin bruises. A blood test shows a prolonged bleeding time and activated partial thromboplastin time (APTT), while platelet count and prothrombin times are all normal. The most likely diagnosis is:

A. Von Willebrand disease
B. Liver disease
C. Disseminated intravascular coagulation
D. Congenital afibrinogenaemia
E. Glanzmann's thrombasthenia

4. Painful leg

A 22-year-old Caucasian woman presents with a 1-day history of a painful right leg which is erythematous on appearance and tender on palpation. She states that she has had this problem many times in the last few years and her family has also suffered from similar problems. Her grandmother died of a pulmonary embolism. The most likely diagnosis is:

    A. Antithrombin deficiency
    B. Factor V Leiden mutation
    C. Protein S deficiency
    D. Lupus anticoagulant
    E. Protein C deficiency

5. Shortness of breath

A 44-year-old Asian female presents with a two-month history of shortness of breath and lethargy. She denies any intolerance to the cold or any changes in her weight and on examination appears slightly pale. She states that she has recently become a vegetarian. A blood film shows the presence of elliptocytes and blood results show the following:

Haemoglobin	9.9 g/dL
Mean cell volume (MCV)	75 fL
Ferritin	Low

The most likely diagnosis is:

    A. Iron deficiency anaemia
    B. Sideroblastic anaemia
    C. Anaemia of chronic disease
    D. Thalassaemia trait
    E. Hereditary elliptocytosis

6. Malaise (1)

A 47-year-old teacher complains of difficulty maintaining her concentration at work teaching secondary school children. She states that over the last four months she has become increasingly tired and easily fatigued. She has noticed it has become more difficult for her to lift books, rise from her chair and she has also noticed a tingling sensation in her fingers. Examination shows a positive babinski sign and absent reflexes. A blood test reveals the following:

Haemoglobin	10 g/dL
MCV	103 fL

The most likely diagnosis is:

    A. Hypothyroidism
    B. Vitamin B_{12} deficiency
    C. Folic acid deficiency
    D. Liver disease
    E. Alcohol toxicity

7. Malaise (2)

A 55-year-old man complains of a 4-week history of general malaise and fatigue, he has also noticed his trousers have become more loose fitting. A blood test shows the following results:

Haemoglobin	12 g/dL
MCV	90 fL
Platelet count	250×10^9/L
WBC	10×10^9/L
Serum iron	10 μmol/L
Total iron-binding capacity	40 μmol/L
Serum ferritin	160 μg/L

The most likely diagnosis is:

    A. Thalassaemia
    B. Iron deficiency anaemia
    C. Anaemia of chronic disease
    D. Macrocytic anaemia
    E. Aplastic anaemia

8. Fatigue

A 43-year-old woman suffers from Crohn's disease. A blood test shows the following results:

Haemoglobin	10.5 g/dL
MCV	120 fL
Platelet count	300×10^9/L

The most likely diagnosis is:

A. Vitamin B_{12} deficiency
B. Iron deficiency
C. Hypothyroidism
D. Folic acid deficiency
E. Anaemia of chronic disease

9. Collapse

A 45-year-old man collapses at home and is brought to accident and emergency. He has a fever at 39.5°C and blood pressure is 90/60 mmHg, although he is in a lucid state. Bruises can be seen on his skin which he remembers being present before he fell. Blood tests show the patient to have a normocytic anaemia with a low platelet count and increased fibrin split products. The most likely diagnosis is:

A. Warm autoimmune haemolytic anaemia
B. Cold autoimmune haemolytic anaemia
C. Paroxysmal nocturnal haemoglobinuria
D. Disseminated intravascular coagulation
E. Thalassaemia minor

10. Microcytic anaemia

A 23-year-old Asian man presents to his GP complaining of shortness of breath following exercise. He has always been a little unfit and decided to start going to the gym but noticed that even after 4 weeks he is still quite short of breath. He denies any coughing or wheezing and on examination you notice mild pallor but the patient says he has always been slightly pale in colour. Investigation results are given below:

Haemoglobin	12 g/dL
MCV	70 fL
Serum iron	14 umol/L
Ferritin	60 ug/L
Transferrin saturation	35 per cent
Mean cell haemoglobin	22 pg
Haemoglobin electrophoresis	HbA2 increased

The most likely diagnosis is:

    A. α thalassaemia trait
    B. Anaemia of chronic disease
    C. β thalassaemia trait
    D. Haemoglobin H disease
    E. Iron deficiency anaemia

11. Iron store

A 29-year-old woman complains of a 1-week history of weakness and malaise, she has recently become a vegetarian and eats mostly green vegetables and drinks lots of tea during the day. She is apyrexial and has a C-reactive protein (CRP) <5. You suspect an abnormality of the patient's iron stores. What is the most appropriate investigation to determine iron store levels?

    A. Bone marrow biopsy
    B. Serum ferritin
    C. Serum transferrin
    D. Total iron binding capacity
    E. Serum iron

12. Peripheral blood smear

A 60-year-old man presents with abdominal pain and a cupful of haematemesis. On examination he is noted to have ascites, hepatomegaly and a very enlarged spleen extending to the right iliac fossa. His initial blood tests reveal a leukoerythroblastic picture with a haemoglobin of 8, white cell count (WCC) of 3 and platelets of 120. A diagnosis of myelofibrosis is made. What is most likely to be seen on the peripheral blood smear?

   A. Schistocytosis
   B. Sickle cells
   C. Spherocytes
   D. Dacrocytes
   E. Target cells

13. Blood transfusion complications

A 65-year-old woman suffers significant bleeding during a difficult bowel resection and is prescribed three units of blood after the operation is completed. It is the first time she has required a blood transfusion and her details are checked carefully. Approximately 4 hours after the transfusion the patient feels acutely unwell and complains of fever, chills and a dry cough. Blood pressure is 110/80 mmHg, temperature 38°C and oxygen saturation is 94 per cent. The most likely diagnosis is:

   A. Immediate haemolytic transfusion reaction
   B. Febrile non-haemolytic transfusion reaction
   C. Delayed haemolytic transfusion reaction
   D. IgA deficiency
   E. Transfusion-related lung injury

14. Limb numbness

A 52-year-old woman presents complaining of a two-month history of increasing fatigue and numbness in both of her arms and legs. She lives at home with her husband and has found it difficult coping with the daily activities of living. She suffers from hypothyroidism which is well controlled with thyroid replacement medication. A peripheral blood smear shows hypersegmented neutrophils. A blood test reveals the following:

Haemoglobin	10 g/dL
Mean corpuscular volume	110 fL
Platelets	150×10^9/L

Liver function tests:

ALT	25 IU/L
AST	27 IU/L
GGT	22 IU/L
ALP	100 IU/L
Urea	5 mmol/L
Creatinine	100 µmol/L

The most likely diagnosis is:

  A.   Thrombotic thrombocytopenic purpura
  B.   Iron deficiency
  C.   Folic acid deficiency
  D.   Liver disease
  E.   Pernicious anaemia

15. Bleeding abnormality

During a busy ward round you are asked to visit a patient the consultant has not had an opportunity to see. The only details you are given are that the patient is female and was admitted the previous day with bleeding abnormalities, you are given the results of her blood investigations:

Prothrombin time	Unaffected
Partial thromboplastin time	Prolonged
Bleeding time	Prolonged
Platelet count	Unaffected

What is the most likely diagnosis?

- A. Factor V deficiency
- B. Warfarin therapy
- C. Glanzmann's thrombasthenia
- D. Bernard Soulier syndrome
- E. Von Willebrand disease

16. Fever

A 14-year-old girl is brought to clinic by her parents who have been worried about a fever the patient has had for the last week. The patient looks pale and unwell. Blood tests reveal a neutropenia with normal red blood counts (RBCs) and platelets. A bone marrow exam reveals no abnormalities. The patient has been otherwise fit and well. There is no organomegaly or lymphadenopathy. The most likely diagnosis is:

- A. Acute myeloid leukaemia
- B. Aplastic anaemia
- C. Acute lymphoblastic leukaemia
- D. Bacterial infection
- E. Thrombotic thrombocytopenic purpura

17. Pruritus

A 65-year-old man presents with a chronic history of headaches and occasional dizziness. He hesitantly mentions that he experiences severe pruritus, especially after hot showers and baths. Blood pressure is 160/85 mmHg. A full blood count (FBC) reveals a haemoglobin of 20 g/dL, MCV of 94 fL, platelet count of 470×10^9/L and WBC count of 7.8×10^9/L

The most likely diagnosis is:

- A. Polycythemia vera
- B. Idiopathic erythrocytosis
- C. Essential thrombocythaemia
- D. Myelofibrosis
- E. Chronic myeloid leukaemia

18. Auer rods

A 29-year-old woman complains of tiredness, especially during activity. On examination the patient appears pale. Auer rods and schistocytes can be seen on peripheral blood smear. The patient is referred for a bone marrow biopsy and the extracted cells are sent for cytogenetic analysis. The most likely results are:

A. t(8:21)
B. t(15;17)
C. t(9:22)
D. t(14;18)
E. t(8;14)

19. Massive splenomegaly

In which of the following dieases is a massive splenomegaly not a characteristic feature?

A. Infectious mononucleosis
B. Thalassaemia
C. Chronic myeloid leukaemia
D. Kala-azar
E. Polycythaemia rubra vera

20. Glucose-6-phosphate dehydrogenase deficiency

A 27-year-old man presents with increasing tiredness and shortness of breath. A macrocytic anaemia with reticulocytes is discovered on blood tests and smear. Genetic analysis reveals the patient has glucose-6-phosphate dehydrogenase deficiency. What cell type is most likely to have been seen on the blood smear?

A. Target cells
B. Pencil cells
C. Spherocytes
D. Elliptocytes
E. Schistocytes

21. Heinz bodies

A 33-year-old man travels to South Africa to take part in a safari. On arriving, the patient takes his antimalarial tablets. A few days into his course he becomes ill complaining of shortness of breath, pallor and bloody urine. Blood tests reveal anaemia and reduced haematocrit, while a blood smear shows the presence of Heinz bodies. The most likely diagnosis is:

A. Hereditary elliptocytosis
B. Glucose-6-phosphate dehydrogenase deficiency
C. Hereditary spherocytosis
D. Autoimmune haemolytic anaemia
E. Microangiopathic haemolytic anaemia

22. Sickle cell anaemia

An 18-year-old African man presents with worries about his general health stating that hypertension and sickle cell anaemia are present in his family history. The patient denies any shortness of breath, chest pain, digit or limb changes. Blood pressure is 124/77 mmHg. What test would be appropriate to investigate sickle cell anaemia?

A. Ham's test
B. Coombs' test
C. Schilling test
D. Metabisulfite test
E. Osmotic fragility test

23. AML and ALL differentiation

A young patient presents with features of anaemia, neutropenia and thrombocytopenia. A large number of blasts are present on bone marrow biopsy. Which investigation would help differentiate between acute myeloid leukaemia (AML) and acute lymphoblastic leukaemia (ALL)?

A. Myeloperoxidase stain
B. Sudan black B
C. Tartrate-resistant acid phosphatase stain
D. Leukocyte alkaline phosphatase
E. Auramine O stain

24. Polycythaemia rubra vera

A 47-year-old woman presents complaining of dark stools and painful fingers on both hands. She appears plethoric and complains of severe itching, often when she is washing. A large liver and spleen is palpable. You suspect features of polycythaemia rubra vera and measure red cell mass and erythropoietin levels among other tests. Which of the following is likely to be most accurate in this patient?

A. Low erythropoietin and low red cell mass
B. Normal erythropoietin and normal red cell mass
C. Raised erythropoietin and low red cell mass
D. Raised erythropoietin and raised red cell mass
E. Low erythropoietin and raised red cell mass

25. Vegetarian patient

A 29-year-old woman presents complaining of shortness of breath, especially when walking up stairs. She is starting to struggle with yoga classes, which were never a problem before. She does not suffer from any medical conditions and takes no regular medication. On examination there is pallor, heart rate is 90 and blood pressure 119/79 mmHg. The patient mentions that she has recently become a vegetarian and in the morning only has time for tea before heading to work. Which of the following would you expect to be increased in this patient?

A. Myoglobin
B. Ferritin
C. Haemoglobin
D. Serum iron
E. Transferrin

26. Anaemia

A 65-year-old man presents with a chronic history of malaise, shortness of breath and paraesthesia in his hands. He appears tired and pale while speaking and on examination his heart rate is 115, respiratory rate 16. A Schillings test is positive while blood tests reveal a macrocytic anaemia and a Coombs test is negative. The most likely diagnosis is:

A. Iron deficiency anaemia
B. Haemorrhage
C. Anaemia of chronic disease
D. Pernicious anaemia
E. Autoimmune haemolytic anaemia

27. Macrocytic anaemia

A 47-year-old woman presents to clinic concerned about her recent ill health. She has noticed over the last three months that she has been suffering from headaches, fatigue and recurrent infections. She notes she has rarely been to the doctor before and otherwise leads a healthy lifestyle. She decided to see a doctor when she noticed petechial rashes appearing on her arms. On examination there is no organomegaly and blood tests reveal an MCV of 105, a pancytopenia with the bone marrow appearing hypocellular on biopsy.

A. Chronic myeloid leukaemia
B. Myeloproliferative disorder
C. Aplastic anaemia
D. Iron deficiency anaemia
E. Acute lymphoblastic anaemia

28. Auer rods

A 65-year-old man presents to you reporting he has become increasingly worried about his lack of energy in the last 2 weeks. He mentions he has been increasingly tired, sleeping for long periods and has suffered from fevers unresponsive to paracetamol. He became increasingly worried when he noticed bleeding orginating from his gums. A blood film shows auer rods, hypogranular neutrophils and stains with Sudan black B. The most likely diagnosis is:

    A. Acute lymphoblastic leukaemia
    B. DiGeorge syndrome
    C. Disseminated intravascular coagulation
    D. Acute myeloid leukaemia
    E. Afibrinogenaemia

29. Chronic myeloid leukaemia

A 70-year-old woman complains of tiredness, fatigue and weight loss. Blood tests reveal an elevated WCC and on examination splenomegaly is palpated. Cytogenetics are positive for the Philadelphia chromosome and the patient is diagnosed with chronic myeloid leukaemia. The most appropriate treatment is:

    A. Hydroxycarbamide
    B. Imatinib
    C. Venesection
    D. Stem cell transplant
    E. Dasatinib

30. Warfarin therapy

A 27-year-old woman who suffers from rheumatic mitral stenosis develops atrial fibrillation. She is placed on warfarin therapy. What is the most appropriate target international normalized raio (INR) range?

    A. <1.0
    B. 1.0–2.0
    C. 2.0–3.0
    D. 3.0–4.0
    E. >5.0

31. Multiple myeloma

A 70-year-old woman complains of a dull pain in her lower back, especially when bending forwards to lift things. She presents after a severe episode in the last 2 days. An x-ray reveals a lumbar compression fracture. Blood tests show a normocytic anaemia and urine electrophoresis reveals a monoclonal gammopathy. A diagnosis of multiple myeloma is made. Which of the following is not a recognized cause of multiple myeloma?

    A. High-dose radiation
    B. Human herpes virus-8 (HHV-8)
    C. HIV
    D. Herbecides and insecticides
    E. Hereditary

32. Hypersplenism investigation

A 44-year-old woman presents with recurrent fever, pallor, malaise and shortness of breath. She has noticed a petechial rash on her skin and small bruises on her arms. A blood test reveals a pancytopenia. During examination, you palpate a large spleen. Which investigation would differentiate between hypersplenism and aplastic anaemia?

    A. Reticulocyte test
    B. Direct Coombs test
    C. Metabisulfite test
    D. Ham's test
    E. Osmotic fragility test

33. Pernicious anaemia

A 66-year-old man presents complaining of a three-month history of weakness, tingling in the limbs and a sore tongue. The patient notes an undesired 5 kg weight loss over 2 weeks. A peripheral blood smear shows a macrocytic anaemia, a Schilling test shows impaired vitamin B_{12} absorption and a diagnosis of pernicious anaemia is made. Which of the following antibodies is most closely associated with pernicious anaemia?

    A. Anti-mitochondrial antibodies
    B. Anti-intrinsic factor antibodies
    C. Anti-gliadin antibodies
    D. Anti-centromere antibodies
    E. Anti-smooth muscle antibodies

34. Leukaemia investigation

A 5-year-old girl presents with her parents who have become concerned about the small petechiae and ecchymoses on her skin. An abdominal examination reveals hepatosplenomegaly. You suspect an acute leukaemia. The most appropriate initial investigation for diagnosis is:

    A. Chromosomal analysis of bone marrow cells
    B. Cytochemical analysis of bone marrow cells
    C. Direct microscopy of bone marrow cells
    D. Electron microscopy
    E. Flow cytometry

35. Bence–Jones protein

A 51-year-old man complains of severe, diffuse back pain. An x-ray finds several lytic lesions in the vertebra alongside hypercalcaemia. Bence–Jones protein is detected in the urine. What is a Bence–Jones protein?

    A. IgG antibody
    B. IgA antibody
    C. IgE antibody
    D. Light chain
    E. IgM antibody

ANSWERS

Blood group

1 D The ABO blood groups are the most important of all the blood groups when considering blood donation and blood types. All red blood cell membranes have a common glycoprotein and fucose stem, adding a sugar residue may then create a blood group which is A, B, AB, etc. Group O blood has only the glycoprotein and fucose stem with no A or B sugars. Genetically, groups A and B are dominant while group O is recessive. Since both parents here are rhesus positive the child must also be rhesus positive, therefore (E) cannot be correct. The table below demonstrates that the child may be either AB positive (A), BB positive (B), AO positive (C) or BO positive. AA positive (D) is the correct rhesus state but cannot be the correct blood type of the patient (see table below). It is important to note that in reality AO positive and AA positive would be called simply A positive.

Blood types	A → B	
B	AB	BB
O	AO	BO

Blood transfusion

2 D In a patient requiring a blood transfusion, it is imperative to be sure of prescribing a safe blood type. The blood group type denotes the antigens that are present on the patient's red blood cells but also the opposing antibodies the patient has in their plasma. A patient who is blood group A (AA or AO) will have group A antigens on their red blood cells but anti-B antibodies. Similarly, a patient who is blood group B (BB or BO) will have group B antigens on their red blood cells but anti-A antibodies. If this patient were group B negative then giving group A negative blood (E) would cause a potentially fatal cross-reaction. Group AB patients have no opposing antibodies in their plasma while group O patients have anti-A and anti-B. In this emergency scenario, since the next of kin is unsure of the patient's blood type, the safest blood group to give is group O negative (D). The O negative blood will have no antigens for the patient's immune system to potentially react with and there is no danger of rhesus sensitization which would occur in group O positive blood (A). If the patient were indeed group B negative, then B negative blood (C) would be the safest blood type to give. Group B positive (B) should be avoided because of the rhesus state (see table below).

Blood group	Antigens on RBC	Antigens in plasma
A	A	Anti-B
B	B	Anti-A
AB	AB	None
O	O	Anti-A and Anti-B

Epistaxis

3 A   Von Willebrand disease (A) affects an important glycoprotein present in the blood plasma. In response to various stimuli, such as endothelial damage, von Willebrand factor (vWF) is released from cells and platelets. Its main function is to facilitate the adhesion of platelets to endothelial cells which are often exposed in vascular injury, it also acts to stabilize factor VIII. In vWF deficiency the most common symptoms include nosebleeds, bruising, gum bleeding and prolonged bleeding from minor wounds. Laboratory tests can be used to investigate bleeding disorders and include prothrombin time (PT), activated partial thromboplastin time (APTT), bleeding time, platelet counts and thrombin time (TT). A prolonged PT (>16–18s) suggests abnormalities in the common (factors I, II, V, X) or extrinsic pathway (factor VII). A prolonged APTT (>30–50s) suggests abnormalities in the common (factors I, II, V, X) or intrinsic pathway (factors VIII, IX, XI, XII). Importantly, factor VII does not cause any anomalies in APTT times. A prolonged TT suggests fibrinogen deficiency while abnormal bleeding times suggest platelet deficiencies. In liver disease (B) the PT, APTT, bleeding time and platelet counts would be abnormal alongside peripheral stigmata of liver disease. Disseminated intravascular coagulation (C) causes abnormalities of PT, APTT, bleeding time and platelets. In congenital afibrogenaemia (D), the PT, APTT, TT and bleeding times would be abnormal while the platelet count would be normal. Glanzmann's thrombaesthenia (E), a platelet abnormality whereby glycoprotein IIb/IIIa is absent preventing platelet bridging with fibrinogen, the bleeding time is significantly prolonged while PT, APTT and platelet counts are normal.

Painful leg

4 B   This patient is suffering from deep vein thrombosis (DVT) and appears to have a history of recurrent DVTs, the occurrence of which at a young age is suggestive of an inherited disorder of coagulation. Factor V Leiden (B) is a mutation of factor V which makes it resistant to the action of protein C. The increased presence of factor V therefore creates a procoagulant state predisposing to pathology such as DVTs. Factor V Leiden is one of the most common causes of an inherited procoagulant state, present in approximately 5 per cent of the Caucasian population. Although protein C (E), protein S (C) and antithrombin deficiency (A) would also cause a procoagulant state, they are much rarer. Lupus anticoagulant (D) antibodies cross-react with phospholipids and can be associated with patients with systemic lupus erythematosus (SLE). The antibodies also create a procoagulant state and patients may suffer from arterial and venous thrombosis.

Shortness of breath

5 A This patient is suffering from iron deficiency anaemia (A). The classic symptoms of anaemia include tiredness, shortness of breath and pallor. Signs can include koilonychia (spoon-shaped nails), while a blood film may show elliptocytes and hypersegmented neutrophils. Sideroblastic anaemia (B) is an abnormality whereby, despite the availability of iron, the body is unable to utilize it due to a genetic anomaly or in relation to the myelodysplastic syndrome. The ferritin is low here, therefore this cannot be the correct answer although a microcytic anaemia does occur. The three important causes of microcytic anaemia are iron deficiency anaemia, anaemia of chronic disease and thalassaemia trait. Ferritin helps to distinguish iron deficiency anaemia from the other causes. In anaemia of chronic disease (C), which can be caused by long-term illnesses such as rheumatoid arthritis, the action of cytokines interrupt iron homeostasis in red blood cells. As a result, iron is unable to leave red blood cells or ferritin stores so that ferritin measurements are classically normal or high. In thalassaemia trait, a genetic abnormality of the globin chains creates abnormal haemoglobin. The haemoglobin and MCV are therefore also reduced, however ferritin usually remains normal. In hereditary elliptocytosis (E), the majority of red blood cells are oval-shaped, predisposing to haemolytic anaemia. However, this does not present as microcytic anaemia.

Malaise (1)

6 B This patient has a macrocytic anaemia, the most common causes of which include vitamin B_{12} and folic acid deficiency, liver disease, alcohol toxicity and hypothyroidism. Vitamin B_{12} is important in DNA synthesis and maintaining the neurological system. In vitamin B_{12} deficiency (B), patients usually present with derangements in tissues with high cell turnover, such as the gastrointestinal system, epithelial surfaces and bone marrow. Symptoms therefore include weakness, fatigue, glossitis and changes in bowel habit. The classic triad of tiredness, glossitis and paraesthesia is not always present but strongly suggests B_{12} deficiency. Neurological consequences of B_{12} deficiency typically includes peripheral neuropathy, optic atrophy, dementia and subacute combined degeneration of the spinal cord (pyramidal tract weakness). Patients therefore present with paraesthesia, muscle weakness, visual impairments, psychiatric disturbance and difficulty walking. Folic acid is also important in DNA synthesis and in folic acid deficiency (C) many of the same features as described in B_{12} deficiency are present, such as fatigue and weakness.

However, neurological symptoms are not as prominent and patients tend to have a history of malnutrition. Hypothyroidism (A) can present very similarly to patients with anaemia. Symptoms such as fatigue, tiredness and weakness are common to both pathologies. In hypothyroidism, a macrocytic anaemia is also present, however neurological symptoms tend to differ. In hypothyroidism, pseudomyotonic reflexes tend to occur whereby a prolonged relaxation phase occurs. Liver disease (D) and alcohol abuse can cause a macrocytic anaemia presentation. However, in liver disease, there are other peripheral stigmata such as gynaecomastia, spider naevia, caput medusae, etc). In alcohol abuse, malnutrition may cause anaemia or direct toxicity to the bone marrow. There is usually a history of alcohol abuse and other features, such as Wernicke's encephalopathy, can develop.

Malaise (2)

7 C   This patient is suffering from anaemia of chronic disease (C). The blood test values show a normocytic anaemia, normal platelet count and serum iron, increased ferritin concentration and reduced total iron binding capacity (TIBC). In anaemia of chronic disease, an underlying disease causes an inflammatory process involving cytokines to occur. Factors such as CRP and erythrocyte sedimentation rate (ESR) are raised. The effect of these cytokines is to interrupt the homeostasis of iron. Erythropoietin is inhibited, iron is unable to flow out of red blood cells, ferritin production is increased and RBC death is increased. The impact of these actions causes anaemia with raised ferritin levels and, if prolonged, serum iron is also eventually reduced. By definition, in iron-deficiency anaemia (B), the serum iron is reduced as well as the MCV, which is not the case here, there is also an increase in the TIBC. In anaemia of chronic disease, protein production can be reduced such that this increase does not occur. A macrocytic anaemia (D) would be accompanied by an increased MCV while aplastic anaemia (E) is unlikely in light of the normal platelet and white blood cell count. In thalassaemia, the haemoglobin and MCV are reduced but serum iron, ferritin and transferrin can be normal.

Fatigue

8 A   This patient is suffering from vitamin B_{12} deficiency (A). Her blood test shows a macrocytic anaemia. In iron deficiency anaemia (B) there is usually a microcytic anaemia. Vitamin B_{12} and folate deficiency (D) are the most common causes of a macrocytic anaemia. Crohn's disease can involve the terminal ileum which is where vitamin B_{12} is absorbed, folate is absorbed in the proximal duodenum. Hypothyroidism (C) is unlikely as the classic symptoms of thyroid pathology, such as changes in weight, appetite and intolerance to room temperature, etc., are not present. In anaemia of chronic disease (E), a normocytic or microcytic blood film is more typical.

Collapse

9 D   This patient is suffering from disseminated intravascular coagulation (DIC)
(D), which may have resulted from an infection, in this case causing
septicaemia. DIC is characterized by the systemic activation of the
coagulation system such that fibrin deposition occurs usually within the
microvasculature. RBCs are damaged when crossing such fibres and
coagulation factors and platelets are also consumed predisposing to severe
bleeding. DIC has various causes. In this case a systemic inflammatory
response such as occurs in sepsis is the most likely underlying cause.
Thalassaemia (E) tends to produce chronic normocytic or microcytic
anaemia without serious bleeding risk. In paroxysmal nocturnal
haemoglobinuria (C), there is a defect in an essential cell membrane protein
causing intermittent release of haemoglobin, it is believed acidosis during
the night increases the degree of haemoglobinuria, hence the term
'nocturnal'. There does not tend to be consumption of coagulation factors.
Haemolytic anaemia produces a macrocytic anaemia, in warm antibody
disease (A) IgG binds to the red cell membrane, while in cold antibody
disease (B) it is IgM. There is no impact upon coagulation factors.

Microcytic anaemia

10 C   This patient is suffering from a microcytic anaemia with normal iron
parameters. The differential diagnoses of a microcytic anaemia include
iron deficiency anaemia, anaemia of chronic disease and thalassaemia
disease. The normal iron parameters eliminate iron deficiency anaemia (E)
while serum iron tends to be low and ferritin tends to be high in an anaemia
of chronic disease (B). This leaves a disease of thalassaemia, α thalassaemia
trait (A) usually results from gene deletion on chromosome 16
(β thalassaemia is coded on chromosome 11). There are two α globin genes
from each parent so that adults have a total of four α globin genes. A
single or double deletion causes a mild, usually asymptomatic anaemia
known as $\alpha+$ and $\alpha-$ disease, respectively. Haemoglobin H disease (D)
involves three α deletions causing a significant anaemia beginning in
childhood with target cells, Heinz bodies and splenomegaly. In β
thalassaemia trait (C) points to mutations of a single β globin gene allele.
This causes a mild microcytic anaemia, electrophoresis shows an increased
haemoglobin A2.

Iron store

11 B   Iron deficiency can be an important cause of anaemia in patients. In this
case vitamin B_{12} and folic acid are less likely to be important given the
patient's diet, however tea is alkaline and reduces the body's ability to
effectively absorb iron. Measuring the patient's serum ferritin (B) provides
an accurate reflection of the body's iron stores since the serum ferritin

originates from the storage pools in the bone marrow, spleen and liver. Be aware that ferritin measurements are only accurate when CRP is normal since both ferritin and CRP are acute phase reactants. The serum transferrin (C) level reflects the levels of protein that bind to iron and transports it around the body and is usually 33 per cent saturated, hence not providing the most accurate level of iron. The serum iron level (E) is a poor reflection of iron stores since this can change dependent on disease states. In iron deficiency anaemia, the serum iron and iron stores are low, however in anaemia of chronic disease iron stores are increased yet the serum iron level is reduced. The total iron binding capacity (D) specifically saturates transferrin in order to measure the iron-carrying capacity in the body rather than iron stores and so would not be appropriate here. A bone marrow biopsy (A) is a very sensitive test since iron staining reflects iron stores in macrophages. However, it is both expensive and invasive and therefore not the most appropriate test compared to serum ferritin.

Peripheral blood smear

12 D Dacrocytes (D), more commonly known as tear-drop cells, are strongly indicative of myelofibrosis. Sickle cells (B) occur due to homozygous haemoglobin S which causes cell sickling on polymerization. Schistocytes (A), more commonly known as fragmented red cells, can be seen in a number of conditions such as haemolytic anaemia or disseminated intravascular coagulation. Spherocytes (C) are commonly seen in haemolytic anaemia or in congenital disease, such as hereditary spherocytosis. Target cells (E) can be indicative of obstructive jaundice, liver disease, haemoglobinopathies and hyposplenism.

Blood transfusion complications

13 E This patient has suffered a complication of blood transfusion, specfically tissue-related lung injury (TRALI) (E). This can be a life-threatening complication whereby within 2–6 h after transfusion an inflammatory process causes sequestration of neutrophils within the lungs and antibodies that form against the donor's white blood cells and then attack the patient's lungs which share the HLA antigens. Patient symptoms can include fever, hypotension, cyanosis and pulmonary oedema on x-ray. An immediate haemolytic transfusion reaction (A) occurs due to the immune destruction of transfused cells by the patient's immune system. Symptoms include hypotension, tachycardia, nausea, abdominal pain and loin pain within 24 h of transfusion. These symptoms are similar to a delayed haemolytic reaction (C), but this typically occurs more than 24 h after transfusion. In IgA deficiency (D) patients develop antibodies to IgA during their first exposure to a blood transfusion, an anaphylactic-type reaction then occurs if the patient is retransfused with bronchospasm, laryngeal oedema and hypotension occurring. Febrile non-haemolytic transfusion reaction (B) occurs due to white cell antibodies reacting with the leukocytes present in the blood transfusion. Patients usually have a history of blood transfusions or pregnancy. Patients usually present with fever, rigors and discomfort.

Limb numbness

14 E This patient is suffering from a megaloblastic anaemia due to vitamin B_{12} deficiency secondary to pernicious anaemia. In a macrocytic anaemia two important differentials include folate and vitamin B_{12} deficiency. Folate deficiency (C) is commonly associated with alcohol disease as it is required to metabolize alcohol, poor diet and skin disease. Hypersegmented neutrophils can be associated with B_{12} or folic acid deficiency, some studies have also found relations with iron deficiency anaemia, however neurological deficits such as limb paraesthesia and numbness are more characteristic of vitamin B_{12} deficiency. Pernicious anaemia (E) is an autoimmune disease whereby antibodies bind intrinsic factor produced by the parietal cells in the gastric fundus. Intrinsic factor is essential in the absorption of vitamin B_{12} via the ileum. Associated conditions can include thyroid disease which compound symptoms of anaemia. Iron deficiency anaemia (B) is characterized by a microcytic anaemia rather than a macrocytic anaemia, which is present in this case. A thrombotic thrombocytopenic purpura (A) is defined by fever, transient neurologic abnormalities, thrombocytopenia, haemolytic anaemia and acute renal failure, which are not present in this case. Liver disease (D) can produce a macrocytic anaemia, however there would likely be other accompanying abnormalities such as jaundice, clotting anomalies, as well as deranged liver function tests, which are not present here.

Bleeding abnormality

15 E Investigations of the vascular system can provide essential information and support a diagnosis made alongside the ever important history and examination. Blood vessel abnormalities can be detected using the bleeding time, this investigation alongside platelet counts is also helpful in determining platelet dysfunction. Investigations of the coagulation cascade can be shown by the PT which reflects the extrinsic pathway and the PTT which measures the intrinsic pathway. This patient is likely to be suffering from Von Willebrand's disease (E) whereby Von Willebrand factor, important in platelet adhesion and Factor VIII function, is deficient. Patient's therefore have normal PT and platelet counts but bleeding time and PTT are abnormal. In Factor V (A) deficiency, the PT and PTT are prolonged while bleeding time and platelet counts would be unaffected. These findings are also found in Factor X deficiency, vitamin K deficiency and warfarin therapy (B). In Glanzmann's thrombaesthenia (C) platelets lack glycoprotein IIb/IIIa therefore fibrinogen bridging between platelets is disrupted, bleeding time is therefore the only abnormal result. In Bernard

Soulier syndrome glycoprotein Ib, a receptor for Von Willebrand factor, is deficient therefore clot formation is disrupted and again only bleeding time would be affected.

Fever

16 D This patient is likely suffering from a dangerous septicaemia shown by the presence of fever alongside a neutropenia. Urgent broad spectrum antibiotics should be administered. In an acute myeloid leukaemia (A) or acute lymphoblastic leukaemia (C), a bone marrow examination would show more than 20 per cent myeloblasts or lymphoblasts, respectively. Although the WCC can be variable, a neutropenia, anaemia and thrombocytopenia is associated with AML and ALL. An aplastic anaemia (B) is a failure of the bone marrow and presents with a hypocellular bone marrow and pancytopenia. A thrombotic thrombocytopenic purpura (E) is the pentad of fever, thrombocytopenia, microangiopathic haemolytic anaemia, renal failure and neurological symptoms.

Pruritus

17 A This patient is most likely suffering from polycythaemia vera (A), one of the myeloproliferative disorders. A V167F mutation in the JAK2 kinase causes uncontrolled stem cell proliferation, usually of the RBC cell line. Patients usually present with headaches, dizziness and, in severe cases, stroke. Hypermast cell degranulation can cause severe pruritus characteristically after hot baths/showers (aquagenic), as well as peptic ulcers. Patients may also present with gout (due to elevated cell turnover), splenomegaly and plethora. An idiopathic erythrocytosis (B) is an isolated erythrocytosis with no change in WBC or platelets, there is a high risk of AML progression. Essential thrombocythaemia (C) tends to occur in middle-aged and elderly patients, causing a thrombocytosis of dysfunction platelets which are often in excess of 600×10^9/L. Haemoglobin, WCC and haematocrit tend to be preserved. Myelofibrosis (D) describes the fibrosis of the bone 'marrow due to abnormal megakaryocytes which produce excess fibrosing factors. Extramedullary haemopoiesis occurs as compensation causing massive splenomegaly and hepatomegaly while WCC, platelets and haemoglobin initially increase, then are reduced. Chronic myeloid leukaemia (CML) (E) is characterized by a hypercellular bone marrow, elevated granulocytes and white cells.

Auer rods

18 B This patient is suffering from an acute promyelocytic leukaemia, a subtype (M3) of AML. It is due to t(15;17) translocation (B) which causes the proliferation of promyelocytes. The most worrisome complication is diffuse intravascular coagulation, potentially leading to massive haemorrhage. The t(8;21) (A) abnormality is part of the acute myelogenous leukaemia disorders (M2 variant) and is associated with variable WCC, anaemia, neutropenia and thrombocytopenia. The t(9;22) (C) translocation occurs in CML and in 95 per cent of patients is associated with the Philadelphia chromosome. Patients have elevated WCC, basophils, neutrophils and myelocytes with a hypercellular bone marrow. A t(14;18) (D) karyotype occurs in follicular lymphoma, a tumour of follicles consisting of centrocytes. A t(8;14) (E) abnormality occurs in Burkitt's lymphoma secondary to a latent Epstein–Barr (EBV) infection and usually affects the maxilla or mandible.

Massive splenomegaly

19 A Infectious mononucleosis (A), secondary to EBV, is usually an acute limited disease which is asssociated with fever, weight loss and malaise giving rise to mild splenomegaly only. CML (C) causes an accumulation of proliferated myeloid cells, the treatment of thalassaemia (B) involves splenectomy thereby reducing the accumulation of dysfunctional globin chains. Polycythaemia rubra vera (E) can cause an accumulation of RBC which are usually filtered at the spleen. Kala-azar (D) is caused primarily by *Leishmania donovani*, parasites which enmesh themselves with the spleen and other parts of the reticuloendothelial system causing massive splenomegaly.

Glucose-6-phosphate dehydrogenase deficiency

20 E Schistocytes (E), fragments of red blood cells, are the strongest indicator of red blood cell haemolysis. Target cells (A) have an accumulation of haemoglobin at their centre with pallor around them. They are indicative of obstructive jaundice, hepatic pathology, haemoglobinopathy and hyposplenism. Pencil cells (B) are hypochromic variations of elliptocytes (D), the former occurring in iron deficiency while the latter occurs in both hereditary elliptocytosis and iron deficiency anaemia. Spherocytes (C) usually occur in hereditary spherocytosis and haemolytic anaemia.

Heinz bodies

21 B This patient is most likely suffering from glucose-6-phosphate dehydrogenase deficiency (G6PD) (B). This is an important enzyme which maintains levels of glutathione, an important protective factor against oxidative stress. Exposure to drugs such as dapsone or antimalarials such as primaquine can denature haemoglobin which produces Heinz bodies with precipitant haemoglobin. Hereditary elliptocytosis (A) is usually associated with iron deficiency anaemia and is not greatly impacted by an additional stressor such as oxidant influences. Hereditary spherocytosis (C) occurs due to a defect in the cell membrane protein spectrin which predisposes such cells to become accumulated within the spleen and more fragile. Autoimmune haemolytic anaemia (D) is due to autoimmune mediated attacks upon RBCs, usually through the action of autoantibodies or complement. Microangiopathic haemolytic anaemia (E) is characterized by anaemia and schistocytes on blood smear produced from the shearing of RBCs upon fibrin meshes formed in the small vasculature, which most often forms due to increased activation of the coagulatory system.

Sickle cell anaemia

22   D   Sodium metabisulfite (D) can be added to blood smears to mimic accelerated deoxygenation. RBCs with high haemoglobin S concentrations undergo sickling in a reduced oxygen environment. Further investigation would be needed to differentiate homozygous and heterozygous sickle cell disease. Ham's test (A) is used to diagnose paroxysmal nocturnal haemoglobinuria. The Schilling test (C) is used to investigate vitamin B_{12} deficiency. The Coomb's test (direct) (B) is used to investigate causes of autoimmune haemolytic anaemia. The osmotic fragility test (E) is used to investigate hereditary spherocytosis.

AML and ALL differentiation

23   C   Sudan black B (B) preferentially stains myeloblasts against lymphoblasts and so is useful in the differentiation of AML and ALL. Myeloperoxidase staining (A) is important in the investigation of extramedullary leukaemia. Tartrate-resistant acid phosphatase stain (C) is used to diagnose hairy cell leukaemia. Leukocyte alkaline phosphatase (D) is useful in a range of conditions, it is elevated in polycythaemia rubra vera, essential thrombocytosis and myelofibrosis while in paroxysmal nocturnal haemoglobinuria and CML it is reduced. Auramine O stain (E) is used to stain for acid-fast bacteria such as mycobacterium and is not used in haematological investigations.

Polycythaemia rubra vera

24   E   Since polycythaemia rubra vera is a point mutation abnormality, the bone marrow produces excess myeloid lineage cells. This feeds back negatively upon erythropoietin production from the renal cells, such that a raised red cell mass but low erythropoietin level (E) is measured. In a renal cell cancer, erythropoietin levels may be uncontrollably raised causing a correspondent increase in red cell mass (D). Conversely, renal failure causes a reduction in erythropoietin therefore red cell mass can be lowered (A). In bone marrow failure raised erythropoietin levels have no impact on increasing red cell mass (C). In the absence of disease, erythropoietin and red cell mass are at homeostatic levels (B).

Vegetarian patient

25 E This patient is most likely suffering from iron deficiency anaemia given her change to vegetarian diet, although there are many foods with good iron content such as green vegetables and whole grain cereals. However, most ingested iron is not absorbed by the body, an acidic pH increases absorption while an alkaline pH reduces it. The characteristic symptoms of iron deficiency anaemia are shortness of breath, pallor and malaise. Transferrin (E) is the principal iron carrying protein in the body. In iron deficiency anaemia, iron-binding capacity increases to compensate the reduced intake. Although haemoglobin (C) and myoglobin (A) contain iron, they are likely to be reduced in iron deficiency anaemia. Similarly, the iron stores of the body are ferritin (B) and over time these will be consumed if intake decreases, as does the serum iron (D).

Anaemia

26 D This patient is most likely suffering from pernicious anaemia (D) whereby antibodies bind to gastric parietal cells reducing B_{12} absorption through deficiency of intrinsic factor. Vitamin B_{12} deficiency can cause a megaloblastic anaemia which presents with an increased MCV on blood tests. Diseases of the small bowel can compound this anaemia such as coeliac's and Crohn's disease. Blood loss (B) is likely to have caused a positive faecal occult blood test and usually presents with a normocytic anaemia. Iron deficiency anaemia (A) and anaemia of chronic disease (C) usually cause a microcytic anaemia. Although autoimmune haemolytic (E) anaemia can cause a macrocytic anaemia, a Coomb's test would be positive.

Macrocytic anaemia

27 C This patient is most likely suffering from aplastic anaemia (C) where there is failure of the bone marrow causing a pancytopenia and hypocellular bone marrow with increasing proportions of fatty tissue. A macrocytosis is strongly suggestive in the background of pancytopenia of aplastic anaemia as the body compensates with the production of fetal haemoglobin which is larger than RBCs. Patients usually present with features of missing cell lineages, such as symptoms of anaemia, infections and bleeding from thrombocytopenia. Iron deficiency anaemia (D) is characterized by shortness of breath, pallor and tiredness. Bleeding and infections are not prominent features. In chronic myeloid leukaemia (A), there is active production of dysfunctional cells, therefore white cells, platelets and granulocytes are raised and the bone marrow is hypercellular. A myeloproliferative disorder (B), active production of mature myeloid cells are produced and so a pancytopenia is not a feature. An analysis of the bone marrow in an acute lymphoblastic anaemia (E) would show more than 20 per cent lymphoblasts.

Auer rods

28 D This patient is suffering from an acute myeloid leukaemia (D). There are many mutations that cause the disorder and it can occur in young or old patients, peak presentations tend to be in middle-aged males. Blood investigations may show a variable WCC, anaemia, thrombocytopenia and neutropenia. A blood smear may have auer rods and leukoerythroblastic cells. ALL (A) may have a similar count to AML although the lymphoblasts are usually seen on blood smear and stain with Periodic acid achiff stain. DiGeorge's syndrome (B) is a genetic disorder caused by a deletion at 22q11, young patients present with cardiac anomalies (Tetralogy of Fallot's), abnormal facies, thymic aplasia, cleft palate and hypocalcaemia. Disseminated intravascular coagulation (C) is a consumptive coagulopathy which does not feature auer rods. Congenital afibrinogenemia (E) is characterized by blood clotting disorder rather than increased predispositions to infections.

Chronic myeloid leukaemia

29 B Chronic myeloid leukaemia occurs due to the reciprocal translocation of chromosome 9 (Abl) and 22 (BCR) causing the BCR/ABL fusion gene, otherwise termed the Philadelphia chromosome, which has uncontrolled tyrosine kinase activity. Treatment begins with imatinib (B), a tyrosine kinase inhibitor which blocks the activity of BCR/ABL. Over time, the action of multiple drug resistance proteins which pump out imatinib and a change in the shape of the active site of BCR/ABL cause resistance. Dasatinib (E) and eventually stem cell transplantation (D) are then required for treatment. Hydroxycarbamide (A) is a chemotherapy drug used primarily in the treatment of polycythaemia rubra vera alongside venesection (C) to reduce viscosity and haematocrit.

Warfarin therapy

30 C The INR is the ratio between the prothrombin time compared to a control sample and provides a means of monitoring bleeding risk. The normal INR is between 0.9 and 1.3 (B), an INR <1.0 (A) suggests a high thrombotic risk. The SIGN guidelines state a patient suffering from rheumatic mitral valve disease with/without atrial fibrillation should have a target INR of 2.5 with a range between 2.0 and 3.0 (C). An INR between 3 and 4 (D) would be appropriate in a patient with lupus anticoagulant syndrome or suffering from venous thromboembolism. It would also be appropriate following a mitral valve replacement with a metallic valve where a high INR is important. An INR >5.0 (E) indicates a high bleeding risk.

Multiple myeloma

31 E Although multiple myeloma has been reported in some cases of first degree relatives and identical twins, no evidence for hereditary (E) passage of disease exists. Radiation (A) has been shown to increase the risk for multiple myeloma. Farmers using herbicides, insecticides, benzene and organic solvents (D) are also reported to have an increased risk for myeloma. HHV-8 (B) is shown to be present in the dendritic cells originating from the bone marrow of myeloma sufferers while chronic untreated HIV (C) is also associated with increased myeloma risk.

Hypersplenism investigation

32 A The reticulocyte test (A) would show reduced counts in aplastic anaemia while it is raised in hypersplenism. The metabisulphite (C) can be added to blood smears to mimic accelerated deoxygenation. RBCs with high haemoglobin S concentrations undergo sickling in a reduced oxygen environment and therefore this is a useful test for sickle cell anaemia. Ham's test (D) is used to diagnose paroxysmal nocturnal haemoglobinuria. The direct Coomb's test (B) is used to investigate causes of autoimmune haemolytic anaemia. The osmotic fragility test (E) is used to investigate hereditary spherocytosis.

Pernicious anaemia

33 B Pernicious anaemia is an autoimmune disease whereby anti-intrinsic factor antibodies (B) bind intrinsic factor produced by the parietal cells in the gastric fundus. Intrinsic factor is essential in the absorption of vitamin B_{12} via the ileum. Associated conditions can include thyroid disease which compound symptoms of anaemia. Anti-mitochondrial antibodies (A) are associated with primary biliary cirrhosis, anti-gliadin antibodies (C) are associated with coeliac disease. Anti-centromere antibodies (D) are associated with limited and occasionally diffuse scleroderma. Anti-smooth muscle antibodies (E) are associated with autoimmune hepatitis.

Leukaemia investigation

34 C In order to diagnose an acute leukaemia, defined as ≥20 per cent of bone marrow cells being blasts, an examination of a bone marrow aspirate under microscopy (C) is necessary. Flow cytometry (E) is useful in distinguishing AML from ALL. Electron microscopy (D) has a reduced role with advanced immunotyping techniques available. (A) and (B) are useful investigations once a leukaemia is confirmed.

Bence Jones protein

35 D Myeloma cells produce monoclonal antibodies and/or light chains (D), called M-proteins and Bence–Jones proteins, respectively. The M proteins are heavy chains and can be IgG (A) and IgA (B) or rarely IgM (E), IgE (C) and IgD. The antibodies and light chains will be of a single class, either kappa or lambda. IgA production predisposes to the hyperviscosity syndrome.

SECTION 8: NEUROLOGY

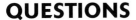

QUESTIONS

1. Limb weakness

A 66-year-old woman complains of stiffness and weakness climbing stairs. She has a history of hypertension and diet-controlled type 2 diabetes. On examination, there is mild upper arm weakness, hip flexion is 4–/5 bilaterally, with bilateral wasting and flickers of fasciculations in the right quadriceps. Knee extension is 4/5. Dorsiflexion and plantar flexion are strong. Brisk knee and ankle reflexes are elicited, as well as a positive Hoffman's and Babinski's sign. Sensory examination and cranial nerves are normal. Her BM is 8.9, her pulse is regular and her blood pressure is 178/97. What is the most likely diagnosis?

A. Myasthenia gravis
B. Diabetic neuropathy
C. Myositis
D. Motor neurone disease
E. Multiple sclerosis (MS)

2. Lesion localization (1)

A 23-year-old man is stabbed in the neck. Once stabilized, his MRI shows a right hemisection of the cord at C6. What is the expected result of this injury?

A. Paralysed diaphragm
B. Absent sensation to temperature in the left hand
C. Paralysis of the left hand
D. Absent sensation to light touch in the left hand
E. Brisk right biceps reflex

3. Multiple sclerosis treatment

A 23-year-old woman complains that her right leg has become progressively stiff and clumsy over the last couple of weeks. She is worried as she has not been able to go to work for the last 4 days. On examination, tone is increased and there is a catch at the knee. She has six beats of clonus and an upgoing plantar. Power is reduced to 3-4/5 in the right leg flexors. There is no sensory involvement and the rest of the neurological exam is normal other than a pale disc on opthalmoscopy. On further questioning, she admits that she has had two episodes of blurred vision in her right eye in the last two years. Each lasted a couple of weeks from which she fully recovered. What is the most appropriate initial treatment?

A. A non-steroidal anti-inflammatory drug (NSAID)
B. Interferon-beta
C. Bed rest
D. Methotrexate
E. A course of oral steroids

4. Lesion localization (2)

A 78 year old right-handed male collapses and is brought into accident and emergency. He seems to follow clear one-step commands but he gets very frustrated as he cannot answer questions. He is unable to lift his right hand or leg. He has an irregularly irregular pulse and his blood pressure is 149/87. He takes only aspirin and frusemide. What is the most likely diagnosis?

    A. Left cortical infarct
    B. Right internal capsule infarct
    C. Left cortical haemorrhage
    D. Left internal capsule haemorrhage
    E. Brainstem haemorrhage

5. Glasgow Coma Scale

A 19-year-old woman collapses at a concert and is witnessed to have a tonic-clonic seizure lasting 2 minutes. When the paramedics arrive and ask her questions, she mumbles but no-one can understand what she is saying. Only when the paramedic applies pressure to her nailbed does she open her eyes and reach out with her other hand to rub her nail and then push him away. What is her Glasgow Coma Scale (GCS)?

    A. 12
    B. 11
    C. 10
    D. 9
    E. 8

6. Risk factors in stroke

A 79-year-old man is admitted with left hemiparesis. CT reveals a middle cerebral artery infarct. What is his most significant risk factor for stroke?

    A. Hypertension
    B. Smoking
    C. Family history
    D. Diabetes
    E. Cholesterol

7. Multiple sclerosis prognosis

A 42-year-old woman presents with ataxia. Gadolinium-enhanced MRI reveals multiple subcortical white matter lesions as well as enhancing lesions in the cerrebellum and spinal cord. She is diagnosed with MS. Two months later she develops optic neuritis. What feature is associated with a milder disease course?

    A. Her age of 42
    B. Her initial presentation of ataxia
    C. Her female gender
    D. The interval between the two episodes of two months
    E. Her MRI scan appearance

8. Seizure (1)

A 71-year-old man with atrial fibrillation is seen in clinic following an episode of syncope. He describes getting a poor night's sleep and, as he got out of bed in the morning, feeling dizzy for a couple of seconds before the lights dimmed around him. He was woken a couple of seconds later by his wife who had witnessed the event. She says he went pale and fell to the floor and his arms and legs jerked. After waking, he was shaken but was 'back to normal' a few minutes after the event. His medication includes aspirin, atenolol and frusemide. What is the most likely diagnosis?

    A. Vasovagal syncope
    B. Orthostatic hypotension
    C. Cardiogenic syncope
    D. Transient ischaemic attack (TIA)
    E. Seizure

9. Headache (1)

A 41-year-old man complains of terrible headache. It started an hour ago, without warning, while stressed at work. It affects the right side of his head. He scores it '11/10' in severity. When asked, he agrees that light does bother him a little. He had a similar episode six months ago, experiencing very similar headaches over 2 weeks which resolved spontaneously. On observation, he looks quite distressed and prefers to pace up and down, unable to sit still. What is the diagnosis?

    A. Subarachnoid haemorrhage
    B. Tension headache
    C. Intracerebral haemorrhage
    D. Migraine
    E. Cluster headache

222 Section 8: Neurology

10. Visual loss

A 49-year-old man complains of sudden onset, painless unilateral visual loss lasting about a minute. He describes 'a black curtain coming down'. His blood pressure is 158/90, heart rate 73 bpm. There is an audible bruit on auscultation of his neck. His past medical history is insignificant other than deep vein thrombosis of his right leg ten years ago. The most likely diagnosis is:

    A. Retinal vein thrombosis
    B. Retinal artery occlusion
    C. Amaurosis fugax
    D. Optic neuritis
    E. Acute angle glaucoma

11. Stroke treatment

A 77-year-old woman is admitted to hospital with a urinary tract infection. She receives antibiotics and seems to be responding well. On the fourth day she is eating her lunch when she suddenly drops her fork. She calls for the nurse who notices the left side of her face is drooping. What is the best next course of action?

    A. CT head
    B. Thrombolysis
    C. MRI head
    D. Aspirin
    E. Place nil by mouth

12. Contraindications for thrombolysis

A 71-year-old right-handed male is brought in by ambulance at 17:50 having suffered a collapse. His wife came home to find him on the floor unable to move his right arm or leg and unable to speak. Her call to the ambulance was logged at 17:30. He has a past medical history of well-controlled hypertension, ischaemic heart disease and atrial fibrillation for which he is on warfarin. He had a hernia repair three months ago and his brother had a 'bleed in the brain' at the age of 67. What is the absolute contraindication to thrombolysis in this male?

    A. Family history of haemorrhagic stroke
    B. History of recent surgery
    C. Time of onset
    D. Current haemorrhagic stroke
    E. Warfarin treatment

13. Spinal claudication

A 69-year-old man presents to clinic with a six-month history of progressive lower back pain which radiates down to his buttock. He found the pain was exacerbated while taking his daily morning walk and noticed that it eased going uphill but worsened downhill. He stopped his daily walks as a result and he now walks only slowly to the shops when he needs to, taking breaks to sit down and ease the pain. He has a history of hypertension, diabetes and prostatic hyperplasia. What is the diagnosis?

A. Peripheral vascular disease
B. Osteoporotic fracture
C. Spinal stenosis
D. Sciatica
E. Metastatic bone disease

14. Difficulty walking and writing

A 31-year-old woman presents to accident and emergency with progressive difficulty walking associated with lower back pain. A few days ago she was tripping over things, now she has difficulty climbing stairs. She describes tingling and numbness in both hands which moved up to her elbows, she is unable to write. On examination, cranial nerves are intact but there is absent sensation to vibration and pin prick in her upper limbs to the elbow and lower limbs to the hip. Power is 3/5 in the ankles and 4–/5 at the hip with absent reflexes and mute plantars. Her blood pressure is 124/85, pulse 68 and sats 98 per cent on air. She has a past medical history of type I diabetes and recently recovered from an episode of food poisoning a month or two ago. What is the diagnosis?

A. MS
B. Guillain–Barré syndrome (GBS)
C. Myasthenia gravis
D. Diabetic neuropathy
E. Infective neuropathy

15. Parkinson's associated symptoms

A left-handed 79-year-old man presents with a troublesome resting tremor of his left hand. The tremor is evident in his writing. He has also noticed his writing is smaller than it used to be. He complains he has difficulty turning in bed to get comfortable and his wife complains that he sometimes kicks her in the middle of the night. When he gets out of bed in the morning he feels a little woozy, but this resolves after a while. On examination, he blinks about three times a minute and his face does not show much emotion. Glabellar tap is positive. He has a slow, shuffling gait. He has difficulty stopping, starting and turning. He holds his feet slightly apart to steady himself. When you pull him backwards, he is unable to right himself and stumbles back. Which of the signs and symptoms is not commonly associated with parkinsonism?

    A. Postural instability
    B. Rapid eye movement (REM) sleep disturbance
    C. Hypomimia
    D. Broad-based gait
    E. Autonomic instability

16. Migraine treatment

A 33-year-old woman attends her six-month follow-up appointment for headache. They are migrainous in nature but whereas she used to have them every few months, over the last three months she has experienced a chronic daily headache which varies in location and can be anywhere from 3–7/10 severity. Her last migraine with aura was two months ago. She takes co-codamol qds and ibuprofen tds. What is the best medical management?

    A. Stop all medication
    B. Start paracetamol
    C. Start sumatriptan
    D. Start propranolol
    E. Continue current medication

17. Seizure (2)

A 17-year-old girl is brought into accident and emergency with generalized tonic-clonic seizure. Her mother had found her fitting in her bedroom about 20 minutes ago. The ambulance crew handover state that her sats are 96 per cent on 15 L of oxygen and they have given her two doses of rectal diazepam but she has not stopped fitting. What is the most appropriate management?

    A. Lorazepam
    B. Phenobarbital
    C. Intubation
    D. Call ITU
    E. Phenytoin loading

18. Phenytoin levels

A 72-year-old man with known epilepsy and hypertension is admitted with pneumonia. His drug history includes aspirin, phenytoin, bendroflumethiazide and amlodipine. His heart rate is 67, blood pressure 170/93, sats 96 per cent on 2 L of oxygen. Neurological examination is normal. His doctor requests blood tests including phenytoin level. What is the correct indication for this test?

   A. Routine check
   B. Ensure levels are not toxic
   C. Confirm patient compliance
   D. Ensure therapeutic level reached
   E. Reassure the patient

19. Seizure (3)

A 23-year-old woman is seen in clinic for recurrent funny turns. She is not aware of them, but her family and friends have noticed them. They say she looks around blankly, then starts picking at her clothes and sometimes yawns, then she comes back after a minute. She can get drowsy after these episodes. What seizure type does this patient describe?

   A. Absence
   B. Tonic clonic
   C. Simple partial
   D. Complex partial
   E. Generalized

20. Dermatomes (1)

You are asked to perform a lower limb peripheral neurological examination on a 45-year-old diabetic male. The patient has normal tone, 5/5 power, normal plantars and proprioception. However, you notice that the patient does not respond to any sensory stimulus on the medial side of the right lower leg. Which dermatome is affected?

   A. L1
   B. L2
   C. L3
   D. L4
   E. L5

21. Lesion pattern location (1)

On examination, a patient has 5/5 power in all muscle groups of his upper limbs, 0/5 power in all the muscle groups of his lower limbs. Cranial nerves are intact. Where is the lesion?

    A. Muscle
    B. Neuromuscular junction
    C. Peripheral nerves
    D. Spinal cord
    E. Brain

22. Dermatomes (2)

On examination, a patient has 5/5 power in his upper limbs, 0/5 power in his lower limbs. Further examination reveals a sensory level at the umbilicus. Cranial nerves are intact. Where is the lesion?

    A. C4
    B. T4
    C. T10
    D. L1
    E. L3

23. Lesion pattern location (2)

A patient is unable to move his right arm or leg. When asked to smile, the left side of his mouth droops. Where is the lesion?

    A. Left motor cortex
    B. Right motor cortex
    C. Left brainstem
    D. Right brainstem
    E. Cervical spine

24. Visual pathway lesion

A light is shone into a patient's right eye and it constricts. When moved to the left eye, the left eye constricts. When moved back to the right eye, the right eye dilates. What is the diagnosis?

    A. Afferent lesion
    B. Efferent lesion
    C. Relative afferent lesion
    D. Relative efferent lesion
    E. Normal

25. Myasthenia gravis

A 55-year-old woman complains of double vision. She finds that she is more tired than usual and has difficulty climbing stairs, especially when they are very long. She has difficulty getting items off high shelves at work and lately even brushing her hair is a problem. During the consultation, her voice fades away during conversation. Reflexes are present and equal throughout. Which sign or symptom is most indicative of myasthenia gravis?

    A. Proximal weakness
    B. Normal reflexes
    C. Diplopia
    D. Fatigability
    E. Bulbar symptoms

26. Lambert–Eaton syndrome

A 55-year-old woman complains of double vision. She finds that she is tired all the time and has difficulty climbing stairs. She has difficulty getting items off high shelves at work. Reflexes are absent but elicited after exercise. Shoulder abduction is initially 4–5 but on repeated testing is 4+/5. What pathology is associated with this female's diagnosis?

    A. Thyrotoxicosis
    B. Peptic ulcer
    C. Diabetes
    D. Stroke
    E. Lung cancer

27. Cranial nerve palsy

On observation, a patient has a left facial droop. On closer examination his nasolabial fold is flattened. When asked to smile, the left corner of his mouth droops. He is unable to keep his cheeks puffed out. Eye closure is only slightly weaker compared to the right and his forehead wrinkles when he is asked to look up high. What is the diagnosis?

    A. Right middle cerebral artery stroke
    B. Parotid gland tumour
    C. Left internal capsule stroke
    D. Bell's palsy
    E. Cerebellar pontine angle tumour

28. Opthalmoplegia

A female presents with diplopia. On closer examination, when asked to look right, her left eye stays in the midline but her right eye moves right and starts jerking. What is the diagnosis?

    A. Myasthenia gravis (MG)
    B. Vertigo
    C. Cerebellar syndrome
    D. MS
    E. Peripheral neuropathy

29. Neurological signs

A neurologist is examining a patient. She takes the patient's middle finger and flicks the distal phalanx, her thumb contracts in response. What sign has been elicited?

    A. Chvostek's
    B. Glabellar
    C. Hoffman's
    D. Tinel's
    E. Babinksi's

30. Dementia

A 69-year-old man is taken to his GP by his concerned wife. She complains that he has not been himself for the last year. He has slowly become withdrawn and stopped working on his hobbies. Now she is concerned that he often forgets to brush his teeth. She has noticed he sometimes struggles to find the right word and this has gradually become more noticeable over the last couple of months. She presented today because she was surprised to come home to find him naked and urinating in the living room last week. He has a history of hypertension and is an ex-smoker. The most likely diagnosis is:

    A. Depression
    B. Frontotemporal dementia
    C. Alzheimer's disease
    D. Vascular dementia
    E. Lewy Body disease

31. Upgoing plantars

Which of the following is not a cause of absent ankle jerks and up-going plantars?

    A. Freidreich's ataxia
    B. B_{12} deficiency
    C. MS
    D. Cord compression
    E. Motor neurone disease

32. Gait abnormality

A patient has difficulty walking. His gait is unsteady. He seems to have difficulty raising his right leg and swings it round in an arc as he walks. He holds his right arm and wrist flexed. What type of gait does this patient exhibit?

A. Hemiplegic
B. Scissoring
C. High stepping
D. Spastic
E. Stomping

33. Visual fields

A patient is admitted with a stroke. On examination of her visual fields, she is unable to see in the right lower quadrant of her field. Where is the lesion?

A. Optic chiasm
B. Left parietal lobe
C. Right temporal lobe
D. Right optic radiation
E. Left optic nerve

34. Dizziness

A 43-year-old woman presents with dizziness to accident and emergency. It started suddenly this morning, she awoke with a headache and the dizziness started when she sat up in bed. She describes the room spinning for a couple of minutes. It settles if she keeps still, but returns on movement. There is no tinnitus or deafness, but some nausea and no vomiting. The most likely diagnosis is:

A. Brainstem stroke
B. Benign paroxysmal positional vertigo
C. Ménière's disease
D. Vestibular neuronitis
E. Migraine

35. Dermatological manifestations

A 40-year-old woman seen in clinic has multiple fleshy nodules and several light brown, round macules with a smooth border on her back, arms and legs. There are also freckles under her arms. What is the underlying disorder?

A. Neurofibromatosis type I
B. Neurofibromatosis type II
C. Tuberous sclerosis
D. Hereditary haemorrhagic telangectasia
E. Sturge–Weber syndrome

36. Imaging

A 19-year-old man is admitted with a GCS of 12. He was doing push ups when he complained of a sudden-onset, severe headache and collapsed. What would you expect on his CT?

    A. Convex haematoma
    B. Midline shift
    C. Crescent-shaped haematoma
    D. Blood along the sulci and fissures
    E. Intraventricular blood

37. Stroke territories

A 60-year-old man presents with visual problems and dizziness. The dizziness started suddenly, he sees the room spinning around and he has noticed he keeps bumping into things on his right. His blood pressure is 159/91, heart rate 72. On examination, there is nystagmus and dysdiadochokinesia. Where is his stroke?

    A. Temporal lobe
    B. Left parietal lobe
    C. Right parietal lobe
    D. Anterior circulation
    E. Posterior circulation

38. Paraesthesia

A 45-year-old man presents with a 5-day history of progressive tingling and numbness of his hands and feet. He insists that he has never had this problem before and that he was perfectly fine a week ago. Over the last 2 days he has had some difficulty walking but mostly he complains about difficulty rolling up cigarettes. On examination, there is mild symmetrical distal weakness, mild gait ataxia and dysdiadochokinesia. He smokes 30 cigarettes a day and drinks 1–2 bottles of wine. He has a family history of hypertension and his 63-year-old mother has type 2 diabetes, whom over the last year has complained of numbness and burning in her feet. He self-discharges. A week later, his symptoms have peaked. He displays moderate distal weakness and numbness to his knees, after which he turns a corner and his symptoms start to slowly resolve. What is the diagnosis?

    A. Miller Fisher syndrome
    B. Alcoholic neuropathy
    C. Chronic idiopathic demyelinating polyneuropathy
    D. Charcot Marie Tooth disease
    E. GBS

39. Headache (2)

A 28-year-old junior doctor has been complaining of a headache for the last 24 hours. It started gradually, intensifying slowly and involving the entire cranium, but over the last couple of hours she has noticed that turning her head is uncomfortable. She feels generally unwell and prefers to lie in a dark room. Her boyfriend has noticed that she seems irritable. On examination, she exhibits photophobia and there is neck stiffness. There is no papilloedema. Close examination of her skin reveals no rashes. Kernig's sign is negative. A lumbar puncture (LP) reveals low protein, normal glucose and lymphocytosis. What is the diagnosis?

    A. Viral meningitis
    B. Migraine
    C. Aseptic meningitis
    D. Bacterial meningitis
    E. TB meningitis

40. Loss of balance

A 36-year-old woman presents to clinic with neurological symptoms. On examination, she is able to stand with her feet together. Upon closing her eyes, however, she is unable to keep her balance. What is the diagnosis?

    A. Diabetes
    B. Cerebellar problem
    C. Alcohol abuse
    D. Proprioceptive problem
    E. Visual problem

ANSWERS

Limb weakness

1 D   This woman presents with upper (brisk reflexes, upgoing plantar) and lower (fasciculations) motor neurone signs. Motor neurone disease (MND) (D) presents with mixed upper and lower motor neurone signs and importantly no sensory involvement. In this case, there is involvement of two regions (arms and legs). Bulbar signs, such as tongue wasting and fasciculation, often help make the diagnosis. Myositis (C) affects the muscle, resulting in tenderness, wasting and fasciculation but no upper motor neurone (UMN) signs. Although the patient is diabetic, neuropathies (B) result in lower motor neurone (LMN) signs only. These may be motor and/or sensory. Typically, diabetes results in a peripheral neuropathy, most commonly sensory. The proximal distribution of weakness would be in keeping with myasthenia (A), but not the UMN signs. There is no mention of fatigability, which is a key feature. MS (E) in this age group is less common and an inflammatory disorder of the central nervous system would not result in LMN signs.

Lesion localization

2 B   Hemisection of the cord is also known as Brown–Séquard syndome. This results in ipsilateral paralysis and loss of light touch and vibration sensation and contralateral loss in pain and temperature below the point of the lesion. The spinothalamic tracts cross at the level of the cord, so sensation to pain and temperature is lost in the contralateral limbs (B). C3, 4, 5 keep the diaphragm alive (A), so breathing should be preserved. As the right corticospinal tract has been severed, the right, ipsilateral hand would be paralysed (C) as well as the right leg. The left dorsal columns carry light touch fibres from the left limb (D). They have been unaffected by the injury. C6 is responsible for the biceps reflex and would be lost (E). Reflexes distal to the lesion would be brisk.

Multiple sclerosis treatment

3 E   The subacute onset of upper motor neurone signs on a background of episodes of optic neuritis in a young woman makes relapsing–remitting MS the likely diagnosis. The diagnosis of MS hinges on the presence of multiple central nervous system (CNS) lesions separated by time and space. These manifest in either signs/symptoms or as enhancing white matter lesions on gadolinium-enhanced MRI. There is no specific role for NSAIDs in MS (A). Even if the patient complained of pain, it would be important to ensure its origin. NSAIDs would not be appropriate for neuropathic pain. This patient may be eligible for a disease-modifying drug such as interferon beta (B) or glatiramer acetate, as she has a relapsing–remitting course and recent symptoms, but this would not be the most immediate treatment. These drugs reduce the number of relapses experienced by one-third over two years and are expensive. Long-term effects on morbidity are currently unclear. Bed rest alone (C) is inappropriate as this patient would benefit from a course of steroids as she has disabling symptoms. Oral steroids (E) have been shown to be as effective as intravenous steroids, although patients tend to be admitted for IV treatment. They reduce the length of the relapse so the patient would recover quicker, but have no effect on number of relapses or accumulation of disability. There is no evidence for methotrexate (D) in relapsing–remitting MS.

Lesion localization

4 A This male has most likely suffered a left cortical infarct (A), probably as a result of an embolus secondary to atrial fibrillation. Treatment with warfarin would have reduced his annual risk of stroke from roughly 5 to 1 per cent. It is a left-sided infarct because of the contralateral (right) hemiparesis and dysphasia (involvement of the dominant cortex). It is not a capsular (B and D) or brainstem (E) event as the patient has an expressive dysphasia which implies involvement of Broca's area which is cortical. It is more likely to be ischaemic than haemorrhagic (C). Roughly 80 per cent of strokes are infarcts, 20 per cent haemorrhagic and in this case there is a plausible embolic explanation coupled with only mild hypertension. Haemorrhagic strokes tend to occur in younger patients with severe hypertension and a family history (pointing to an anatomical anomaly). However, they cannot be differentiated clinically and a CT is required to confirm the stroke subtype.

Glasgow Coma Scale

5 D The GCS is frequently used to assess level of consciousness. The lowest score is 3, the highest 15. A score of 8 or below is classified as coma. GCS is assessed by evaluating eye (1–4), verbal (1–5) and motor (1–6) response. Clinically, it is best to assess for the highest possible score and work down. So, if a patient is not opening their eyes spontaneously, assess whether they respond to verbal command and only then to pain. In this case, E = 2 (responds to pain), V = 2 (incomprehensible sounds), M = 5 (localizes to pain), giving this patient a GCS of 9/15. It is important to carefully monitor her GCS, like most measurements a trend is more useful than a one-off assessment.

Risk factors in stroke

6 A The three most important risk factors for stroke are hypertension, hypertension and hypertension (A)! INTERSTROKE, a recent large case–control study evaluating risk factors for stroke, has shown that ten risk factors are associated with 90 per cent of the risk of stroke and that of these modifiable risk factors, hypertension is the most important for all stroke subtypes and is a particularly dangerous risk factor for intracerebral haemorrhage. Other risk factors include smoking (B), lipids (E) and diabetes (D) which promote atherosclerosis. Poor diet, lack of regular activity and increased waist–hip ratio are as significant risk factors as smoking. Unmodifiable risk factors include increasing age (by far the most significant), male sex, family history (C) and ethnicity (higher in Blacks and Asians). Patients in atrial fibrillation have an annual stroke risk of 5 per cent. This can be lowered to 1 per cent by anticoagulating with warfarin, aiming for an international normalized ratio (INR) of between 2 and 3 (avoid confusion with aspirin which is an antiplatelet). Stroke is the third most common cause of death in England (after heart disease and cancer) and is more often disabling than fatal, so primary and secondary prevention are crucial.

Multiple sclerosis prognosis

7 C   In this woman's case, all of the features except her gender (C) point to a more aggressive disease course. Although it is close to impossible to predict an individual patient's outcome, features of a better prognosis include onset under 25 years (A), optic neuritis or sensory, rather than cerebellar symptoms on initial presentation (B), a long interval (>1 year) between relapses (D) and few lesions on MRI (E). Full recovery from relapses is also a positive feature. Progressive MS carries a poorer prognosis compared to relapsing–remitting MS.

Seizure

8 B   This man most likely experienced an episode of orthostatic or postural hypotension (B) where syncope occurs as a result of reduced cerebral perfusion as the patient moves from lying to standing. Symptoms are similar to vasovagal in that the patient may become pale and describe 'the lights or sound dimming'. Perfusion is restored after the patient collapses and unconsciousness lasts no more than seconds or a couple of minutes with full recovery. However, vasovagal epsiodes (A) can be brought on by sleep or food deprivation, hot or emotional environments, Valsalva manoeuvre (such as straining) and are not as closely related to position. Syncope while lying down is more suggestive of cardiac syncope or seizure activity. It is important to rule out cardiac causes of syncope (C) which may be heralded by chest pain or palpitations. Arrhythmias or aortic stenosis may be the underlying cause. TIAs (D) are a very rare cause of syncope. Seizures (E) may be triggered by lack of sleep. They may be heralded by an aura, typically visual or olfactory. There may be urinary incontinence, tonic-clonic movements, tongue-biting and cyanosis during the event. However, jerky movements may occur in syncope of any cause. This alone does not equate to a seizure.

Headache

9 E Cluster headache (E) is more common in men and is classically excruciating, unilateral headache associated with autonomic features such as miosis, ptosis, conjunctival injection, tearing, sensation of nasal congestion and facial flushing. Timing is important, headaches occur in clusters of multiple episodes over a couple of weeks, then resolve spontaneously only to reoccur months to years later. They are not associated with aura or signs of raised intracranial pressure. Although the headache is severe and of acute onset in this instance, with possible photophobia, there is nothing in the stem to suggest raised intracranial pressure, such as papilloedema, nausea and vomiting or meningism, such as nuchal rigidity (A). More importantly, he has had similar episodes in the past. The timing and autonomic symptoms point to cluster headache. Tension headache (B) is classically associated with stress, reported as a tight band around the head and is much more benign. Intracranial haemorrhage (C), depending on location, is likely to cause focal signs or, especially if posterior fossa, signs of raised intracranial pressure and coning. Hypertension is an important risk factor. Migraine (D) classically is heralded by an aura and is associated with nausea and vomiting with osmo- (smell), phono- (sound) and photophobia. Patients prefer to curl up in a dark, quiet room, whereas patients with cluster headache feel the need to move around.

Visual loss

10 C This man gives a classical description of amaurosis fugax (C), painless, unilateral visual loss of short duration described as 'a black curtain descending', caused by retinal artery emboli, with a likely cardiac source as a consequence of atrial fibrillation.

Retinal artery (B) and vein (A) occlusion are also painless and of sudden onset, but they typically occur in older patients and result in prolonged visual loss. Amaurosis fugax may herald retinal artery occlusion which is confirmed on ophthalmoscopy showing oedema and a cherry red macula. It is also a complication of giant cell (temporal) arteritis. Retinal haemorrhages and cotton wool spots are typically seen in retinal vein occlusion. Optic neuritis (D) is associated with MS and patients complain of painful, blurred vision. Acute angle glaucoma (E), again seen in older patients, presents with painful, blurred vision. Patients describe 'seeing haloes around things'.

Stroke treatment

11 E This patient has suffered a stroke. This is a medical emergency. As she is within the 3-hour window for thrombolysis (B), she must be assessed immediately. However, thrombolysis is only useful in ischaemic stroke and can severely worsen haemorrhagic stroke. It is impossible to clinically tell the difference with certainty; she therefore warrants urgent imaging. Haemorrhages are much easier to detect on CT (A) as blood shows up white (hyperdense), plus there is easier access to CT unlike MRI (C) which is not always available. If thrombolysis is contraindicated, 300 mg of aspirin (D) is given in the case of ischaemic stroke. Option (E), however, is the most appropriate next step as removing her lunch is a quick, simple intervention that may prevent the complication of aspiration pneumonia. The nurse can then call the doctors or put out a thrombolysis call.

Contraindications for thrombolysis

12 C This man presents with a stroke. It is clinically impossible to tell with certainty whether it is ischaemic or haemorrhagic (D) which is why he needs a CT to differentiate between the two. However, the time of onset is unclear and therefore it is not possible to determine whether he is outside the 3-hour time window for thrombolysis (C). Neither warfarin treatment (E) nor family history of haemorrhagic stroke (A) are absolute contraindications although they would be taken into consideration. INR should be <1.7. The absolute contraindications for thrombolysis are: onset of symptoms more than 3 hours ago, seizures at presentation, uncontrolled blood pressure (over 180/110), previous intracranial bleed, lumbar puncture in the last week, ischaemic stroke or head injury in the last three months, active bleeding (not menstruation), surgery (B) or major trauma (including CPR) within the last 2 weeks or non-compressible arterial puncture within the last week.

Spinal claudication

13 C This man gives a good history of spinal claudication (C), lower back pain and sciatica on walking. The pain worsens when the spine is extended (walking, especially downhill, and improves when flexed, going uphill, sitting). It is caused by narrowing of the spinal canal as a result of spondylosis (degenerative disease). Intermittent claudication from peripheral vascular disease (A) can be similar in timing, worse on walking and relieved by rest, but the pain comes from ischaemic muscles, typically calf or buttock, and has no relation to the incline. There is nothing to suggest osteoporotic fracture (B), and in addition, his sex is protective for osteoporosis. Sciatica (D) presents as sharp pain shooting down the posterior leg and occurs as a result of impingement of the nerve roots forming the sciatic nerve. It is a symptom rather than a diagnosis. Metastatic bone disease (E) could result in spinal stenosis or sciatica but in itself does not explain the patient's exact symptoms and there is nothing else to suggest malignancy in the stem such as constitutional symptoms or a nodular prostate.

Difficulty walking and writing

14 B This woman presents with an ascending polyneuropathy. Her symptoms start distally and progress proximally, giving a glove and stocking distribution. Both sensory and motor neurones are involved. This is consistent with Guillain–Barré (B), an inflammatory disorder of the peripheral nerves often preceded by an infection such as campylobacter gastreoenteritis. Multiple sclerosis (A) is an inflammatory disorder of the central nervous system resulting in upper motor neurone signs – this patient's reflexes are absent. Myasthenia gravis (C) is a disorder of the neuromuscular junction and although it results in lower motor neurone signs, there is no sensory involvement and the weakness is greater in proximal muscles and commonly involves the cranial nerves resulting in droopy eyelids, difficulty speaking and swallowing. A key feature is fatigability as the stores of acetylcholine are used up. Although this woman is diabetic and has a polyneuropathy, her symptoms progress too quickly. Diabetic neuropathy (D) takes time to develop and, although there are different types, most commonly results in a distal sensory neuropathy of the feet. Vibration and pain are most affected which is why they may have a stomping gait and develop ulcers. Infective neuropathies (E) include Lyme disease from ticks and leprosy which is uncommon in developed countries and she has no history of travel.

Parkinson's associated symptoms

15 D This man presents with many symptoms of parkinsonism. However, the parkinsonian gait is typically narrow-based, not broad (D). Parkinson's is a disease of dopaminergic neurone loss in the nigrostriatal pathways and results in the triad of bradykinesia, rigidity and tremor. A fourth sign to look out for is postural instability (A). This can be elicited by asking the patient to steady himself and pulling him backwards. During REM sleep (B), the brain is active but muscles are paralysed (thus associated with dreaming). In Parkinson's disease (PD), muscles may be active allowing patients to act out their dreams, resulting in kicking, yelling, etc. Hypomimia (C) is the technical term for mask-like facies or reduced facial expression. Symptoms of autonomic dysfunction (E) are common and include constipation, postural hypotension and sexual dysfunction. Very prominent autonomic symptoms may suggest Shy–Drager's, a type of multiple system atrophy (which in turn is one of the Parkinson's plus syndromes).

Migraine treatment

16 A This woman has developed analgesia (rebound) headache as a result of over-using co-codamol and ibuprofen. Starting paracetamol (B) would result in overdose as it is already contained in co-codamol. The treatment is to withdraw analgesics (A) which initially will worsen the headache (the patient should be prepared for this) but in the long run will alleviate it. It is not advisable for headache patients to take simple analgesia more than 2 days a week. Once she is off the analgesia, it will be easier to discern the effect of her migraines. She may require abortive sumatriptan (C) to be taken as soon as the headache starts or prophylactic beta blockers (D) taken daily. Continuing her current medication (E) will not improve matters.

Seizure

17 E Status epilepticus is a serious condition of continuous seizure activity lasting more than 30 minutes. The mortality rate is one in five. This girl has been fitting for at least 20 minutes despite two doses of diazepam so must urgently be loaded with phenytoin (E) and monitored closely. ITU (D) should be alerted in case phenytoin does not stop the seizure in which case phenobarbital (B) can be considered, but the phenytoin should be given first. Ultimately, general anaesthetic and intubation (C) may be required. There is increasing evidence that lorazepam (A) is more effective than diazepam, but in this case the patient has already had two doses of benzodiazipine so the next step is phenytoin infusion.

Phenytoin levels

18 C Routine measurement of phenytoin levels (A) is not good practice, they should be ordered with a question in mind. They can be helpful either for adjustment of phenytoin dose or looking for toxicity or patient compliance. Phenytoin levels are useful when adjusting the dose to avoid toxicity as phenytoin has zero-order kinetics (once elimination reaches saturation rates, it cannot be cleared any faster so a small change in the dose may result in high blood levels), but there is no reason to change this patient's dose. There is no reason to suspect phenytoin toxicity either (B) as there are no signs or symptoms such as nystagmus, diplopia, dizziness, ataxia, confusion. However, his high blood pressure may be caused by non-compliance with his medication (C). Although target levels exist (D), they are imprecise and not applicable to all patients. Seizures may be well controlled with low levels, thus phenytoin should be adjusted according to the clinical picture and not levels. Levels are not helpful in reassuring the patient in this situation (E), although they often inappropriately reassure the doctor who requests them.

Seizure

19 D This woman has complex partial seizures (D) which start focally in the brain (classically temporal lobe) and by definition result in reduced awareness. Patients do not remember the seizure, unlike simple partial seizures (C) where consciousness is maintained. Automatisms typically characterize complex partial seizures where patients carry out repetitive and seemingly purposeless actions such as chewing, lip-smacking, picking and fumbling. Absence and tonic-clonic are types of generalized seizures (E). Absence seizures (A) typically occur in children and last seconds. Children are reported as 'staring blankly'. Seizures can be difficult to detect as they can be subtle, short-lived and the child is unaware of them. Tonic-clonic (previously called grand mal) (B) are the classic seizures where patients fall to the ground unconscious and then go through a tonic (tensing) then clonic (jerking) phase lasting seconds to minutes, typically associated with tongue-biting and incontinence and post-ictal drowsiness. Complex partial seizures may subsequently generalize but this has not been reported by this patient. Carbamazepine, lamotrigine and valproate are first-line monotherapy.

Dermatomes

20 D The dermatomes of the lower leg are important to know when performing a lower limb neurological examination. If the upper leg is divided into three equal thirds from the greater trochanter to the knee L1 (A), L2 (B) and L3 (C) correspond to these dermatome areas. If the lower leg is split into two sides down to the ankle, the medial side of the leg corresponds to dermatome L4 (D), while L5 (E) extends from the lateral side of the lower leg down to the dorsum of the great toe.

Lesion pattern location

21 D From these limited options, spinal cord (D) is most likely. There is a stark difference between power in upper and lower limbs making generalized processes affecting muscle, neuromuscular junction and peripheral nerves less likely. Muscle (A) or neuromuscular junction (B) lesions tend to have a proximal distribution, while a peripheral neuropathy (C) would have a distal predilection. For a brain lesion (E) to affect both legs, the lesion would have to be in the midline of the frontal cortex (think back to the homunculus), thus sparing the upper limbs. This is much rarer than a lesion transecting the cord (either thoracic or lumber in this case) to result in paraplegia.

Dermatomes

22 C Like the previous question, this patient is paraplegic. The lesion can be in the thoracic or lumbar cord. A sensory level helps further identify the location of the lesion. Dermatomes overlap and are not always consistent. You do not need to be able to delineate every dermatome but it is useful to have a general idea of certain levels such as: C4 shoulders (A), T4 nipples (B), T10 umbilicus (C), L1 pockets (D), L3 knee (E) (see Figure 8.1).

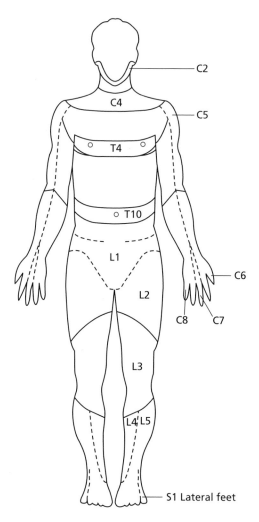

Fig. 8.1 Dermatomes (from Koppel and Naparus (2008) *Thinking Medicine: Structure your knowledge for success in medical exams*, Cavaye, with permission).

Lesion pattern location

23 C It is useful to divide the body into the areas such as: face/arms/legs, left/ right, proximal/distal. This allows a rapid diagnosis of where the lesion might be. This patient shows crossed signs. The left side of the face is affected but so is the right side of his body. Therefore, if the lesion were cortical, there would have to be two lesions to explain this (A and B). As his face is involved, there has to be a lesion above the spinal cord (E). Crossed signs tend to suggest brainstem involvement (if only one lesion is responsible). In this case a left brainstem lesion (C) would affect cranial nerves exiting on that side (LMN left-sided droop) and the cortical spinal tracts as they descend which then go on to cross at the medulla (UMN right arm and leg weakness). A right brainstem (D) lesion would cause the opposite. Please note that this is a general rule of thumb and lesions do not always result in textbook deficits.

Visual pathway lesion

24 C This is the swinging torch test. To recap the pathways, CN II (optic nerve) is the afferent limb that detects light, CN III (occulomotor nerve) is the efferent limb which results in pupillary constriction. Light enters the right eye, is picked up by the right CN II and triggers off both right (direct) and left (consensual) CN III responses. By eliciting the direct light response as described in the vignette, this shows that the afferent and efferent pathways of the right and left eye are grossly intact. Subtleties can be picked up by comparing the two against each other. This is done by moving the light (stimulus) from one eye to the other. If the right optic nerve is damaged but still functioning (for example in optic neuritis), the direct and consensual response will appear normal. However, moving the light from the intact left optic nerve to the damaged right optic nerve will result in reduced detection of the stimulus, thus causing the right eye to abnormally dilate in response to light. This is not a normal response (E). This is called a relative afferent pupillary defect (RAPD) (C). It is relative to the other eye, and afferent because CN II (the optic nerve) is the afferent limb (A) of the reflex. The efferent limb (B and D) is CN III which is intact (see Figure 8.2).

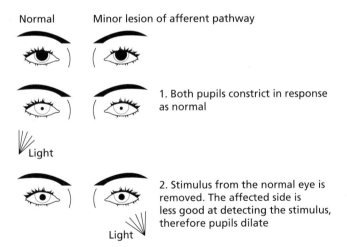

Fig. 8.2 Swinging light test/RAPD (from Koppel and Naparus (2008) *Thinking Medicine: Structure your knowledge for success in medical exams*, Cavaye, with permission).

Myasthenia gravis

25 D Disease of the muscle and neuromuscular junction can be similar. Both generally tend to affect proximal muscles (A). Cranially, this may result in ptosis and ophthalmoplegia (C) as well as bulbar symptoms (E) such as dysphagia and hypophonia. In both cases, reflexes (B) and muscle bulk tend to be preserved or, if severe and longstanding, reduced. A key clinical feature that differentiates myopathies and MG is fatigability (D). As patients with myasthenia use their muscles, they exhaust the supply of acetylcholine, resulting in increasing weakness. This can be elicited by asking the patient to repeatedly abduct and adduct one arm and compare it to the other arm that has remained at rest. Alternatively, you can ask the patient to count to 100 and their voice will fatigue, or ask them to do squats or test neck flexion.

Lambert–Eaton syndrome

26 E In contrast to MG, patients with Lambert–Eaton myasthenic syndrome (LEMS) experience increased strength upon repetition. LEMS is a rare disease caused by autoantibodies against the voltage-gated calcium channels on the presynaptic motor nerve terminal. It is a paraneoplastic disorder, most often associated with small-cell lung cancer (E), although a variety of underlying malignancies may be the culprit. LEMS may be difficult to differentiate from MG clinically, an EMG is key for diagnosis as well as testing for autoantibodies and searching for underlying malignancy. MG is associated with other autoimmune disease such as thyrotoxicosis (A), haemolytic and pernicious anaemia, connective tissue disease, as well as thymomas, which is why a thymectomy is often performed. Neither MG nor LEMS are directly associated with petic ulcer, diabetes or stroke (B, C, D).

Cranial nerve palsy

27 A The patient presents with a CN VII (facial) palsy. The key feature here is forehead sparing which implies an upper motor neuron lesion. This excludes Bell's palsy (D) and parotid gland (B) or cerebellar pontine angle (CPA) tumours (E) as these would affect the lower motor neuron. In the case of CPA tumours, there is likely to be cerebellar, CN V and CN VIII involvement too. The most common cause of a lower motor neuron CN VII palsy is Bell's palsy which is idiopathic and a diagnosis of exclusion. It is treated conservatively with lubricating eye drops and taping down the eye at night to avoid corneal ulcers. Medically, steroids should be given within 48 hours of onset along with acyclovir. Most patients will recover, although around 10 per cent may be left with permanent deficits. An upper motor neuron facial palsy is most commonly due to stroke. In this case, the left-sided symptoms point to a right hemisphere lesion (A, and not C).

Opthalmoplegia

28 D This patient has an intranuclear opthalmoplegia (INO). This means that there is a problem in the communication between CN VI (abducens) of the right eye and CN III (occulomotor) of the left eye. Normally these nuclei communicate via the medial longitudinal fasciculus in order to maintain conjugate gaze. This keeps the eyes aligned on the same spot. If they are not aligned, double vision occurs. In this patient's case, there is a lesion in the medial longitudinal fasciculus (MLF). To look right, she abducts her right eye, but as the MLF is affected, she is unable to direct the left eye to adduct to maintain conjugate gaze. This results in diplopia. The right eye which has abducted fully develops compensatory nystagmus as the left eye has failed to adduct. Note that the problem is not in the oculomotor nerve or medial rectus. The vestibulo-occular reflex would be intact, i.e. if the patient were to keep her eyes fixed on a target and move her head left, her left eye would adduct normally. Multiple sclerosis (D) is a common cause of INO. MG (A) often results in ophthalmoplegia (paralysis of one or more extraocular muscle), but this affects the neuromuscular junction, not the MLF. Cerebellar syndromes (C) would result in nystagmus but not ophthalmoplegia. Peripheral neuropathies (E) are not directly associated with opthalmoplegia or nystagmus. Vertigo (B) is a symptom, not a diagnosis. It is the illusion of movement (i.e. a subjective sensation of movement where there is none). It is best elicited by asking the patient if they see the room moving. This clearly differentiates it from the vague report of 'dizziness' (see Figure 8.3).

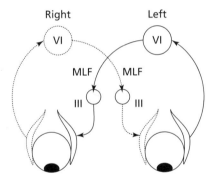

Fig. 8.3 Internuclear ophthalmoplegia (from Koppel and Naparus (2008) *Thinking Medicine: Structure your knowledge for success in medical exams*, Cavaye, with permission).

Neurological signs

29 C The neurologist has elicited a positive Hoffman's reflex (C) suggestive of upper motor neurone disease. It would have been negative if the thumb had not contracted in response to flicking the patient's distal phalanx. Chvostek's sign (A) is contraction of the face on stimulation of the facial nerve over the masseter. This is seen in hypocalcaemia. The glabellar tap (B) is an insensitive test for parkinsonism where the doctor taps above the bridge of the nose and the patient continues to blink. A normal response is to desensitize to the stimulus and stop blinking. Tinel's sign (D) can be elicited by tapping a nerve such as the ulnar nerve at the elbow, resulting in a tingling sensation in the distribution of the nerve. This is a sign of nerve compression. It is also useful in carpal tunnel syndrome by tapping over the median nerve at the wrist. Babinski's reflex (E) is extension and outward fanning of the toes in response to a firm stimulus of the outer soles. It is suggestive of upper motor neurone disease.

Dementia

30 B The patient has developed a change in their behaviour. They are initially negative symptoms: withdrawal and disinterest in hobbies (as opposed to positive symptoms such as hallucinations). This would be compatible with depression (A) were it not for the development of word finding difficulties and disinhibition. These localize the problem to the temporal and frontal lobes, respectively (B). Although he is hypertensive, the progression has been gradual as opposed to the classically step-wise progression of vascular dementia (D), often these patients have had vascular events. There are no extra-pyramidal (parkinsonian) features to suggest Lewy Body disease (E). Alzheimer's disease (C) tends to affect memory and language before personality. There may be a family history, especially in someone this age, but becomes increasingly common with age. It is important to note that dementias are definitively diagnosed on biopsy/ autopsy, but this is rarely done. Differentiating between the dementias on clinical grounds can be difficult. Brain imaging may help visualizing subcortical infarcts and cortical atrophy.

Upgoing plantars

31 C Causes of absent ankle jerks and upgoing plantars is a common question as it implies both upper and lower motor neuron involvement. The more common single causes include cord compression (D) involving both the cord (UMN) and nerve ganglia/roots (LMN) as well as subacute combined degeneration of the cord (B). Other more common causes include the presence of more than one pathology, e.g. stroke (UMN) with superimposed peripheral neuropathy (LMN) – usually in a diabetic patient. Motoneurone disease (E) consists of a mixture of UMN and LMN signs without any sensory involvement. In Friedrich's ataxia (A), both cord and peripheral nerve involvement accompany cerebellar degeneration. These patients also have sensory loss, pes cavus and may have complications such as diabetes and hypertrophic cardiomyopathy. Multiple sclerosis (C) may cause a mixture of pyramidal signs (UMN), sensory loss (dorsal columns) and ataxia (cerebellum), but will never involve the LMN.

Gait abnormality

32 A This patient has a hemiplegic gait (A). There is asymmetrical weakness involving the right upper and lower limb. His flexors are stronger than his extensors in the upper limb while the extensors are stronger than the flexors in the lower limb. This may be complicated by increased tone (spasticity) and, if longstanding, contractures. This is a typical pyramidal (or UMN) pattern. As a result, the patient circumducts his leg in order to walk as he cannot flex his hip properly to take a step. Technically, this should be termed 'hemiparetic' rather than 'hemiplegic' gait, as paresis refers to weakness while plegia implies paralysis. If there were complete paralysis, they would not be able to walk. Hemiparesis is typically as a result of contralateral hemispheric lesions, e.g. stroke, tumour or abscess. UMN lesions result in spasticity (D), but this particular gait is best described as hemiplegic. Bilateral lower limb spasticity, seen in cerebral palsy and cord lesions (multiple sclerosis), results in scissoring (B). The legs are stiff and the adductors are stronger than abductors, resulting in the legs crossing over with each step. High stepping gaits (C) are seen in foot drop as the patient is unable to dorsiflex the ankle so must lift their knee high to avoid their foot dragging on the ground. Stomping gaits (E) are seen in patients with sensory peripheral neuropathy, e.g. diabetics. By banging their foot down, vibrations travel up the leg where they can be detected by intact nerves, returning their joint position sense.

Visual fields

33 B A lesion in the left parietal lobe (B) results in a right lower quadrantanopia. Quadrantanopias and hemianopias are contralateral to the lesion. Temporal (C) and parietal lesions result in upper and lower quadrantanopias, respectively. Complete optic radiation lesions (D) result in hemianopia. Lesions at the optic chiasm (A), such as pituitary tumours and craniopharyngiomas, result in a bitemporal hemianopia. Optic nerve lesions (E) result in ipsilateral monocular visual loss. Note: when laterality is mentioned, always clarify contra/ipsilateral to what, e.g. the signs, the lesion.

Dizziness

34 B Benign paroxysmal positional vertigo (BPPV) (B) is a disorder of the vestibular system. If the calcium carbonate crystals in the semicircular canals dislodge, they can send conflicting information with regards to head position, resulting in vertigo. Vertigo is triggered by movement, starts suddenly and lasts minutes to seconds. Eliciting the timeline of symptoms is particularly important. Although the sudden onset may suggest a stroke (A), it would not spontaneously resolve and return specifically on movement. Because the brainstem is a small area with many neural structures, a lesion here would most likely result in accompanying deficits. Ménière's (C) disease is often accompanied by tinnitus, hearing loss and a sensation of increased ear pressure. Vertigo lasts from minutes to hours. It is thought to be due to excessive endolymph. Vestibular neuronitis (D) is of uncertain aetiology and has a similar time course to Ménière's; however hearing is not affected. Migraine sufferers (E) have an increased incidence of vertigo which may occur with or without headache. In this case, the headache is not a central feature and the story is more consistent with BPPV.

Dermatological manifestations

35 A This question explores dermatological manifestations of neurological disease (neurocutaneous syndromes). This patient has neurofibromatosis type I (A), previously known as von Recklinghausen disease. She has café-au-lait spots, axillary freckling and neurofibromas. Lisch nodules (hamartomas on the iris) may also be evident, although a slit lamp may be required to see them and patients are at increased risk of optic glioma. Neurofibromatosis type II (B) patients less commonly display cutaneous signs, and if so tend to be much milder. It is associated with bilateral acoustic neuromas leading to deafness. Both types are autosomal dominant as is tuberous sclerosis. Patients with tuberous sclerosis (C) may have ash-leaf macules (hypopigmented macules), Shagreen patches (plaques with an orange peel texture often seen in sacrolumbar region) and adenoma sebaceum (clusters of pink papules on cheeks and chin). There is a strong association with epilepsy and benign tumours. Hereditary haemorrhagic telangiectasia (D) also known as Osler–Weber–Rendu disease, as the name suggests is associated with telangectasia, epistaxis and vascular disorders of the CNS. Sturge–Weber syndrome (E) patients may have facial port-wine stains and intracranial lesions and calcification which result in epilepsy, hemiplegia and mental retardation. All five syndromes are genetic, and all have distinct mutations on different chromosomes. There is no association between any of these conditions.

Imaging

36 D Convex (lenticular) haematomas (A) are seen in extradural haemorrhages as the blood is trapped between the dura and the skull. These most commonly occur as a result of trauma and rupture of the middle meningeal artery. Crescent-shaped haematomas (C) indicate the blood is between the dura and arachnoid. Subdural haemorrhages occur as a result of bleeding from bridging veins, more commonly seen in the elderly and alcoholics as the veins are stretched from cerebral atrophy. Blood along the sulci and fissure (D) indicates that it is located between the arachnoid and the pia. Subarachnoid haemorrhages present clinically as a thunderclap headache which may be associated with reduced GCS and seizures. All intracranial haemorrhages require discussion with a neurosurgeon in case surgical evacuation of the clot is indicated (although it often is not). Signs that point to increased severity of bleed include midline shift (B), which indicates increased intracranial pressure, and intraventricular bleeding (E).

Stroke territories

37 E The temporal lobe (A) is involved in memory (note: bilateral lesions required for memory to be affected), Meyer's loop of the visual pathway also pass here and lesions could result in a contralateral upper quadrantanopia. The left parietal lobe (B) is involved in language; lesions here could result in aphasia, acalculia, agnosia, agraphia and/or right–left confusion. Lesions in the right parietal lobe (C) may result in neglect (visual, sensory or motor). The patient is not blind. They are physically able to see but fail to attend to the left hemifield. Strokes in the anterior circulation (D) include those to the anterior and middle cerebral arteries which supply the frontal, temporal and parietal lobes. The posterior circulation (E) supplies the brainstem, cerebellum (coordination) and occipital lobe (vision). This would be consistent with the vertigo, right hemianopia, nystagmus and ataxia that is suggested in the vignette. Dysdiadochokinesia is the cerebellar sign of difficulty performing rapidly alternating movements.

Paraesthesia

38 E The key is in the timing: speed of onset, time to peak and resolution. This is why it is crucial to elicit a clear timeline of events. This man has an acute peripheral polyneuropathy (both sensory and motor involvement). The timing is consistent with GBS (E). Chronic idiopathic demyelinating polyneuropathy (CIDP) (C) has a slower rate of onset and resolution over months, if indeed it does resolve, and patients are also prone to relapse. Miller Fisher syndrome (A) is a variant of GBS, exhibiting the classic triad of ophthalmoplegia, ataxia and areflexia. Although the patient shows ataxia, this could be related to his alcohol intake. The neuropathy in Miller Fisher syndrome classically starts proximally with involvement of the eyes and face (the opposite of GBS where deficits starts distally and work their way proximally). Alcoholic neuropathy tends to progress slowly and may resolve slowly on abstinence. In rarer cases, it is acute. Charcot Marie Tooth disease is a hereditary neuropathy, symptoms start much earlier in life and it is often accompanied by a family history. His mother may have diabetic neuropathy which has developed later in life. This man's lifestyle needs to be addressed in terms of advice, as well as support, to prevent future disease.

Headache (2)

39 A This is clearly a picture of meningitis. Although migraine (B) results in headache associated with photophobia and irritability, the overall picture with abnormal LP along with neck stiffness suggests meningitis. Basic signs of meningitis that you should always look for include: photophobia, neck stiffness, Kernig's sign (patient's leg is held flexed at the hip and knee and there is pain and resistance on subsequent knee extension – not particularly sensitive but useful if present). The analysis of cerebrospinal fluid (CSF) is very helpful in its diagnosis, although the history and clinical picture give a good indication. Viral meningitis is much less severe than bacterial meningitis which can progress rapidly to septicaemia and its complications (signs include septic shock: hypotension and tachycardia, reduced urine output, vasodilatation and a non-blanching petechial rash – you will not find it unless you look for it). If bacterial meningitis is a possibility, antibiotics should be given as soon as possible while the exact diagnosis is made. TB meningitis tends to be more indolent and there may be a history of exposure. The CSF results below give it away:

	In essence	Cells	Protein	Glucose
Bacterial	Low glucose, neutrophilia	Neutrophils	↑/N	↓
Viral	High protein, lymphoycytosis	Lymphocytes	↑↑N	
TB/fungal	Low glucose, lymphocytosis	Lymphocytes	↑/N	↓
SAH	High RBC	RBC	++	++
		Some WBC	↑/N	N

Loss of balance

40 D The test performed is Romberg's test. It is positive in patients with proprioceptive loss (D). Central postural control is maintained by three systems, the vestibular, visual and proprioceptive. Patients with cerebellar problems (B) may find it difficult to stand with their feet together despite maintaining their eyes open. This is not a positive Romberg's test. Romberg's test is complete when patients close their eyes, thus removing visual cues. If a patient has problems with joint position sense, they will no longer be able to maintain their balance. Romberg's test does not diagnose visual problems (E). Diabetes (A) and alcohol (C) may each cause peripheral neuropathies and diminished joint position sense. However, beware of offering an underlying cause for the proprioceptive problem without enough information. By definition, D is the better answer as it includes both these and many other causalities.

SECTION 9: ONCOLOGY

QUESTIONS

1. Weakness (1)

A 62-year-old woman presents to accident and emergency with a 1-day history of sudden onset back pain and difficulty walking. She has not opened her bowels or passed urine for the previous day. She has a past medical history of breast cancer, diagnosed two years earlier and staged as T2N1M0 disease with oestrogen receptor positive status. She has been treated for her cancer with a wide local excision and axillary node clearance, followed by radiotherapy, chemotherapy and tamoxifen. On examination, there is reduced tone in the lower limbs. Power is diminished throughout the lower limbs, but especially on hip flexion. There is reduced sensation below the L1 dermatome. What is the most appropriate diagnostic investigation?

    A. A full set of bloods, including bone profile
    B. Computed tomography (CT) thorax, abdomen and pelvis
    C. Magnetic resonance imaging (MRI) spine
    D. Bone scan
    E. Positron emission tomography (PET) CT

2. Weakness (2)

A 62-year-old woman with metastatic breast cancer, including bone metastases, presents to accident and emergency with sudden onset back pain and difficulty walking. An urgent MRI of the spine confirms cord compression at the level of L1–L2. What is the most appropriate initial management?

    A. Surgical decompression of spinal cord
    B. Dexamethasone
    C. Radiotherapy
    D. Chemotherapy
    E. Physiotherapy

3. Pyrexia

A 60-year-old man with metastatic adenocarcinoma of the lung, who has finished two cycles of palliative cisplatin/pemetrexed chemotherapy, presents with a 2-day history of fever and lethargy. On examination, he is pyrexial with a temperature of 38.8°C. What is the most appropriate next step?

    A. Blood cultures
    B. Urgent full blood count
    C. Urgent chest x-ray
    D. Start empirical broad spectrum antibiotics
    E. Prescribe paracetamol

4. Hypercalcaemia (1)

A 50-year-old woman with T2N2M1 squamous cell carcinoma of the tongue has been electively admitted for her third cycle of palliative cisplatin/5-fluorouracil chemotherapy. She has known metastasis to the T3 vertebrae and the ribs. Since her last cycle of chemotherapy she has been very lethargic and constipated. Upon checking her bloods you discover that her corrected calcium levels are 2.95 mmol/L. The most appropriate treatment is:

A. Administering the chemotherapy
B. Intravenous rehydration and pamidronate
C. Calcitonin
D. Delaying the chemotherapy and advising the patient to minimize calcium intake
E. Intravenous rehydration alone

5. Hypercalcaemia (2)

A 50-year-old woman presents to accident and emergency complaining of excessive lethargy. In addition, she mentions that she has been constipated. On examination, there are clinical features of dehydration. Blood tests have revealed a corrected calcium of 3.3 mol/L. Her chest x-ray shows bilateral streaky shadowing throughout both lung fields. She is given 3 L of saline in 24 hours after admission. The following day her blood tests are repeated and her corrected calcium level is now 3.0 mmol/L. Results of parathyroid hormone levels and thyroid function tests are still awaited. What is the most appropriate management?

A. Intravenous saline rehydration
B. Intravenous saline rehydration and pamidronate
C. Pamidronate
D. Calcitonin
E. Intravenous saline rehydration plus calcitonin

6. Terminology

A 74-year-old man with T2N0M0 squamous cell carcinoma of the tongue is currently undergoing hyper-fractionated radiotherapy with curative intent. He has had no previous surgery. This type of therapy is best described by which of the following terms:

A. Adjuvant
B. Neoadjuvant
C. Palliative
D. Radical
E. Brachytherapy

7. Tumour markers

A 57-year-old woman with adenocarcinoma of the sigmoid colon with liver metastasis is attending for cycle six of her palliative FOLFOX chemotherapy. Which tumour marker can be measured in the blood test to indicate the effect of the chemotherapy?

    A. α-fetoprotein (αFP)
    B. β-human chorionic gonadotrophin (β-hCG)
    C. CA 19-9
    D. CA 125
    E. CEA

8. Testicular cancer

A 22-year-old man with testicular cancer has undergone an inguinal orchidectomy. Histology has confirmed teratoma. A preoperative CT staging scan has shown involvement of the para-aortic lymph nodes. Which of the following treatments is the best post-operative option?

    A. Chemotherapy (bleomycin, etoposide, cisplatin)
    B. Lymph node dissection
    C. Radiotherapy to affected lymph nodes
    D. Chemo-radiotherapy
    E. Surveillance using tumour markers.

9. Oesophageal carcinoma

A 60-year-old man has presented to the gastroenterology outpatient clinic with a four-month history of progressive dysphagia. The patient reports a weight loss of 9 kg in the same time period. He has suffered from gastro-oesophageal reflux disease for the past 10 years. At endoscopy, a 5 cm malignant stricture is seen at the lower end of the oesophagus and biopsies are taken. Histological analysis is most likely to reveal:

    A. Squamous cell carcinoma
    B. Small cell carcinoma
    C. Adenocarcinoma
    D. Leiomyoma
    E. Gastrointestinal stromal tumours

10. Skin cancer

A 70-year-old man presents to his GP having noticed a slowly enlarging 'spot' on his left cheek. On examination, there is a well-circumscribed, skin-coloured nodular lesion on the left cheek with some overlying small blood vessels visible. The most likely diagnosis of this lesion is:

A. Basal cell carcinoma
B. Squamous cell carcinoma
C. Nodular malignant melanoma
D. Superficial spreading malignant melanoma
E. Basal cell papilloma

11. Lung cancer (1)

A 62-year-old electrician has presented to accident and emergency with a sudden decline in his exercise tolerance. He mentions that he can only walk 5 yards and that he has had a persistent cough with some haemoptysis over the previous month. A chest x-ray confirms a right-sided pleural effusion, which is then drained. A repeat x-ray shows a round shadow in the right perihilar region. Subsequent bronchoscopy and biopsy confirms small cell carcinoma. Which of the following statements is most true about small cell carcinomas of the lung?

A. They are sensitive to chemotherapy
B. Two-year survival of disease confined to the lung is 50 per cent
C. They are more common than non-small cell lung carcinomas
D. They are not associated with cigarette smoking
E. They most commonly arise from the periphery of the lung

12. Lung cancer (2)

A 68-year-old man presents to his GP complaining of increasing shortness of breath. He has noticed deterioration in his exercise tolerance, particularly while mowing the lawn. He has a past history of squamous cell carcinoma of the lung for which he finished radiotherapy treatment a year ago. On examination, there are fine inspiratory crackles in the right lung base. The most likely cause of his shortness of breath is:

A. Recurrence of the cancer
B. Pneumonitis
C. Pulmonary oedema
D. Pulmonary fibrosis
E. Chronic obstructive pulmonary disease (COPD)

13. Breast cancer

A 39-year-old woman has undergone a wide local excision for a 0.5 cm ductal carcinoma of her right breast. Sentinel node biopsy, histology and staging scans have confirmed the disease as T1N0M0. Histology has confirmed the cancer as oestrogen and progesterone receptor positive. Which of the following statements is most accurate regarding this female's treatment options?

    A. She should receive radiotherapy
    B. She is not suitable for radiotherapy
    C. She is not suitable for tamoxifen therapy
    D. She requires no further treatment
    E. She should be considered for cetuximab therapy

14. Pain control (1)

A 51-year-old man with a recent diagnosis of pancreatic carcinoma with metastases to the liver and omentum is about to commence gemcitabine chemotherapy. Prior to his first cycle he mentions that he is getting increasing severe abdominal pains. He is currently taking paracetamol for this, which eases the pain but is now becoming less effective. The most appropriate analgesia for this patient is:

    A. Fentanyl patch
    B. Oral morphine sulphate solution as required
    C. Morphine sulphate tablets
    D. Codeine phosphate
    E. Codeine phosphate plus paracetamol

15. Pain control (2)

A 48-year-old woman with a recent diagnosis of metastatic cancer of unknown primary, including metastasis to the sacral and thoracic spine, is currently being treated for lower back pain with regular paracetamol, diclofenac and oral morphine solution. She is receiving additional oral morphine solution rescue doses for her breakthrough pain. On review of her drug chart, she has received 60 mg of oral morphine solution over the past 24 hours. Which of the following is the most appropriate escalation for this patient's pain management?

    A. 30 mg of morphine sulphate tablets, twice daily with 10 mg oral morphine solution, as required
    B. 5–10 mg of oral morphine solution, as required
    C. 10 mg of oral morphine solution, six times a day
    D. 30 mg of morphine sulphate tablets, twice daily
    E. 18 mg of diamorphine via a continuous subcutaneous syringe driver

16. Headache

A 58-year-old male with known small cell lung cancer presents to accident and emergency with a 5-day history of severe headache and recurrent vomiting. He has recently commenced chemotherapy for small cell carcinoma of the lung. On examination of the visual fields, there is a left inferior homonymous quadrantinopia. The most important diagnostic investigation is:

A. Urea and electrolyte blood tests
B. CT head
C. CT thorax, abdomen and pelvis
D. Lumbar puncture
E. Chest x-ray

17. Anaemia

A 64-year-old man presents to accident and emergency following a collapse. He describes a blackout, subsequently regaining consciousness when on the floor. He presently feels well and describes no other symptoms. However, he mentions that he has unintentionally lost some weight over the past few months. There is no past medical history. Blood tests reveal a haemoglobin level of 9 g/dL with a mean cell volume on 71 fL. The most appropriate next investigation of this patient is:

A. Flexible sigmoidoscopy
B. Endoscopy
C. Colonoscopy
D. Endoscopy and colonoscopy
E. Profile of tumour markers

18. Skin reaction

A 57-year-old man with metastatic adenocarcinoma of the lung is attending for cycle three of his palliative pemetrexed/cisplatin chemotherapy. During his cisplatin infusion, he noticed his arm becoming painful, swollen and red at the cannula site. The most likely cause of this is:

A. Cellulitis
B. Venous thrombosis
C. Extravasation of chemotherapy
D. Adverse drug reaction
E. Normal chemotherapy reaction

19. Electrolyte imbalance (1)

A 55-year-old woman with metastatic pancreatic cancer attends the oncology clinic prior to her second cycle of chemotherapy. She tolerated her first cycle well but her husband mentions that there have been occasions where she has been confused. Her urea and electrolyte blood tests reveal a serum sodium of 116 mmol/L. All other results were within the normal range. The chemotherapy is delayed and a urine specimen is sent off. This reveals a urine osmolality of 620 mmol/kg. The most likely cause of the hyponatraemia is:

    A. Water overload
    B. Diabetes insipidus
    C. Addison's disease
    D. Syndrome of inappropriate anti-diuretic hormone (ADH)
    E. Renal impairment

20. Electrolyte imbalance (2)

A 55-year-old woman with metastatic pancreatic cancer attends the oncology clinic prior to her second cycle of chemotherapy. She tolerated her first cycle well, but her husband mentions that there have been occasions where she has been confused. Her urea and electrolytes on this occasion reveal a serum sodium of 116 mmol/L. All other results were within the normal range. The chemotherapy is delayed and a urine specimen is sent off. This confirms a diagnosis of syndrome of inappropriate ADH (SIADH). The most appropriate treatment is:

    A. Intravenous infusion of 5 per cent dextrose
    B. Intravenous infusion of normal saline
    C. Intravenous infusion of hypertonic saline
    D. Desmopressin
    E. Fluid restriction to 1 L per day

21. Electrolyte imbalance (3)

A 60-year-old man with metastatic adenocarcinoma of the lung, who has finished two cycles of palliative cisplatin/pemetrexed chemotherapy, presents with a 2-day history of nausea and vomiting. On examination, he is tachycardic with a blood pressure of 105/60 mmHg. Blood tests show a urea of 15 mmol/L and a creatinine of 180 µmol/L. Results from a week earlier showed a urea of 4.0 mmol/L and a creatinine of 90 µmol/L. All other blood tests and arterial blood gas results are within the normal range. What is the most appropriate initial management of this patient?

    A. Oral fluid rehydration
    B. Intravenous fluid rehydration
    C. Urgent renal ultrasound scan
    D. Haemodialysis
    E. CT scan of kidneys, ureter and bladder

22. Electrolyte imbalance (4)

A 65-year-old woman who is currently receiving chemotherapy for acute myeloid leukaemia is found on blood testing to have urea of 10.1 mmol/L, creatinine of 190 mol/L, potassium of 6.1 mmol/L, phosphate of 8.5 mg/dL and corrected calcium of 2.00 mmol/L. The patient is asymptomatic. Her electrolyte levels were normal prior to the start of treatment. What is the most likely cause of this electrolyte disturbance?

    A. Tumour lysis syndrome
    B. Hypovolaemia
    C. Haemolytic uraemic syndrome
    D. Neutropenic sepsis
    E. Disease progression

23. Cutaneous manifestation of cancer

A 56-year-old man with gastric cancer presents to his GP complaining of a lump in his belly button. On examination, there is a palpable nodule at his umbilicus. This sign is referred to as:

    A. Sister Mary Joseph nodule
    B. Krukenberg tumour
    C. Acanthosis nigricans
    D. Peutz–Jeghers syndrome
    E. Paget's disease

24. Facial flushing (1)

A 62-year-old man with known metastatic small cell carcinoma of the lung has presented to accident and emergency with sudden onset shortness of breath and arm and hand swelling. On examination, his face appears plethoric and Pemberton's sign is positive. What is the most likely diagnosis?

    A. Pancoast's tumour
    B. Horner's syndrome
    C. Superior vena cava obstruction
    D. Facial oedema
    E. Malignant pleural effusion

25. Facial flushing (2)

A 55-year-old man has presented to his GP complaining of several episodes of spontaneous facial blushing. In addition, he mentions he has had several episodes of watery diarrhoea. On examination of the cardiovascular system, giant v waves are noted on observation of the jugular venous pressure. In addition, a pansystolic murmur is heard in the lower sternal edge on inspiration. Examination of the gastrointestinal system reveals an enlarged, irregular, non-tender liver edge. What is the most likely diagnosis?

A. Superior vena cava obstruction
B. Carcinoid tumour
C. Carcinoid syndrome
D. Phaeochromocytoma
E. Conn's syndrome

ANSWERS

Weakness (1)

1   C   Spinal cord compression represents an oncological emergency and should be suspected in a patient presenting with this history. Cancers most likely to metastasize to the spine and thus cause spinal cord compression include breast, lung, thyroid, prostate and renal. Examination findings in cord compression include a sensory level, lower motor neuron signs at the level of the compression and upper motor neuron signs below the level of the compression. However, in acute compression, as in the case outlined, lower motor neuron signs may be seen below the level of the compression. The investigation of choice in cord compression is an MRI spine (C) and this should be performed promptly. CT of the thorax, abdomen and pelvis (B), bone scan (D) and PET CT (E) are useful for the staging of cancers but are not used to identify cord compression. Blood tests (A) may be helpful as patients with bony metastases may have raised calcium levels, which may require correction. However, they are not used to diagnose cord compression.

Weakness (2)

2   B   Spinal cord compression is an oncological emergency that requires urgent treatment. Initial management should include administering dexamethasone (B) and contacting oncology and neurosurgical teams. Subsequent treatment of the cord compression includes spinal radiotherapy (C) or neurosurgical decompression (A) and options must be discussed with the relevant teams. The patient should be initially kept flat, with neutral spine alignment, including log-rolling while being nursed. Therefore, physiotherapy (E) is an inappropriate answer here. However, physiotherapy has an important role once spinal stability is ensured to rebuild strength. Chemotherapy (D) is not a treatment for cord compression.

Pyrexia

3   B   In patients who are actively undergoing chemotherapy and present with a fever, neutropenic sepsis must be suspected. This is an oncological emergency where the neutrophil count drops below 1.0×10^9/L and prompt management is required as sepsis may become life-threatening. Patients with suspected neutropenic sepsis must receive initial treatment with empirical broad-spectrum antibiotics (D) while other investigations are being organized. However, it is important to request an urgent full blood count (FBC) (B) and take blood cultures (A) before antibiotics are started because this can guide further management if the organism causing sepsis is resistant to the initial antibiotics. Local guidelines may vary in their choice of initial antibiotic but an example is ceftazidine. Following blood cultures and commencement of antibiotic therapy, further investigations should be organized without delay. An urgent full blood count (B) is required to check the neutrophil count. A source of sepsis should also be sought and chest x-rays (C) and urine analysis organized. Paracetamol (E) can be administered for symptomatic relief. Patients with neutropenic sepsis should be transferred to a side room with barrier nursing maintained.

Hypercalcaemia (1)

4 B Hypercalcaemia is an important problem in cancer patients. Patients with multiple myeloma are especially likely to develop hypercalcaemia. Causes of hypercalcaemia in cancer include lytic bone metastasis or secretion of PTH-like hormones by the tumour. While patients may be asymptomatic, they can also present with lethargy, anorexia, constipation, polydipsia, polyuria, confusion and weakness. The treatment of hypercalcaemia of this level in patients with cancer is with rehydration and administration of bisphosphonates, such as pamidronate (B). Administration of chemotherapy (A) is likely to be beneficial, as it will help control the underlying malignancy. However, the immediate emergency should be addressed first. Calcitonin (C) has limited use in the treatment of hypercalcaemia as it is short-lived, painful upon administration and causes diarrhoea. Delaying the chemotherapy and advising the patient to avoid calcium (D) is inappropriate as it neither addresses the underlying problem nor treats the oncological emergency. While intravenous rehydration (E) is important, a bisphosphonate is required in malignant hypercalcaemia to provide treatment of raised calcium levels. It is worth noting that patients with hypercalcaemia associated with malignancy have a poor prognosis.

Hypercalcaemia (2)

5 A Acute hypercalcaemia is an emergency that requires prompt treatment. Patients may present with lethargy, anorexia, constipation, polydipsia, polyuria, confusion and weakness. The treatment of acute hypercalcaemia is saline, saline and more saline! Four to six litres of saline may be required on the first day, with ongoing aggressive rehydration on subsequent days. Bisphosphonates (B) and (C) should be reserved for hypercalcaemia of malignancy. In the case outlined, the underlying cause of the hypercalcaemia is unknown. The most common causes of hypercalcaemia are hyperparathyroidism and malignancy. However, the parathyroid hormone levels are outstanding. In light of the raised calcium, the chest x-ray findings should raise the suspicion of sarcoid or possible lymphangitis carcinomatosis. While a diagnosis of sarcoid must be confirmed with histology, hypercalcaemia in sarcoidosis is an indication for corticosteroid therapy. Therefore, this patient can be given a steroid challenge. If the calcium levels fall following this, it is suggestive of sarcoid. Administering bisphosphonates, however, would complicate the process of making the diagnosis of sarcoid as any correction in calcium following steroid therapy may have been produced by the bisphosphonate. Calcitonin (D) and (E) is seldom used in hypercalcaemia as it has a short-lived action and is painful upon intravenous administration.

Terminology

6 D Treatment with curative intent is known as radical therapy (D). Adjuvant therapy (A) is treatment given following surgical resection of a cancer. The aim of such therapy is to reduce the chances of recurrence. Neoadjuvant therapy (B) is treatment given before surgery to reduce the size of a tumour and thus facilitate its removal. Palliative therapy (C) is given to those patients where cure is not possible and treatment aims are to reduce the tumour load and thus increase life expectancy and quality of life. Brachytherapy (E) is a form of radiotherapy where the radiation source is placed within or adjacent to the area requiring treatment. Examples of cancers where brachytherapy is used are cervical or prostate cancer.

Tumour markers

7 E Tumour markers can be used for screening purposes, disease staging, assessing response to therapy and assessing disease recurrence. Carcinoembryonic antigen (CEA) (E) is associated with colorectal cancers and thus is the correct answer here. α-fetoprotein (A) is raised in hepatocellular carcinoma and teratomas. β-hCG (B) is raised in seminomas, teratomas and choriocarcinomas. CA 19-9 (C) is raised in pancreatic carcinoma. CA 125 (D) is raised in ovarian cancer. It is important to note that the tumour markers are nonspecific and the tumour markers listed may be raised by other malignancies or non-cancerous pathologies. For example, CEA may be raised by gastric cancer, pancreatic cancer, cirrhosis, pancreatitis and smoking.

Testicular cancer

8 A Testicular tumours can be germ cell tumours (95 per cent) and non-germ cell tumours (5 per cent). Germ cell tumours include seminomas (most commonly affecting the 30–65 year age group) and teratomas (most commonly affecting the 20–30 year age group). Non-germ cell tumours include Leydig cell tumours, Sertoli cell tumours and sarcomas. The treatment of testicular cancer has advanced a great amount and metastatic testicular cancer is often curable. The Royal Marsden staging of testicular cancers is as follows:

Stage 1 – confined to testis

Stage 2 – lymph node involvement below the diaphragm

Stage 3 – lymph node involvement above the diaphragm

Stage 4 – extra-lymphatic involvement

Seminomas are very radiosensitive. Therefore, stage 1 and 2 seminomas are usually treated with inguinal orchidectomy plus lymph node radiotherapy. More advanced seminomas are treated with inguinal orchidectomy plus BEP (bleomycin, etoposide, cisplatin) chemotherapy. Metastatic teratomas are usually treated with inguinal orchidectomy plus bleomycin, etoposide, cisplatin (BEP) chemotherapy. Tumour markers may be useful in assessing reponse to therapy. Alpha-fetoprotein (α-FP) and beta human-chorionic gonadotrophin (β-hCG) is raised in approximately 70 per cent of teratomas. β-hCG is elevated in 15 per cent of seminomas.

This patient has been diagnosed with metastasis to the para-aortic lymph nodes. Therefore, postoperatively, the treatment that provides the highest chance of cure is chemotherapy (A). Lymph node dissection (B) is not performed as BEP chemotherapy gives the highest chance of cure. Radiotherapy (C) would be sensible for low stage seminomas. Chemo-radiotherapy (D) is not performed in testicular cancer. Surveillance with tumour markers (E) is inappropriate as the disease is known to have spread.

Oesophageal carcinoma

9 C All of the mentioned histological types of cancer can occur in the oesophagus. The two most common types are adenocarcinoma and squamous cell carcinoma. Adenocarcinoma (C) usually affects the lower third of the oesophagus while squamous cell carcinoma (A) affects the upper two-thirds. While squamous cell carcinoma was the most common type of oesophageal cancer in western and developing worlds, the incidence of adenocarcinoma of the oesophagus has risen dramatically in the western world in the last four decades. Thus, adenocarcinoma of the oesophagus is currently the most common histological type of this cancer in the western world. The incidence of oesophageal carcinoma in the developed world is highest in Caucasian men. The strongest risk factor for oesophageal adenocarcinoma is symptomatic gastro-oesophageal reflux disease. Therefore, due to the patient in question, the history of gastro-oesophageal reflux disease and the endoscopic position of the cancer, the most likely histological type is adenocarcinoma. Squamous cell carcinoma still remains the dominant type of oesophageal malignancy in Asian countries and risk factors include excess alcohol intake and smoking. Small cell carcinomas (B), leiomyomas (D) and gastrointestinal stromal tumours (E) are rare tumours of the oesophagus.

Skin cancer

10 A Basal cell carcinomas (A) are the most common skin malignancy and occur on the sun-exposed areas, particularly the head and neck. They can present as slow-growing papules or nodules with overlying telangectasia. The well-demarcated border is often described as a 'pearly, rolled edge'. Basal cell carcinomas are slow growing and almost never metastasize but, if left untreated, may cause disfiguring injury by eroding into structures. For this reason, basal cell carcinomas are sometimes referred to as 'rodent ulcers'. Squamous cell carcinomas (B) occur in sun-exposed areas and present as an ulcerated lesion with irregular, hard, raised edges. If left untreated, squamous cell carcinomas can metastasize. Malignant melanoma (D) is a particularly deadly form of skin cancer as they spread early and metastatic disease is difficult to control. Nodular malignant melanoma (C) is the most aggressive variant and presents as a growing pigmented nodule, which may bleed and ulcerate. Superficial spreading malignant melanoma is the most common variant and presents as a flat, irregularly pigmented lesion with irregular edges. Basal cell papillomas (E) are also known as seborrhoeic warts and are benign, irregular, warty, superficial lesions.

Lung cancer (1)

11 A The most common cause of death from cancer in the UK is due to lung cancer. Bronchial carcinoma can be divided into small-cell carcinoma and non-small cell carcinoma. Non-small cell carcinoma includes squamous cell carcinoma, adenocarcinoma, large cell carcinoma and alveolar cell carcinoma. Small cell carcinomas of the lung are highly aggressive and have often disseminated at presentation. However, they are sensitive to chemotherapy (A) and, with treatment, median survival is increased from three months to one year. Due to its aggressive nature, the long-term survival of these cancers is poor, with a 25 per cent survival of limited disease (disease confined to the lung) at two years. Therefore, answer (B) is incorrect. Small cell carcinomas account for 20–30 per cent of bronchial cancers, while the rest are non-small cell carcinomas. Of these, squamous cell carcinomas are the most common. Therefore, answer (C) is incorrect. Answer (D) is incorrect as cigarette smoking is the most significant aetiological factor in the development of bronchial cancers. Finally, small cell carcinomas usually arise from the peri-hilar region of the lung. Adenocarcinomas occur more commonly in the periphery. Thus, answer (E) is also incorrect.

Lung cancer (2)

12 D Radiotherapy works by generating free radicals, which can then cause damage to DNA. Cancer cells have impaired ability to repair the damage and thus the cell undergoes cell death. The short- and long-term side effects of radiotherapy are dependent on where the treatment is being directed. In the case of the lungs, acute side effects include erythema and moist desquamation of the overlying skin and pneumonitis (B). The longer-term side effects of radiotherapy to the lung fields include pulmonary fibrosis (D). While recurrence of the cancer (A) should be kept in mind, the presence of the fine inspiratory crackles should alert pulmonary fibrosis as the answer. End-inspiratory crackles are a sign of pulmonary oedema (C), but they would be bibasal. Both lung cancer and COPD (E) have smoking as their prominent aetiological factor. However, there are no signs or symptoms in this case that suggest COPD would be the cause of the breathlessness.

Breast cancer

13 A This is a difficult question for the budding oncologist. The treatment options for breast cancer include surgery, radiotherapy, chemotherapy and endocrine therapy. The female in this question has early disease. For such patients, breast-conserving surgery (i.e. wide local excision) is now favoured and has been shown to achieve equivalent local control and survival to mastectomy. Radiotherapy (A) is recommended for all patients who have had wide local excisions and reduces the risk of local recurrence. Therefore, option (B) is incorrect. Radiotherapy may also be given post-mastectomy for tumours that have a high risk of local recurrence (such as large tumours, multifocal lesions, axillary lymph node involvement, high-grade tumours or proximity to surgical margins). Chemotherapy should be considered in all early breast cancer patients under the age of 70. In those above the age of 70, there is no clear evidence for or against the use of chemotherapy, but it should be considered for high-risk patients, with the advantages and disadvantages of chemotherapy evaluated for each specific patient. Chemotherapy in breast cancer is now being used on a neoadjuvant basis, to shrink a large operable cancer for which breast conserving surgery may then be possible in place of mastectomy. Tamoxifen is an oestrogen-receptor antagonist and is given to patients who have oestrogen and/or progesterone receptor positive disease. Therefore, the woman in the question should receive tamoxifen, making answers (C) and (D) incorrect. Finally, cetuximab (E) is a monoclonal antibody, which targets the epidermal growth factor receptor. It is used in colorectal and head and neck cancers, but not breast cancer.

Pain control (1)

14 E Managing pain relief well is a crucial element of oncology, as uncontrolled pain adds a significant burden of disease to patients and can be prevented with appropriate management. Prescribing pain relief should follow the World Health Organizations (WHOs) pain relief ladder as follows:

Step 1 – Non-opioid analgesia, e.g. paracetamol, NSAIDs

Step 2 – Weak opioid analgesia, e.g. codeine, tramadol

Step 3 – Strong opioids, e.g. morphine, diamorphine, fentanyl

Here, the patient remains poorly controlled with non-opioid analgesia. Therefore, the next step on the pain relief ladder would involve the addition of a weak opioid analgesic such as codeine. While codeine phosphate can be started alone, it is likely to be more effective when used with regular paracetamol. Therefore, answer (E) is the correct answer. Fentanyl patches (A), oral morphine sulphate solution (B) and morphine sulphate tablets (C) are strong opioids and should be started if weak opioids are ineffective. Patients on regular analgesia must be reviewed regularly for pain control and side effects of analgesia. For example, in this question, starting codeine phosphate (D) is likely to have a constipating effect and laxatives should be started if needed.

Pain control (2)

15 A This question requires an in-depth knowledge of opioid analgesia. Pain relief should follow the WHOs pain relief ladder, where strong opioids, such as morphine, are started for pain that is not relieved by non-opioid and weak opioid pain relief. To begin with, opiate-naive patients can be started on oral morphine solution, 5–10 mg every 4 hours. Breakthrough pain between these regular doses must be rescued by an equal dose of oral morphine solution as required. Once a 24-hour requirement of morphine is established, the dose can be given as a modified release preparation (morphine sulphate tablets) in two divided doses. A sixth of the total daily morphine dose should be given as required (used a maximum of every 4 hours) for breakthrough pain. The patient in the question has used 60 mg of oral morphine solution in 24 hours. This can be divided into two doses of 30 mg of modified release preparation of morphine given with 12-hour intervals. A sixth of the total daily dose of morphine for breakthrough pain is 10 mg. Therefore, answer (A) is the correct answer. Using 5–10 mg of oral morphine solution (B) will not provide any background pain relief to prevent the pain. The slower half-life of the 30 mg morphine sulphate tablets will provide a better background pain relief than 10 mg of oral morphine solution six times a day (C). In addition, this option does not allow any cover for breakthrough pain. Similarly, answer (D) does not address the breakthrough pain. Finally, answer (E) is incorrect as oral analgesia must also be favoured when possible. The dose conversion of morphine to diamorphine can be calculated using the BNF.

Headache

16 B In a patient presenting with a headache, vomiting and focal neurology on examination, a space-occupying lesion should be suspected. In light of the diagnosis of small cell carcinoma, brain metastases must be considered (small cell lung carcinomas are known to metastasize to the brain). Therefore, the most important diagnostic investigation is an urgent CT head (B). Subsequent treatment options include steroid therapy, radiotherapy or surgery. Urea and electrolyte blood tests (A) should be sent off, particularly as small cell lung carcinomas are associated with electrolyte imbalance and neurological symptoms. However, due to the focal neurology on examination, a space-occupying lesion must be sought urgently. A CT thorax, abdomen and pelvis (C) may be useful in assessing the extent of spread and response to treatment, but it will not help identify an underlying brain lesion. Similarly, a chest x-ray (E) is unlikely to be useful in this setting. Lumbar puncture (D) in this setting is contraindicated due to the features of raised intracranial pressure (headache, vomiting and focal signs). Carrying out this procedure in this setting may result in fatal herniation of the brainstem through the foramen magnum.

Anaemia

17 D The patient in the case outlined has presented with a microcytic anaemia. The most common cause of a microcytic anaemia is iron deficiency. In pre-menopausal women, the most common cause of iron deficiency anaemia is menstrual blood loss. However, blood loss from the gastrointestinal tract is the most common cause in men and post-menopausal women. Therefore, the case outlined in this question should raise the suspicion of a gastrointestinal cancer, such as gastric or colonic carcinoma. Colorectal cancer is more prevalent in males and the peak age of onset is in patients aged over 70 years. Therefore, this must be kept in mind for a patient such as this. Left-sided colonic lesions may commonly present with change in bowel habit, PR bleeding, abdominal pain or bowel obstruction. However, caecal and right-sided colonic lesions are often asymptomatic. Similarly, gastric cancers may also be asymptomatic. While non-malignant gastrointestinal causes such as oesophagitis, gastritis, gastric erosions and coeliac disease can cause iron-deficiency anaemia, there must be a low threshold of suspicion for cancer. Therefore, the correct answer in this case is endoscopy and colonoscopy (D). Flexible sigmoidoscopy (A) is limited in that it does not view the whole of the large bowel. This is particularly important in this case as the patient does not have any gastrointestinal symptoms. Endoscopy (B) and colonoscopy (C) alone are not the correct answers as blood loss may come from the upper or the lower gastrointestinal tract, as explained. Profile of the tumour markers (E) may be useful but endoscopy and colonoscopy are the investigations of choice as they allow direct visualization of a lesion and intervention and biopsy if necessary.

Skin reaction

18 C Extravasation of chemotherapy (C) is describing the inadvertent administration of drugs into the surrounding tissues rather than into a vein. This may be caused by a displaced cannula. Depending on the agent being administered, the degree of injury may range from a mild skin reaction to skin necrosis and thus, it requires urgent attention. The chemotherapy infusion should be stopped, the arm elevated and the affected area marked. A senior doctor should be informed and the guidelines on extravasation for that particular agent should be checked. Cisplatin is classified as an exfoliant, which can cause inflammation and shedding of the skin. A cold pack should be applied and advice of a plastic surgeon sought. Saline washout of the extravasation site may be necessary in this case. Acute onset of cellulitis (A) after administration of chemotherapy is an unlikely answer. Cancer patients are at higher risk of venous thrombosis (B) and all patients attending hospital should have a venous thromboembolism risk assessment and prescription of a low-molecular weight heparin if required. In this situation though, it is more likely that extravasation has caused the pain and swelling, particularly in light of the skin reaction. Since this is his third cycle of chemotherapy, an adverse drug reaction (D) is unlikely. You are not expected to know the details of managing extravasation of chemotherapy. However, it is important to know that such a reaction after administration of chemotherapy is not normal (E) and senior attention should be sought.

Electrolyte imbalance (1)

19 D Small cell carcinoma of the lung, prostate cancer, cancers of the thymus, pancreatic cancers and lymphomas may cause SIADH (D). ADH acts on the collecting tubules of the nephrons to cause reabsorption of water. Therefore, in SIADH, excess reabsorption of water results in a low serum osmolality (<260 mosmol/kg) but a high urinary osmolality (>500 mosmol/kg). Symptoms of SIADH vary and include confusion, nausea and irritability. When the serum sodium concentration drops below 115 mmol/L, the patient is at risk of seizures and comas. Water overload (A) will cause hyponatraemia but the urine will also be dilute. Diabetes insipidus (B) is a cause of hypernatraemia. Addison's disease (C) is a cause of hyponatraemia, as the adrenocortical insufficiency results in loss of the action of the mineralocorticoids on the distal convoluted tubule of the nephron where they normally cause reabsorption of sodium and loss of potassium. Therefore, patients with Addison's disease may have a low serum sodium but a raised serum potassium. In addition, the urinary osmolality in Addison's disease is not over 500 mosmol/kg. Finally, renal impairment (E) may cause hyponatraemia. However, the urea and creatinine on the urea and electrolytes would be deranged.

Electrolyte imbalance (2)

20 E The treatment of SIADH should always include management of the underlying cause. However, early correction of the hyponatraemia should be sought to provide symptomatic relief and prevent any serious complications. Fluid restriction (E) is the initial treatment of choice and, if tolerated, may be enough to correct the sodium. If fluid restriction is not effective or cannot be maintained by the patient, demeclocycline can be given. This works by inhibiting the action of vasopressin on the collecting ducts, thus preventing reabsorption of water. Five per cent dextrose (A) is a hypotonic solution and infusion is likely to make the hyponatraemia worse. Administration of normal saline (B) or hypertonic saline (C) can be given in severe cases. However, frequent monitoring of the urea and electrolytes is important to ensure that the sodium is not corrected any quicker than 1–2 mmol/L per hour. If correction is done faster than this, there is a risk of central pontine myelinolysis. Desmopressin (D) is the treatment for diabetes insipidus.

Electrolyte imbalance (3)

21 B The history, examination findings and rapid decline in renal function seen on blood tests demonstrate acute renal failure. The acute renal failure in this question is pre-renal, i.e. caused by kidney hypoperfusion, secondary to fluid loss. With swift intravenous fluid rehydration (B), the renal impairment is usually reversible. On the other hand, if fluid repletion is delayed or inadequate, acute tubular necrosis may occur with subsequent irreversible intrinsic renal damage. Oral fluid rehydration (A) is not correct here as rapid fluid replacement, titrated against the blood pressure, jugular venous pressure (JVP) and blood tests is needed. A renal ultrasound (C) scan may be useful for patients with acute renal failure, particularly when outflow obstruction is suspected. However, it should not delay fluid replacement when hypovolaemia is identified as the cause. Haemodialysis (D) is indicated for patients who develop pulmonary oedema, have persistent hyperkalaemia despite treatment, develop severe metabolic acidosis, uraemic encephalopathy or uraemic pericarditis. CT KUB (E) is the investigation of choice for renal colic and is not appropriate for this setting. When treating patients with pre-renal acute renal failure, an accurate fluid balance should be kept and patients regularly re-examined for signs of fluid overload. Nausea and vomiting are very common side effects of chemotherapy, particularly with platinum compounds such as cisplatin. Therefore, patients on chemotherapy should also receive anti-emetics to prevent this adverse effect. Furthermore, all patients presenting with acute renal failure should have their medications reviewed and any nephrotoxic drugs (such as NSAIDs or ACE inhibitors) stopped. Significantly, the platinum compounds, with the exception of carboplatin, can cause renal damage. Therefore, this patient may require the dose of their chemotherapy to be adjusted for the next cycle or a change in their treatment.

Electrolyte imbalance (4)

22 A Tumour lysis syndrome (A) occurs when there is rapid cell death of neoplastic cells. This may occur when patients with rapidly proliferating cells, such as leukaemia, lymphoma or myeloma, start chemotherapy. This syndrome is characterized by a rise in serum urate, potassium and phosphate and a drop in the calcium. Renal failure may be precipitated and the condition may become life threatening. Hypovolaemia (B) may cause acute renal impairment and can cause a rise in the serum potassium. However, it is unlikely to produce hyperphosphataemia and hypocalcaemia as well. Haemolytic uraemic syndrome (C) is usually caused by *Escherichia coli* 0157 and is characterized by intravascular haemolysis with red cell fragmentation, thrombocytopenia and acute renal failure. The patient has not demonstrated any of the clinical features of sepsis, thus neutropenic sepsis (D) is not the correct answer. The development of this picture of electrolyte imbalance suggests rapid cell death of tumour cells. Thus disease progression (E) is the incorrect answer.

Cutaneous manifestation of cancer

23 A A Sister Mary Joseph nodule (A) is a metastatic deposit from an underlying malignancy. Gastrointestinal or gynaecological cancers may cause a Sister Mary Joseph nodule and it is associated with multiple peritoneal deposits. It was first described by the American surgeon William J Mayo, whose attention had been drawn to the sign by Sister Mary Joseph Dempsey. A Krukenberg tumour (B) is a metastatic ovarian cancer, where the primary is either gastrointestinal or breast. Acanthosis nigricans (C) is seen as thickened, hyperpigmented skin predominantly of the flexures. It has many underlying causes, including insulin-resistant diabetes, hypothyroidism, hyperthyroidism and polycystic ovary disease. The most significant malignant cause of acanthosis nigricans is gastrointestinal tumours. Peutz–Jeghers syndrome (D) has an autosomal dominant inheritance and it consists of mucocutaneous pigmentation on the lips, oral mucosa, palms and soles. It is also associated with gastrointestinal hamartomas, which can undergo malignant change. Paget's disease of the breast (E) is referring to as intra-epidermal spread of an underlying intraductal breast carcinoma to the skin surrounding the nipple.

Facial flushing (1)

24 C Superior vena cava obstruction (C) is an oncological emergency that requires urgent attention. A particularly swift response is needed when there is airway compromise. Superior vena cava obstruction is most commonly associated with lung cancer. However, it may also be caused by other causes of mediastinal masses, including germ cell tumours, lymphomas or goitres, and thrombotic disorders. Patients with superior vena cava obstruction may present with dyspnoea, swollen facies and upper limbs, plethora or headache. On examination, engorged veins over the neck may be seen. In addition, Pemberton's sign may be positive. This is when the arms are raised above the head and there is a resultant increase in the facial plethora, distension of neck veins, elevation of the jugular venous pressure and worsening of the dyspnoea. Pancoasts tumour (A) refers to an apical lung cancer. These can invade into the sympathetic chain causing a Horner's syndrome (B). Clinical features of Horner's syndrome are miosis, ptosis, enophthalmos and ipsilateral anhydrosis. The clinical features of a pleural effusion (E) have not been mentioned in this question, making this an unlikely diagnosis. The treatment of superior vena cava obstruction is with immediate steroids. Subsequent management options include chemotherapy, radiotherapy, chemo-radiotherapy or venoplasty. The features described do not fit in a presentation of facial oedema (D).

Facial flushing (2)

25 C Carcinoid tumours arise from enterochromaffin cells (APUD cells). They most commonly occur in the appendix, ileum or rectum but can occur elsewhere, including other areas of the gastrointestinal tract, ovary, testis or lung. It is often difficult to histologically determine whether carcinoid tumours are benign or malignant. Carcinoid tumours (B) of the gastrointestinal tract are usually asymptomatic but may cause appendicitis, intussusception or obstruction. Carcinoid syndrome (C) refers to carcinoid tumours with liver metastases. These patients are usually symptomatic and may present with spontaneous facial flushing, abdominal pain and watery diarrhoea. Fifty per cent of patients develop cardiac abnormalities, such as tricuspid regurgitation or pulmonary stenosis. Symptoms are produced by the tumours secreting substances such as 5-hydroxytryptamine, bradykinin and histamine. Investigations for carcinoid syndrome should include radiological imaging of the liver metastases and 24-hour urine 5-hydroxyindoleacetic acid. While facial flushing may be seen in superior vena cava obstruction (A), the other features are not seen, making this an unlikely diagnosis. Phaeochromocytoma's (D) are catecholamine-producing tumours, usually of the adrenal medulla. Patients present with features of catecholamine overload such as uncontrolled, episodic hypertension. Conn's syndrome (E) are aldosterone producing adenomas which may present with features of hypokalaemia, polyuria or polydipsia.

SECTION 10: DERMATOLOGY

Questions

QUESTIONS

1. Skin appendages

Which one of the following structures is considered a skin appendage?

- A. Epidermis
- B. Dermis
- C. Pilosebaceous unit
- D. Subcutaneous fat
- E. Cutaneous nerves

2. Cell types of the epidermis

Which of the following cell types are seen in the epidermis?

- A. Merkel cells
- B. Langerhans cells
- C. Melanocytes
- D. Keratinocytes
- E. All of the above cells are present in the epidermis

3. Management of psoriasis

A 56-year-old man, diagnosed with psoriasis three years ago, presents to your clinic with pruritus. His symptoms are not improving despite being prescribed conventional therapy. On examination, you note the presence of erythematous scaly plaques on the extensor surfaces of the knee and elbows. There is no evidence of flexural involvement. The most appropriate treatment is:

- A. Topical retinoid therapy
- B. Topical tar preparations
- C. Topical steroid preparations
- D. Topical vitamin D analogue preparations
- E. Antibiotics

4. Nail changes

You are asked by your registrar to see a 45-year-old Caucasian woman with psoriasis who has presented with suspicious nail changes. Which one of the following nail changes are associated with psoriasis?

- A. Koilonychia
- B. Onycholysis
- C. Beau's lines
- D. Clubbing
- E. Paronychia

5. Atopic dermatitis

A 12-year-old boy who has been suffering from atopic dermatitis for the last ten years presents to you with a 3-day history of severe itching and pus discharge from his left elbow. On examination, you observe lichenification of his left elbow with superimposed excoriations which are weeping a viscous yellow fluid. You take a swab of this discharge. Which one of the following organism growths would you likely expect to be isolated from the swab?

    A. *Corynebacterium* spp.
    B. *Streptococcus pyogenes*
    C. *Propionibacterium acnes*
    D. *Staphylococcus aureus*
    E. *Pseudomonas aeruginosa*

6. Management of atopic dermatitis

A 2-year-old boy who you suspect has atopic dermatitis presents with areas of erythema coupled with itchy blisters on his scalp and cheeks. The most appropriate first-line management is:

    A. Phototherapy
    B. Immunosuppressant ointment
    C. Emollient and steroid ointment
    D. Oral immunosuppressant therapy
    E. Wet wraps

7. Hirsutism

Which one of the following is a cause of hirsutism?

    A. Hypothyroidism
    B. Anorexia nervosa
    C. Penicilliamine
    D. Psoralens
    E. Polcystic ovarian disease

8. Alopecia

A 67-year-old woman presents to you with extensive scalp hair loss which has been getting progressively worse over the last year. You also notice thinning of the eyebrows. The patient's past medical history includes hypertension, left-sided pulmonary embolism one year ago and hypercholesterolaemia. You assess the patient's medication list. Which one of the following drugs could be responsible for causing generalized alopecia?

    A. Aspirin
    B. Warfarin
    C. Simvastatin
    D. Ramipril
    E. Bendroflumethiazide

9. Acanthosis nigricans

A 56-year-old man presents in your clinic with a three-month history of weight loss despite no change in his appetite. The patient has no past medical history and no known drug allergies. On examination, you notice an area of hyperpigmented skin in his left axilla. On palpation, the texture of the area of hyperpigmentation feels velvety. You suspect that the patient has acanthosis nigricans secondary to a possible malignancy. Which one of the following malignancies is most commonly associated with this dermatological presentation?

    A. Lung carcinoma
    B. Testicular carcinoma
    C. Breast carcinoma
    D. Gastrointestinal carcinoma
    E. Prostate carcinoma

10. Contact dermatitis

Contact dermatitis is described as what type of reaction?

    A. Type I hypersensitivity
    B. Type II hypersensitivity
    C. Type III hypersensitivity
    D. Type IV hypersensitivity
    E. Non-allergic

11. Dermatitis herpetiformis (1)

A 24-year-old woman presents to you with a one-month history of intense burning and itch in her buttock area. On examination, you notice patches of small erythematous papulo-vesicular blisters in the patient's buttock area. There is obvious evidence of scratching with some areas of bleeding. The signs are typical of dermatitis herpetiformis. Which one of the following conditions is associated with this dermatological presentation?

A. Inflammatory bowel disease (IBD)
B. Irritable bowel syndrome
C. Coeliac disease
D. Varicella zoster virus
E. Herpes simplex virus

12. Dermatitis herpetiformis (2)

A 33-year-old man with coeliac disease presents with a blistering rash over the elbows and scalp. A diagnosis of dermatitis herpetiformis is made. The most appropriate treatment is:

A. Oral prednisolone
B. Dapsone
C. Non-steroidal anti-inflammatory drugs (NSAIDs)
D. Aciclovir
E. Fluconazole

13. Genodermatoses

A 26-year-old man presents to you with multiple patches of macular hyperpigmentation which have been present since he was an infant but now are increasing in number. In addition he has several small, soft, violaceous nodules on his trunk which tend to catch on clothing causing discomfort. What is the pattern of inheritance in this condition?

A. Autosomal recessive
B. Autosomal dominant
C. X-linked dominant
D. Polygenic
E. No pattern of inheritance

14. Cutaneous hypopigmentation

Which one of the following conditions is a cause of generalized cutaneous hypopigmentation?

A. Phenylketonuria
B. Vitiligo
C. Tuberous sclerosis
D. Leprosy
E. Pityriasis versicolor

15. Painful swellings

A 40-year-old woman presents with a 36-hour history of developing erythematous boils on her trunk. Some of them have burst leaving what seems to be painful wounds on her chest. On examination of the chest you notice three very painful ulcerating wounds with undermined edges and surrounding erythema. The lesions are closely associated with a condition that the patient was diagnosed with 15 months ago. Which one of the following conditions is associated with the above described cutaneous lesions?

A. Vasculitis
B. Sarcoidosis
C. Tuberculosis
D. Crohn's disease
E. Herpes simplex virus

16. Management of pyoderma gangrenosum

Which of the following treatment options would be the most appropriate for a patient with pyoderma gangrenosum?

A. Oral low-dose prednisolone and dressings
B. IV antibiotics and dressings
C. Oral antibiotics and dressings
D. Oral high-dose prednisolone and dressings
E. No treatment required

17. Orogenital ulceration

Which of the following answers from the list below is not a cause of orogenital ulceration?

    A. Ulcerative colitis
    B. Stevens–Johnson syndrome
    C. Syphilis
    D. Reiter's syndrome
    E. Coeliac disease

18. Lupus pernio

A 49-year-old woman presents to you in clinic with blue-red nodules on the nose which resemble lesions seen in lupus pernio. Which one of the following conditions is lupus pernio is associated with?

    A. Rheumatoid arthritis
    B. Systemic lupus erythematosus (SLE)
    C. Sarcoidosis
    D. Tuberculosis
    E. Herpes simplex infection

19. Benign cutaneous tumours

Which one of the following tumours of the skin is not considered to be benign?

    A. Seborrhoeic keratosis
    B. Pyogenic granuloma
    C. Bowen's disease
    D. Epidermal naevi
    E. Histiocytoma

20. Tuberous sclerosis

Following genetic profiling and clinical examination, you diagnose an 18-year-old woman with tuberous sclerosis. She initially presented with cutaneous lesions which were suspicious of this diagnosis. Which one of the following skin lesions is associated with tuberous sclerosis?

    A. Pyoderma gangrenosum
    B. Ash-leaf hypopigmentation
    C. Erythema nodusum
    D. Café-au-lait spots
    E. Erythema multiforme

21. Nutritional deficiencies

Which one of the following nutritional deficiencies is the triad of dermatitis, diarrhoea and dementia associated with?

A. Vitamin C deficiency
B. Vitamin B_1 deficiency
C. Protein malnutrition
D. Nicotinic acid deficiency
E. Vitamin B_6 deficiency

22. Cutaneous bacterial infection

A 45-year-old woman presents to you with a 3-day history of an ovoid patch of tender erythema, on the posterolateral aspect of her left calf, which has been increasing in size. She recalls injuring her left leg a week ago while gardening. On examination, the patient is afebrile and on inspection of the left calf, the patch of erythema measures roughly 3×3 cm with poorly demarcated edges. On palpation the zone of erythema is warm and very tender. Full blood count reveals a white cell count of 20.1 with a neutrophil count of 15.0. Which of the following organisms is the most likely cause of this condition?

A. *Corynebacterium minutissimum*
B. *Staphylococcus aureus*
C. *Clostridium perfringens*
D. *Staphylococcus epidermidis*
E. *Streptococcus pneumoniae*

23. Treatment of cellulitis

A 68-year-old man is diagnosed with right forearm cellulitis. You are asked to start the patient on treatment and he has no known drug allergies. Which one of the following antibiotics would be the most appropriate choice in this scenario?

A. IV clindamycin
B. Oral clindamycin
C. IV flucloxacillin
D. Oral flucloxacillin
E. Oral erythromycin

24. Apple jelly nodules

A 56-year-old man presents with two lesions on his neck which have been increasing in size over the last three months. On examination you notice two firm brown-coloured nodular lesions on the anterior aspect of the neck. The nodules give an 'apple-jelly' appearance on diascopy. The patient is systemically well. The most appropriate treatment is:

A. Oral flucloxacillin
B. Oral rifampicin, pyrazinamide, isoniazid and ethambutol
C. IV vancomycin
D. Oral erythromycin
E. Oral rifampicin and pyrazinamide

25. Cutaneous malignancies (1)

A 75-year-old man presents to your clinic with a dark lump on his forehead which has been increasing in size over the last 6 weeks. He first noticed the lump, which initially appeared as a small pinkish-red patch of skin, over a month ago. On examination you observe a 1×2 cm hyperpigmented nodule with everted edges and a centrally, deep, ulcerated red base. Which one of the following is the most likely diagnosis?

A. Basal cell carcinoma
B. Squamous cell carcinoma
C. Actinic keratoses
D. Keratoacanthoma
E. Bowen's disease

26. Cutaneous malignancies (2)

A 49-year-old woman is diagnosed with a malignant melanoma which was excised from her right leg. She has been doing some research on the internet regarding the different types of malignant melanoma. Which one of the following variants of malignant melanoma is considered to be the most common?

A. Nodular melanoma
B. Lentigo maligna melanoma
C. Acral melanoma
D. Superficial spreading melanoma
E. Subungual melanoma

27. Prognosis in malignant melanoma

A 40-year-old woman who you referred for excision biopsy of a suspected malignant melanoma on her right leg returns for a follow up of her results. The results of the biopsy return confirming a superficial spreading melanoma with a Breslow thickness of <1 mm. What five-year survival rate does a Breslow thickness of <1 mm correspond to?

A. 50 per cent
B. 60–75 per cent
C. 75–80 per cent
D. 80–96 per cent
E. 95–100 per cent

28. Cutaneous malignancies

A 67-year-old woman presents to you with pruritic plaques over her chest and back which are erythematous and resemble psoriatic plaques. From the patient's history you suspect that the lesions are malignant. Which one of the following cutaneous malignancies resembles psoriasis in the initial stages?

A. Merkel cell carcinoma
B. Histiocytosis X
C. Kaposi's sarcoma
D. Malignant melanoma
E. Cutaneous lymphoma

29. Leg ulcers

A 63-year-old woman presents to your clinic with a painful wound on her left foot which has not been healing despite regular application of dressings. The patient has a history of peripheral vascular disease. On examination, you observe a 2×1 cm well-demarcated ulcer on the left heel of the foot. The ulcer has a 'punched out' appearance and the base appears necrotic. What is the most likely diagnosis?

A. Arterial ulcer
B. Traumatic ulcer
C. Venous ulcer
D. Neoplastic ulcer
E. Neuropathic ulcer

30. Perioral pigmentation

Which one of the following congenital disorders is associated with perioral pigmentation?

 A. Hereditary haemorrhagic telangiectasia
 B. Neurofibromatosis
 C. Ehlers–Danlos syndrome
 D. Tuberous sclerosis
 E. Peutz–Jeghers syndrome

31. Management of dermatophyte infections

An 18-year-old man presents to you with an itchy scalp which has been present for 2 weeks following a visit at the barber shop. On examination, you notice a 3×3 cm oval area of patchy hair loss in the crown area of the scalp with a ring of erythema. You suspect that the patient has a dermatophytic infection. Which one of the following options would be the most appropriate in treating this condition?

 A. Oral co-amoxiclav
 B. Terbinafine cream
 C. Fusidic acid cream
 D. Acyclovir cream
 E. Oral acyclovir

32. Viral skin infections

Which one of the following viruses is responsible for causing molluscum contagiosum?

 A. Human papilloma virus (HPV)
 B. Herpes simplex virus (HSV)
 C. Pox virus
 D. Varicella zoster virus (VZV)
 E. Human immunodeficiency virus (HIV)

33. Acne vulgaris

A 16-year-old male presents to you with multiple comedones on his face and back. On examination you notice the presence of multiple comedones on the patient's forehead, cheeks and back with peri-lesional erythema. There are no nodules or cysts in these areas. You diagnose the patient with moderate acne. The most appropriate treatment is:

    A. Topical benzoyl peroxide
    B. Oral erythromycin
    C. Topical clindamycin
    D. Oral amoxicillin
    E. Oral isotretinoin

34. Facial rash

A 47-year-old woman presents to clinic with a erythematous, macular, non-tender, 'wing-shaped' rash over the bridge of the nose and cheeks. Which one of the following conditions is responsible for causing this type of facial rash?

    A. Rheumatoid arthritis
    B. Systemic sclerosis
    C. Systemic lupus erythematosus
    D. Dermatomyositis
    E. Psoriatic arthritis

35. Drug-induced SLE-like syndrome

A 47-year-old woman patient presents with a facial, macular 'butterfly rash'. Rheumatological investigations do not reveal that the patient has SLE. You suspect drug-induced SLE-like syndrome and assess her medication history. Which one of the following drugs is most likely to be responsible for this condition?

    A. Trimethoprim
    B. Aspirin
    C. Atenolol
    D. Diclofenac
    E. Lansoprazole

36. Nodular rash

A patient on the ward has a nodule-like rash and you are asked by your registrar to define the meaning of a nodule. From the list below, select the most appropriate definition of a nodule.

A. A well-defined flat area of altered pigmentation
B. A raised well-defined lesion usually less than 0.5 cm in diameter
C. A raised flat-topped lesion which is usually greater than 2 cm in diameter
D. A solid lump greater than 0.5 cm in diameter which may be subcutaneous or intradermal
E. A well-defined pus-filled lesion

37. Erythema multiforme

Which of the following is not a recognized cause of erythema multiforme?

A. Wegener's granulomatosis
B. Herpes simples virus
C. Sarcoidosis
D. Penicillins
E. Idiopathic

38. Erythema nodosum

Which of one of the following answers from the list below is a recognized cause of erythema nodosum?

A. Diabetes mellitus
B. Sarcoidosis
C. Venous insufficiency
D. Pregnancy
E. Trauma

39. Erythema chronicum migrans

Which one of the following conditions is erythema chronicum migrans associated with?

    A. Rheumatoid arthritis
    B. IBD
    C. Sarcoidosis
    D. Lyme disease
    E. SLE

40. Skin changes in diabetes mellitus

Which one of the following skin changes is not typically seen in patients with diabetes mellitus?

    A. Neuropathic ulcers
    B. Necrobiosis lipoidica
    C. Acanthosis nigricans
    D. Lipohypertrophy
    E. Livedo reticularis

ANSWERS

Skin appendages

1 C   The layers of the skin, starting from the surface inwards are the:

- epidermis (A);

- dermis (B), within which the cutaneous nerves (E) reside;

- subcutaneous fat (also known as the hypodermis) (D).

The skin appendages are structures, derived from ectoderm and mesoderm, which are housed within the skin and serve specific functions. These are the:

- hair follicle;

- sebaceous gland;

- apocrine sweat gland;

- eccrine sweat gland;

- nails.

The pilosebaceous unit (C) consists of the hair follicle, the sebaceous gland and arrector pili muscle. In some areas of the body, such as the axilla, the apocrine gland will also form part of the pilosebaceous unit. Therefore (C) is the correct answer here.

Cell types of the epidermis

2 E   The epidermis is comprised of four layers, starting from the surface and working inwards.

1 The cornified (or horny) layer which is defined as an outer, non-nucleated barrier.

2 The granular layer, which is the zone where epidermal nuclei disintegrate.

3 The spinous (or prickle layer) cell layer, where the majority of keratinocytes reside.

4 The basal layer, zone where keratinocytes undergo physiological mitosis.

The cell types found in the epidermis are the keratinocytes (D) (the main cell type), melanocytes (C) (pigment-producing cells found in the basal layer), Langerhans cells (B) (immunologically competent cells that are also found in the dermis) and the Merkel cells (A) (found in the basal layer of the epidermis and member of the amine precursor uptake and decarboxylation system). Therefore all cells mentioned in answers A–D can be seen in the epidermal layer.

Management of psoriasis

3 A Psoriasis, one of the most common dermatological presentations, is a chronic inflammatory skin condition characterized by the presence of well-defined, erythematous plaques with silvery scales, usually present on the extensor surfaces of the elbows, knees, scalp and sacrum. Plaques, without silvery scales, may be present on flexures (e.g. axillae, groin). Associated signs, which may be present, include nail changes, Kobner phenomenon (lesions appearing along sites of traumatic skin injury), Auspitz sign (pinpoint bleeding when scale removed) and systemic signs such as arthropathy (e.g. asymmetrical oligomonoarthritis, arthropathy of the distal interphalangeal joints (DIPs), rheumatoid-like sero-negative polyarthritis, arthritis mutilans and psoriatic spondylitis).

Management is targeted at disease control and includes:

- education;

- stress and alcohol avoidance;

- topical drugs are regarded as the mainstay of therapy (e.g. tar, dithranol, vitamin D analogues, topical steroid and antibiotic/fungal treatment is beneficial in flexural disease).

For psoriasis that is not responsive to conventional therapy (also known as relcalcitrant psoriasis), topical retinoids, phototherapy, oral drugs (e.g. methotrexate, cyclosporin, acitretin, hydroxycarbamide) may be considered.

Parenteral cytokine inhibitors or monoclonal antibodies may be considered for recalcitrant psoriasis unresponsive to systemic therapy mentioned above.

The question states that the patient is unresponsive to conventional therapy. Therefore, the next step would be to consider topical retinoid therapy.

Nail changes

4 B Onycholysis is described as separation of the nail from the nail bed which usually starts from the distal and/or lateral attachment and moves proximally. The causes of onycholysis are:

- skin diseases, such as psoriasis, dermatitis;

- infection (e.g. fungal infections);

- systemic diseases, such as reactive arthritis, hyper-/hypothyroidism;

- trauma;

- idiopathic.

Koilonychia (A) is spooning of the nails which occurs secondary to iron deficiency anaemia. Paronychia (E) can be divided into: (1) Acute; which commonly occurs due to staphylococcal infection and is characterized by acute inflammation of the posterior nail fold with purulent discharge; and (2) Chronic; which usually affects several nails showing loss of the cuticle with tender, bolstered, posterior nail folds. Chronic paronychia may be due to bacteria (e.g. *Pseudomonas pyocanea* or *Proteus vulgaris*) but, more frequently, it is caused by *Candida* (e.g. *Candida albicans*).

Beau's lines (C) are described as self-limiting transverse ridges that occur on the nails. They result from temporary interference with nail formation and are commonly seen during convalescence from a range of diseases (e.g. pneumonia) and conditions associated with prolonged fever. Finger clubbing (D) is described as an increase of the normal nail curve associated with a loss of the normal angle formed between the nail and posterior nail fold. Causes of clubbing are as follows:

- Cardiovascular causes:

  - cyanotic congenital heart disease, endocarditis, atrial myxoma, aneurysms and infected vascular grafts.

- Respiratory causes:

  - bronchogenic carcinoma, chronic lung suppuration (e.g. empyema, abscess, bronchiectasis, cystic fibrosis), fibrosing alveolitis, mesothelioma and tuberculosis.

- Gastrointestinal causes:

  - IBD;

  - cirrhosis;

  - GI lymphoma;

  - coeliac diseases.

- Rare causes:

  - thyroid acropachy;

  - oesophageal carcinoma.

- Idiopathic

Therefore, onycholysis (B) is the nail change associated with psoriasis. Other nail changes associated with psoriasis (with 50 per cent of patients with psoriasis experiencing nail changes) include pitting, thickening and subungual hyperkeratosis.

Atopic dermatitis

5 D 'Eczema' is a term used to describe what is known as dermatitis which, in simple terms, implies inflammation of the skin. Dermatitis can be further categorized into acute, subacute and chronic. Acute dermatitis is characterized by painful, inflamed, oedematous and oozing epidermis with developing vesicles or small blisters. Histologically, areas of gross oedema are seen within the epidermis which results in keratinocytes being pushed apart. Subacute dermatitis is defined as inflamed skin in the presence of visible scales and crust. Histologically, scaling and crusting are seen with epidermal disruption with lymphocytic infiltrate among keratinocytes. Chronic dermatitis can be described as thickened, elevated plaque (can be purple or violaceous in colour) and is known as epidermal acanthosis which is depicted on histology by thickened keratinocyte layer with infiltration of lymphocytes in the papillary dermis. Atopic dermatitis (eczema) is a chronic form of dermatitis with a strong genetic aetiological component (with a family history of atopy in 70 per cent). The condition usually begins in infancy (as early as 6 weeks of age) and is frequently associated with asthma and rhinitis. The condition tends to clear spontaneously between the ages of two and five. However, this may continue into adolescence and adult life, developing into the chronic type characterized by lichenification in the popliteal and antecubital fossae. Infants present with itchy scaly lesions on the scalp, face (with central sparing of the face) and trunk. The cheeks, wrists and hands are usually erythematous and scaling and scratched. Common sites of involvement, in toddlers and older children, are the elbow, knee, buttock flexures, ankles, dorsa of the feet (usually under shoe straps), retroauricular folds and antecubital fossae. There may be involvement of all four limbs with widespread excoriation and secondary infection in severe disease. Diagnosis is made on clinical grounds: Presence of itch for the preceding 12 months coupled with two or more of the following:

- flexural dermatitis;

- onset of less than two years;

- history of asthma or hay fever;

- dry skin.

Patients with atopic dermatitis are prone to staphylococci colonized skin infections. These are not always obvious but will tend to improve symptoms of atopic dermatitis if treated. Although all the mentioned bacteria in answers (A–E) can be isolated on the skin, from the list of answers the most likely answer is (D).

Management of atopic dermatitis

6 C In the first instance, the use of emollients (C) to prevent dry skin coupled with the application of topical steroid preparations, in areas where there is active disease (e.g. erythematous areas), will decrease discomfort and itch. Furthermore, emollients can also reduce the quantity and potency of topical steroids needed.

Other types of therapy include:

- antibiotics, for staphylococcal infections;
- antihistamines, to help control itch;
- wet wraps (E) (special bandaging techniques; wet bandages are applied over either steroid cream or weak antiseptic and then covered with dry stockinet to prevent itching. Alleviates discomfort and provides hydration to skin);
- occlusive bandaging.

For severe atopic dermatitis, the following treatment regimens may be considered:

- phototherapy (A);
- oral immunosuppressant (D) and cytotoxic therapy – not indicated in childhood disease;
- topical immunosuppressant preparations (B) have been shown to be beneficial in children as well as adults.

Therefore, answer (C) is the most appropriate first step in managing this patient.

Hirsuitism

7 E Hirsutism is defined as the growth of excess hair occurring in androgenic-dependent areas (e.g. the abnormal growth of chest or facial hair in women). The causes include:

- polycystic ovarian disease (E);
- adrenal/ovarian tumours;
- Cushing's syndrome;

- acromegaly;

- congenital adrenal hyperplasia;

- androgen/corticosteroid therapy.

Answers (A–D) are known causes of hypertrichosis, which is described as the growth of excess hair in non-androgenic areas and can be congenital or acquired.

Causes include:

- hypothyroidism (A);

- malnutrition;

- anorexia nervosa (i.e. lanugo hair) (B);

- drugs (e.g. cyclosporin, minoxidil, penicillamine, psoralens) (C).

Therefore, answer (E) is the correct option here.

Alopecia

8 B   Although rare, warfarin (B) has been reported to cause hair loss coupled with other anticoagulants such as heparin. Other drugs include cytotoxic drugs (e.g. cyclophosphamide, mercaptopurine derivatives, adriamycin, vinca alkaloids), anti-hyperthyroidism drugs (e.g. thiouracil, carbimazole), anti-tuberculosis drug ethionamide and large doses of vitamin A (and synthetic retinoids) have been reported to cause generalized diffuse alopecia.

Acanthosis nigrans

9 D   Acanthosis nigricans, as described above in the question stem, is commonly associated with gastric carcinoma (D), although it has also been seen in Hodgkin's lymphoma, obesity, acromegaly, diabetes mellitus and thyroid disease.

Contact dermatitis

10 D   Contact dermatitis is an inflammatory condition, induced by direct irritant action of a substance on the skin. It is a very common condition which can occur 4–12 hours after contact with the irritant (e.g. nickel, chromates, lanolin, colophony, rubber). The pattern of contact often gives a clue to the allergen and there is usually a sharp cut-off where contact ends; however, secondary spread elsewhere is frequent (also known as sensitization). Contact dermatitis is a type IV delayed type hypersensitivity reaction (D) which is antibody-independent. Allergic type IV reactions occur as a result of cell-mediated cytotoxicity (e.g. CD4 T cells, mediator release and macrophage activation). Other examples of type IV cell-mediated reactions include tuberculosis and Mantoux test graft rejection. Type I hypersensitivity reactions (A) are IgE-mediated resulting in basophil/mast cell activation leading to vasoactive mediator release leading to anaphylaxis. Type II (cytotoxic) hypersensitivity reactions (B) are mediated by IgG and IgM immunoglobulins. Immunoglobulins + tissue antigen leads to complement activation, cell lysis, opsonization, phagocytosis and inflammation. Examples include transfusion reactions, haemolytic anaemia, haemolytic disease of the new born. Type III (immune complex) hypersensitivity (C) occurs as a result of circulating antibody reacting with free antigen leading to formation of immune complexes. Immune complex deposits lead to complement, mast cell and neutrophil activation. Examples include SLE, RA and glomerulonephritis.

Dermatitis herpetiformis (1)

11 C Dermatitis herpetiformis is a chronic, itchy, blistering skin condition which is seen in patients with gluten-sensitive enteropathy (i.e. coeliac disease). Patients usually experience burning and intense itching in affected areas where the papulo-vesicular blisters are present. Common affected sites are the elbows, scalp, shoulders and ankles. Although the name of the condition suggests association with the herpes simplex virus, this is not the case; the cutaneous inflammation pattern is similar to what is seen in herpes infections. Therefore, answer (C) is the only correct option here.

Dermatitis herpetiformis (2)

12 B A course of dapsone (B), a sulphone antibiotic, will reduce the symptoms of itching. In addition, avoiding gluten-based food may also clear the lesions slowly. Dermatitis herpetiformis does not respond well to systemic steroids (A), although topical steroid-antibiotic preparations have shown benefit. NSAIDs (C) may help with pain but are not considered first-line therapy. Aciclovir (D) and fluconazole (E) are not recommended in the treatment of dermatitis herpetiformis.

Genodermatoses

13 B This patient has neurofibromatosis which can be divided into two types depending on signs (type-1 and type-2). Both forms are autosomal dominant inherited conditions (B). Type-1 neurofibromatosis (also known as von Recklinghausen's disease) is characterized by café-au-lait spots (macular hyperpigmentation) and neurofibromas (gelatinous small violaceous nodules which appear at puberty and may become papillomatous). Other signs which may be present are freckling in the axillary or inguinal regions, optic glioma and Lisch nodules (hamartomas on the iris). Type-2 neurofibromatosis is characterized by café-au-lait spots (but much less than type-1) and bilateral vestibular Schwannomas (characteristic of type-2). Juvenile cataracts (juvenile posterior subcaspular lenticular opacity), which is only seen in type-2, may also be a presenting condition. Neurofibromas, meningiomas and gliomas may also be seen in type-2.

Cutaneous hypopigmentation

14 A Causes of generalized cutaneous hypopigmentation include:

- phenylketonuria (A);
- albinism;
- hypopituitarism.

Causes of localized cutaneous hypopigmentation include:

- vitiligo (B);
- pityriasis versicolor (E);
- postinflammatory skin conditions;
- tuberous sclerosis (C);
- leprosy (D).

Painful swellings

15 D This patient has presented with pyoderma gangrenosum which is described, initially, as indolent boils which rapidly expand, break down and leave large, ulcerated painful areas with a characteristic undermined edge. Associated symptoms may include pyrexia and malaise. Pyoderma gangrenosum may be the first signs of ulcerative colitis, Crohn's disease and rheumatoid arthritis and can be idiopathic in 50 per cent of sufferers. Vasculitis (A), sarcoidosis (B), tuberculosis (C) and cutaneous manifestations of herpes simplex (E) infections are not associated with pyoderma gangrenosum.

Management of pyoderma gangrenosum

16 D Systemic steroid therapy (D) should be prescribed in moderately high doses (e.g. 60–100 mg prednisolone daily) which are gradually reduced as the lesions heal. In addition, the application of non-adherent dressings will encourage wound healing. If a solitary lesion exists, intra-lesional injection with a steroid preparation may be of benefit. For non-healing ulcers surgical curettage ± skin grafting may be performed.

Orogenital ulceration

17 E Orogenital ulceration may be seen in conditions such as inflammatory bowel disease (A), Steven–Johnson syndrome (B), secondary syphilis (C), Behçet's disease, Reiter's syndrome (D) and gonnococcal infection. Orogenital ulceration is not usually seen in coeliac disease (E).

Lupus pernio

18 C Lupus pernio is characterized by the presence of chronic sarcoid plaques resembling blue-red nodular lesions which may be present on the nose, hands (bulbous, sausage-shaped fingers which signify underlying bone cysts) and feet. Granulomatous infiltration of the nasal mucosa and respiratory tract may precede nasal septum destruction. Lupus pernio is one of the cutaneous manifestations of sarcoidosis (C) along with scar sarcoid which are the development of sarcoid granulomas in scars. Low-dose, alternate day systemic steroid therapy may be beneficial in lupus pernio. Rheumatod arthritis (A), SLE (B), tuberculosis (D) and herpes simplex infection (E) are not associated with lupus pernio.

Benign cutaneous tumours

19 C Bowen's disease (C) is a form of intra-epidermal carcinoma *in situ*, which may, if untreated, but rarely, progresses to invasive squamous carcinoma. The condition presents as a solitary, scaling, erythematous plaque which usually appears on the trunk. It is usually mistaken for a patch of psoriasis and is frequently treated as the latter. Seborrhoeic keratosis (A) is a condition of unknown aetiology characterized by a benign proliferation of epidermal keratinocytes which do not progress to malignancy. Lesions are raised and brown in colour and, due to the fact that they tend to grown outwards, they have a 'stuck on' appearance. This condition can be mistaken for malignant melanoma (especially when they are found on the face as flat lesions which resemble lentigo maligna) and, if in doubt, warrant excision. Pyogenic granuloma (B) is a benign tumour which arises from cutaneous vasculature. These lesions tend to appear 1–2 weeks post trauma, commonly from rose thorn injuries on the fingers. Epidermal naevi (D) are linear (often raised) plaques that arise from localized benign proliferations of epidermal keratinocytes. Histiocytoma (E) is described as a benign firm, elevated yellow/brown (flesh coloured) nodule. Histiocytomas tend to appear on the lower leg area and are known to rapidly enlarge. A dimple may develop in the middle of the lesion (secondary to the lesion being squeezed) which is not seen in malignant melanomas.

Tuberous sclerosis

20 B Tuberous sclerosis is an autosomal dominant condition characterized by a triad of cutaneous abnormalities, mental retardation and seizures.

The four main types of skin lesions associated with this condition are:

1   Ash-leaf hypopigmentation – described as multiple oval-shaped areas of hypopigmentation which may be the earliest sign of this condition (B)

2   Periungual fibromata – multiple, hypertrophic nodules around the nails which resemble viral warts

3   Shagreen patches – these are normal-coloured plaques, but have a firmer texture than normal skin, which tend to appear on the trunk

4   Adenoma sebaceum – although the pathological name does not fit the description of these lesions, these are in fact perivascular fibromata which are raised, red papules which appear on the face, especially around the nose

Pyoderma gangrenosum (A) (e.g. seen in inflammatory bowel disease), erythema nodosum (C) (e.g. seen in sarcidosis), café-au-lait spots (D) (e.g. seen in neurofibromatosis) and erythema multiforme (E) (e.g. seen in cutaneous allergic drug reactions) are not associated skin lesions seen in tuberous sclerosis.

Nutritional deficiencies

21 D Nicotinic acid deficiency (D) results in pellagra, a condition associated with dermatitis, diarrhoea and dementia. Nicotinic acid replacement is rapidly curative. Vitamin C (A) deficiency results in scurvy, characterized by bleeding gums, easy bruising and frank purpura. Protein malnutrition (C) results in kwashiorkor which tends to affect infants and is characterized by dry skin (with or without erythematous eruptions), dry, brittle and hypopigmented hair. Signs of oedema and ascites may be present. Vitamin B_1 (B) deficiency results in beriberi (neuropathy and cardiomyopathy) and vitamin B_6 (E) results in neuropathy and in some cases coupled with dermatitis eruptions.

Cutaneous bacterial infection

22 B This patient is suffering from cellulitis, described as a cutaneous infection with deep involvement of the subcutis which commonly affects the lower limbs but may appear anywhere on the body. The infected skin may be raised, is erythematous, hot and tender with poorly demarcated edges. Patients may have accompanying pyrexia and a full blood count may reveal leukocytosis. There may be a history of preceding trauma or insect bite to the affected area. The common organisms that have been reported to cause cellulitis are *Staphylococcus aureus* (B) *and Streptococcus pyogenes*. *Corynebacterium minutissimum* (A) is a bacterial organism responsible for a cutaneous infection called erythrasma which is characterized by an asymptomatic, reddish-brown area of skin, commonly seen in the body flexures (especially in the groin). If left untreated, the condition will spread slowly with well-demarcated edges. *Clostridium perfringens* (C) has been isolated in patients with cellulitis who are less than 24 hours post surgery. The organism produces gas leading to crepitus being felt in the affected areas. *Staphylococcus epidermidis* (D) and *Streptococcus pneumoniae* (E) are not usually cellulitis-causing organisms and are incorrect options.

Treatment of cellulitis

23 C Generally, the use of antibiotics for certain conditions is usually hospital protocol dependent and therefore will vary depending in which hospital one works. The most appropriate answer here would be IV flucloxacillin (C) rather than oral flucloxacillin (D). Intravenous antibiotic therapy is indicated in patients with cellulitis who are pyrexial and have leukocytosis. It is also indicated in elderly patients with co-morbidities (e.g. diabetes, immunosuppression). Otherwise, in patients who do not have a large area of cellulitis and are not pyrexial, oral antibiotic therapy may be indicated. Patients who are allergic to penicillin may be started on clindamycin (A and B) or erythromycin (E), depending on hospital antibiotic protocols.

Apple jelly nodules

24 B This patient is suffering from lupus vulgaris, a cutaneous manifestation of tuberculosis caused by the organism *Mycobacterium tuberculosis*. Lupus vulgaris is the most common form of cutaneous tuberculosis occurring after primary infection in individuals with good natural resistance to the organism. The condition commonly affects females more than males and lesions may be present on the face and neck areas. The lesions appear as brown, firm, translucent nodules which give a characteristic 'apple jelly' appearance on diascopy. If untreated, the nodules tend to spread causing scarring and contractions and in some case may undergo malignant change. Biopsy of these nodules reveal well-formed, tuberculoid granulomata which can be seen in the mid-dermis. Patients with lupus vulgaris should receive full anti-tuberculous drugs (B) for at least one year.

Cutaneous malignancies (1)

25 B The most likely diagnosis here is squamous cell carcinoma (SCC) (B). The majority of SCCs arise in areas of sun-damaged skin (but can appear anywhere on the body), while some may appear in scar tissue. Lesions present as hyperkeratotic, ulcerated (may be deep), expanding nodules with everted edges. They are commonly seen on the back of the hands, face and trunk but may also appear on the edge of scars (e.g. burns scars). Immunosuppressed patients are at risk of developing SCCs. Basal cell carcinomas (BCCs) (A) are slow growing and initially present as reddish-coloured, domed-shaped pearly nodules with a translucent surface and visible dilated surface capillaries. As the lesions expand, the central area tends to ulcerate, leaving a rolled-edge appearance. Actinic keratosis (C) are characterized by scaly, erythematous crusting lesions which tend to occur on the scalp, face and back of hands. They are very common lesions which arise secondary to prolonged sun exposure. Actinic keratoses have the potential to transform into metastasizing squamous carcinoma. Keratoacanthomas (D) are rapidly growing, and usually self-healing, epidermal nodules which possess pathological features indistinguishable from early SCCs. Keratoacanthomas develop as solitary lesions on the face and grow rapidly to a size of 2–3 cm in diameter. The nodule then develops a necrotic centre and heals spontaneously leaving a pitted scar appearance.

Bowen's disease (E) is a form of intra-epidermal carcinoma *in situ*, which may, if untreated, but rarely, progresses to invasive squamous carcinoma. The condition presents as a solitary, scaling, erythematous plaque which usually appears on the trunk. It is usually mistaken for a patch of psoriasis and is frequently treated as the latter.

Cutaneous malignancies (2)

26 D Malignant melanoma is a cutaneous malignancy which is derived from the epidermal melanocyte. There is a high incidence of this condition in white-skinned individuals coupled with a history of prolonged sun exposure (and long hours of strong sunshine). Lesions are commonly seen in the face (in both sexes), the back (common in males) and the leg (in females) and globally it affects men and women equally. The disease starts as a growing/changing area of brown/black coloured skin. In addition, a high index of suspicion is warranted in moles which are growing/changing with irregular edges and varying pigmentation. The Glasgow 7 point checklist (major points: (1) size, (2) shape, (3) colour; minor points: (4) diameter >7 mm, (5) inflammation, (6) oozing/bleeding, (7) itch/odd sensation) or the 'ABCDE' (Asymmetric lesions, Border irregularity, Colour irregularity, Diameter and Evolving) screening tool can be used to identify melanomas, but it is worth noting that not all melanomas have the above characteristics. The four main types of melanoma are superficial spreading (D) (which accounts for 80 per cent of presenting melanomas), nodular melanoma (A), lentigo maligna (B) and acral melanoma (C). Subungual melanoma (E) is a variant of the acral type. If malignant melanoma is suspected, patients are referred, without delay, for diagnostic excision biopsy with a narrow margin of 2–5 mm of normal skin.

Prognosis in malignant melanoma

27 E Breslow thickness (depth) is a prognostic tool, measured during biopsy of suspected melanoma, assessing the level of invasion (in mm) of the melanoma starting from the granular layer of the epidermis to the deepest point. Breslow thickness can also predict whether lymph node metastasis is likely, i.e. the greater the Breslow thickness, the greater chance of there being lymph node metastasis.

Breslow thickness	Approximate five-year survival
<1 mm	95–100 per cent (E)
1–2 mm	80–96 per cent (D)
2.1–4 mm	60–75 per cent (B)
>4 mm	50 per cent (A)

Therefore, in this question, the Breslow thickness is <1 mm, implying that the five-year survival is between 95 and 100 per cent, therefore (E) is the most appropriate answer.

Cutaneous malignancies

28 E Cutaneous lymphomas (E) mostly originate from T-lymphocytes and the most common type is mycosis fungoides which presents initially as pruritic cutaneous plaques which may be confused with psoriasis. Merkel cell carcinoma (A) is a rare malignancy arising from the Merkel cell. They present as non-specific nodules and are usually found on the head and neck areas. They can be surgically excised but carry a poor prognosis (50 per cent of patients develop metastatic spread). Histiocytosis X (B) is a proliferative disorder of the epidermal Langerhans cell. It is a rare condition and patients present with a grey rash on the scalp and body flexures which may resemble seborrhoeic dermatitis. Kaposi's sarcoma (C) (caused by HHV-8) is a malignancy derived from the dermal endothelial cells. This condition may develop in both HIV and non-HIV patients. Lesions are described as brown/purple papular nodules that typically present on the skin, but can appear in the GI or respiratory tract. Malignant melanoma (D) is a cutaneous malignancy which is derived from the epidermal melanocyte. There is a high incidence of this condition in white-skinned individuals coupled with a history of prolonged sun exposure (and long hours of strong sunshine). Lesions are commonly seen in the face (in both sexes), the back (common in males) and the leg (in females), globally it affects men and women equally. The disease starts as a rowing/changing area of brown/black coloured skin. In addition, a high index of suspicion is warranted in moles.

Leg ulcers

29 A The appearance of the ulcer (i.e. 'punched out' appearance, well demarcated and occurring at pressure points of the foot) coupled with the history of pain and peripheral vascular disease makes the diagnosis more likely to be an arterial ulcer (A). The surrounding skin of an arterial ulcer tends to be shiny in appearance, erythematous and hairless. Traumatic ulcers (B), as the name suggests, occur at sites of trauma. Patients usually present following wearing tight shoes or injury and present with ulcers on their toes or margins of the feet. Venous ulcers (C) arise secondary to venous insufficiency and account for approximately 80 per cent of all leg ulcers. They are usually painless and tend to occur in the gaiter area and characteristically around the medial malleolus. Venous ulcers are circumferential, shallow with irregular sloping edges and prominent granulation tissue in the bases. Associated signs include lipodermatosclerosis and hyperpigmentation around the ulcer site. Malignant/neoplastic ulcers (D) may be due to either primary or secondary malignant lesions. Malignant change in pre-existing ulcers may also occur (e.g. Marjolin's ulcers). Some examples of malignant ulcers include SCC, BCC, cutaneous lymphoma and malignant melanoma (primary or secondary lesions).

Neuropathic ulcers (E) tend to occur at high pressure sites (e.g. ball of foot and heel) in patients with peripheral neuropathy or diseases that lead to peripheral neuropathy, such as diabetes. They are usually painless and clinically may be confused with arterial ulcers due to their 'punched-out' appearance.

Perioral pigmentation

30 E Peutz–Jeghers syndrome (E) is the disorder that is characterized by peri-oral pigmentation. The cutaneous features of tuberous sclerosis (D) include angiofibromas, periungual fibromas, shagreen patches and ash-leaf patches. The cutaneous features of neurofibromatosis (B) include café-au-lait spots, axillary freckling and neurofibromas. The cutaneous features of Ehlers–Danlos syndrome (C) are skin fragility, tissue paper scars and skin hyperelasticity. Facial and mucosal telangiectasia is seen in hereditary haemorrhagic telangiectasia (A).

Management of dermatophyte infections

31 B Tinea capitis (also known as scalp ringworm) is characterized, initially, by a well-demarcated pruritic scaling area of hair loss with surrounding erythema. The condition occurs secondary to infection with dermatophyte organisms (e.g. *Trichophyton* spp., *Microsporum* spp.). Other forms of dermatophyte infections include tinea pedis (athletes foot), tinea corporis (body ringworm) and nail infections.

Treatment of cutaneous dermatophyte infections include:

- topical preparations – terbinafine (B), imidazoles;

- oral preparations (which are reserved for severe cutaneous infections involving multiple body sites) – griseofulvin and terbinafine.

Viral skin infections

32 C This is a common benign infection, caused by the pox virus (C), characterized by (pearly) elevated, smooth, reddish papules with a central punctum (all lesions). They are most commonly see on the face and neck but may also appear on the trunk. Multiple lesions are usually found in young patients, whereas in adults, lesions may be isolated to one body site and in the genital area. HPV (A) virus is responsible for warts. HSV (B) is responsible for causing cold sores and genital ulceration. VZV (D) is responsible for causing chicken pox and shingles. Dermatological complications of HIV infection (E) include hairy oral leukoplakia, persistent viral warts (and molluscum contagiosum), persistent HSV infections, severe recurrent candidosis, acute onset psoriasis, severe drug reactions and Kaposi's sarcoma.

Acne vulgaris

33 B Patients with moderate acne (inflammatory lesions present on the face and/or chest and back) can be treated with either topical antibiotic preparations and/or oral antibiotic therapy (e.g. oral erythromycin for four to six months). Patients with extensive acne on the back as well as the face and chest would find it difficult to apply topical preparations in the back area making oral antibiotics more practical and appropriate in this clinical scenario. In conjunction with oral antibiotics, topical antibiotics of the same type may be used but do not show great improvement. Patients with severe acne (i.e. nodules, cysts with scarring) or moderate acne refractory to oral antibiotic therapy should be started on oral synthetic retinoids (e.g. isotretionoin) which shows improvement in 60–70 per cent of patients. Women of child-bearing age should use effective contraception during and even one month after treatment due to high teratogenic effects of the synthetic retionoids.

Facial rash

34 C Cutaneous manifestations of SLE (C) include:

- macular (butterfly) facial rash that tends to spare the nasolabial folds;
- diffuse palmar (and dorsal) hand erythema ± telangiectasia (not like that seen in liver disease);
- patchy/diffuse hairloss.

Rheumatoid arthritis (A), systemic sclerosis (B), dermatomyositis (D) and psoriatic arthritis (E) are not known to cause the classic butterfly rash as seen in SLE.

Drug-induced SLE-like syndrome

35 A Sulphonamides are one of the many drugs that are known to cause drug-induced SLE-like syndrome. The other drugs responsible for this condition include:

- hydralazine;
- methyldopa;
- griseofulvin;
- oral contraceptives;
- penicillins;
- minocycline;
- phenylbutazone;
- procaine amide;
- diphenylhydantoin.

Nodular rash

36 D A nodule is defined as a solid lump greater than 0.5 cm in diameter which can be subcutaneous or intradermal in origin. (A) describes a macule, (B) describes a papule, (C) defines a plaque and (E) describes a pustule.

Erythema multiforme

37 A This is an erythematous disorder characterized by annular, target lesions, which may develop into frank blisters. The severe form of erythema multiforme is known as Stevens–Johnson syndrome and is associated with severe involvement of the eyes and mucosal surfaces. Causes include:

- idiopathic (E) (in approximately 50 per cent of sufferers);
- infections (e.g. HSV (B), EBV, Mycoplasma, Streptococcus);
- vasculitis (e.g. SLE, PAN);
- ulcerative colitis;
- carcinoma and lymphoma;
- sarcoidosis (C);
- pregnancy;
- drugs (e.g. penicillins (D), sulphonamides, co-trimoxazole, salicylates).

Wegener's granulomatosis (A) is not typically associated with erythema multiforme.

Erythema nodosum

38 B Erythema nodosum is described as painful, palpable, dusky blue-red lesions on the lower legs but may also, less commonly, be present on the forearms. Common associated symptoms include general malaise, fever and arthralgia. The lesions tend to resolve in 2–6 weeks. Causes include:

- systemic diseases (e.g. sarcoidosis (B), IBD, leukaemia and lymphoma);
- infections (e.g. streptococcal infections, tuberculosis, leprosy, EBV);
- drugs (e.g. penicillins, OCP, sulphonamides).

Erythema chronicum migrans

39 D Lyme disease (D) is a multisystem condition caused by the spirochaete *Borrelia burgdorferi* and is usually transmitted by the tick *Ixodes ricinus*. After the tick bites an area of skin, patients experience a febrile episode and develop either a papule/raised plaque or erythema surrounding the tick bite. A biopsy of the affected site (and very careful search) may reveal the spirochaete. Treatment is with antibiotics (e.g. oral penicillins or tetracyclines) for a minimum period of 2 weeks.

Skin changes in diabetes mellitus

40 E Neuropathic ulcers (A) are usually painless and tend to occur at sites of pressure (i.e. heel and metatarsal heads) with coexisting peripheral neuropathy. Necrobiosis lipoidica (B) is described as shiny, atrophic, red or yellowish plaques with marked telangiectasia over their surfaces which have a tendency to ulcerate. These are very slow healing ulcers which are not directly related to the severity of the diabetes. Acanthosis nigricans (C) is characterized by hyperpigmentation and hyperkeratosis, most marked in the body flexures. Although associated with malignancy, it is also seen in obesity and endocrine disorders such as diabetes, thyroid disease and acromegaly. Lipohypertrophy (D), a common chronic complication in insulin-dependent diabetes mellitus, is described as hypertrophy of subcutaneous fat at sites of repeated insulin injections that appear as lumps under the skin. These sites may be painful/tender and tend to subside (within a few months) if injections are avoided in those areas. Livedo reticularis (E) is characterized by reticular, cyanotic cutaneous discoloration surrounding pale central areas occurring mostly on the legs, arms, trunk and are more pronounced in cold weather. The condition occurs as a result of capillary dilatation coupled with stagnation of blood which causes the mottled discoloration of the skin. Causes include thrombocythaemia, hyperviscosity, vasculitis, physiological and idiopathic.

SECTION 11:
INFECTIOUS DISEASES

QUESTIONS

1. Fever (1)

A 27-year-old woman, who has recently returned from holiday in Africa, presents to accident and emergency with a 7-day history of fevers, sweats, headache, malaise and lethargy. On examination, her temperature is 39°C. Cardiorespiratory and gastrointestinal examinations are unremarkable. What is the most likely differential diagnosis?

    A. Malaria
    B. Tuberculosis
    C. Influenza
    D. Typhoid
    E. Dengue fever

2. Fever (2)

A 25-year-old woman, who has recently returned from holiday in Africa, presents to accident and emergency with a 7-day history of fevers, sweats, headache, malaise and lethargy. On examination, her temperature is 39°C. A diagnosis of malaria is suspected. What is the investigation of choice to confirm the diagnosis?

    A. Blood cultures
    B. Full blood count
    C. Thick and thin blood films
    D. Ziehl–Nielson stain
    E. Paul–Bunnell test

3. Fever (3)

A 30-year-old man, who has recently returned from holiday in Africa, presents to accident and emergency with a 7-day history of fever, sweats, malaise and lethargy. Thick and thin blood films detect *Plasmodium falciparum*. What is the most appropriate treatment?

    A. Conservative management
    B. Acyclovir
    C. Omeprazole
    D. Chloroquine
    E. Quinine

4. Haemoptysis (1)

A 40-year-old Indian man presents to accident and emergency with a one-month history of haemoptysis. He is a non-smoker. On further questioning, he mentions that he has also been having fevers and night sweats. Chest x-ray shows nodular shadowing in the right upper zone. What is the most likely diagnosis?

    A. Sarcoidosis
    B. Small cell carcinoma of the lung
    C. Primary tuberculosis
    D. Post-primary tuberculosis
    E. Pneumocystis pneumonia

5. Cough

A 54-year-old investment banker presents to accident and emergency with a 5-day history of productive cough of green sputum, fevers and feeling generally unwell. On examination, there is bronchial breathing in the left lower zone. Chest x-ray demonstrates left lower zone consolidation. What is the most likely causative organism?

    A. *Mycoplasma pneumoniae*
    B. *Klebsiella pneumoniae*
    C. *Staphylococcus aureus*
    D. *Haemophilus influenzae*
    E. *Streptococcus pneumoniae*

6. Diarrhoea (1)

A 74-year-old woman patient, who is being treated for chest infection following an elective gastrectomy, develops profuse diarrhoea. A stool sample is collected and microscopy, culture and sensitivity reveal *Clostridium difficile* toxin. What is the most appropriate treatment?

    A. Intravenous co-amoxiclav
    B. Oral metronidazole
    C. Isolate the patient and treat conservatively with intravenous fluids
    D. Isolate the patient and treat conservatively with oral rehydration solution
    E. Prednisolone

7. Diarrhoea (2)

A 23-year-old woman medical student, who has returned home from a trip to India 1 day ago, presents to accident and emergency with profuse watery diarrhoea. This started suddenly and she describes her stool as being profuse and colourless. She is unable to quantify the number of times she has opened her bowels prior to presentation. On examination her pulse is 110 bpm. Cardiorespiratory and gastrointestinal examination are unremarkable. What is the most likely diagnosis?

    A. Cholera
    B. Typhoid
    C. Pseudomembranous colitis
    D. Shigella
    E. Enterotoxigenic *Escherichia coli* diarrhoea

8. Diarrhoea (3)

A 30-year-old woman aid worker, who has returned from a trip to Haiti 1 day ago, presents to accident and emergency with profuse watery diarrhoea. This started suddenly and she describes her stool as being profuse and colourless. On examination her pulse is 120 bpm. What is the most appropriate treatment?

    A. Rehydration with oral rehydration solutions
    B. Rehydration with intravenous fluids
    C. Rehydration with oral rehydration fluids plus metronidazole
    D. Codeine phosphate
    E. Oral azithromycin

9. Diarrhoea (4)

A three-year-old boy presents, with his mother, to his GP with a 2-day history of fevers, vomiting and diarrhoea. His mother mentions that several other children at the nursery have been off sick this week with the same problem. What is the most likely cause?

    A. Enterotoxigenic *E. coli*
    B. Salmonella
    C. Rotavirus
    D. Influenza
    E. Shigella

10. Rash (1)

A nine-year-old boy presents to his GP with a 2-day history of sudden onset itchy rash over his face, scalp, neck and trunk, On examination, his temperature is 38°C and there is a widespread vesicular rash. What is the most likely infective organism?

   A. Epstein–Barr virus
   B. Cytomegalovirus
   C. Varicella zoster virus (VZV)
   D. *Staphlococcus aureus*
   E. Herpes-simplex type 1

11. Rash (2)

A 70-year-old man presents to accident and emergency with a 1-day history of a painful rash across his trunk. He has a past medical history of hypertension and hypercholesterolaemia. On examination, there is a well-demarcated blistering rash on the right side of his trunk. What is the most appropriate treatment?

   A. Oral acyclovir
   B. High dose intravenous acyclovir
   C. Topical steroids
   D. Paracetamol
   E. Amitryptiline

12. Painful rash

A 27-year-old investment banker presents to accident and emergency with a 4-day history of painful rash on his penis and testicles. He also reports feeling generally run down with a fever and myalgia. He returned from a trip to New York a week ago. On examination, there is a painful vesicular rash over his penis and testicles. What is the most appropriate treatment?

   A. Oral acyclovir
   B. High-dose intravenous acyclovir
   C. Oral flucloxacillin
   D. Paracetamol
   E. Glyceryl trinitrate cream

13. Penile discharge

A 22-year-old medical student presents to the GUM clinic with large amounts of yellow-coloured penile discharge and discomfort on urinating. He has just arrived home from his summer holiday in Ibiza. What is the most likely diagnosis?

   A. Chlamydia
   B. Genital herpes
   C. Cystitis
   D. Gonorrhoea
   E. Syphilis

14. Penile lesion (1)

A 30-year-old man presents to his GP with a lesion on his penis, which appeared a week ago. On further questioning, he reports a change in sexual partner 4 weeks ago. He has otherwise been well. On examination, there is a painless hard ulcer on the shaft of the penis. What is the most likely diagnosis?

   A.   Chancroid
   B.   Genital herpes
   C.   Chlamydia
   D.   Primary syphilis
   E.   Secondary syphilis

15. Penile lesion (2)

A 34-year-old man presents to his GP with a painless hard penile ulcer. Venereal Disease Research Laboratory tests and *Treponema pallidum* haemagglutination assay confirm the diagnosis of primary syphilis. What is the most appropriate treatment for this patient?

   A.   Co-amoxiclav
   B.   Acyclovir
   C.   Azithromycin
   D.   Ciprofloxacin
   E.   Procaine penicillin

16. Jaundice (1)

A 45-year-old man presents to accident and emergency, having returned from a holiday to India a week ago. He has subsequently been unwell with nausea and reduced appetite. Over the past 2 days he has become jaundiced. He mentions that his two brothers with whom he went on holiday have also become jaundiced in the last 2 days. On examination, he is apyrexial and there is a palpable liver edge. Liver function tests reveal a raised ALT, AST and bilirubin. All other blood tests are normal. What is the most likely diagnosis?

   A.   Hepatitis A
   B.   Hepatitis B
   C.   Hepatitis C
   D.   Gilbert's syndrome
   E.   Malaria

17. Jaundice (2)

A 40-year-old man presents to accident and emergency having returned from a holiday to India a week ago. He has subsequently been unwell with nausea and reduced appetite. Over the past 2 days he has become jaundiced. On examination, he is apyrexial and there is a palpable liver edge. Liver function tests reveal a raised ALT, AST and bilirubin. A diagnosis of hepatitis A is suspected. What is the most appropriate treatment?

    A. Intravenous hydrocortisone
    B. Pegylated interferon alpha plus ribavirin
    C. Conservative management
    D. Acyclovir
    E. Chloroquine

18. Sore throat

A 19-year-old medical student presents to accident and emergency with a 1-week history of fever, anorexia and a sore throat. On examination, she is pyrexial at 39°C and cervical, axillary and inguinal lymph nodes are palpable. Palatal petechiae are visible within the mouth and her tonsils appear inflamed. A full blood count reveals a lymphocytosis and a blood film reveals the presence of atypical lymphocytes. What is the most likely diagnosis?

    A. Toxoplasmosis
    B. Cytomegalovirus infection
    C. Infectious mononucleosis
    D. Streptococcal sore throat
    E. Influenza

19. Neck stiffness

A 19-year-old medical student presents to his GP during fresher's fortnight. He is complaining of neck stiffness, headache and sensitivity to light. On examination, a non-blanching, petechial rash is observed on the trunk. What is the most appropriate immediate management?

    A. Send the patient to accident and emergency immediately
    B. Send him home with advice to rest and return if the symptoms worsen
    C. Administer 1.2 g of intramuscular benzylpenicillin
    D. Give 500 mg of ciprofloxacin
    E. Take a full set of blood tests

20. Facial swelling

A 19-year-old man presents to his GP with a 4-day history of painful facial swelling, fevers and lethargy. On examination, there is bilateral swelling of his parotid glands. What is the most likely diagnosis?

    A. Measles
    B. Mumps
    C. Influenza
    D. Infectious mononucleosis
    E. Pertussis

21. Rash (3)

A 41-year-old teacher presents to her GP with a 5-day history of fevers, headaches, lethargy and muscle aches. She also mentions that she is developing an expanding red rash on her left thigh. On further questioning, she mentions that she has been on a school camping trip the previous week. She is otherwise fit and well. What is the most likely diagnosis?

    A. Lyme disease
    B. Sarcoidosis
    C. Brucellosis
    D. Syphilis
    E. Erythema ab igne

22. Haemoptysis (2)

A 39-year-old Indian man presents to his GP with a 5-week history of haemoptysis, night sweats and weight loss. Which of the following investigations can be used to confirm the diagnosis of tuberculosis?

    A. Tuberculin skin testing
    B. Blood cultures
    C. Chest x-ray
    D. Ziehl–Nielsen sputum staining
    E. Computed tomography pulmonary angiogram (CTPA)

23. Neck stiffness

A 23-year-old man presents to accident and emergency with a 1-day history of severe headache, discomfort when looking at the lights and neck stiffness. There is a non-blanching rash observed on his trunk. He has recently recovered from chicken pox. On examination he is pyrexial at 39°C. The most likely causative organism is:

    A. *Streptococcus pneumoniae*
    B. *Listeria monocytogenes*
    C. *Neisseria gonorrhoeae*
    D. VZV
    E. *Neisseria meningitidis*

24. Skin lesion (1)

A 51-year-old man presents to accident and emergency with a lesion on his forearm. He mentions that he has spent the past three months travelling around South America and only returned home 3 days ago. While his lesion has been present for a few weeks he was reluctant to see a doctor in South America. On examination, there is a 3×3 cm erythematous ulcer on the left forearm with a raised edge. What is the most likely diagnosis?

    A. Leishmaniasis
    B. African trypanosomiasis
    C. Herpes zoster
    D. Schistosomiasis
    E. Cryptosporidiosis

25. Leishmaniasis

Which of the following statements is most accurate regarding leishmaniasis?

    A. It is transmitted by the anopheles mosquito
    B. Leishmania are bacteria
    C. Leishmaniaisis is usually a self-limiting condition
    D. It is transmitted by the tsetse fly
    E. The presence of Leishman–Donovan bodies confirms the disease

26. Itchy rash (1)

A 24-year-old man presents to accident and emergency with fevers, lethargy, myalgia and a cough. He has also developed an itchy rash on his feet. He returned home from a charity trip to Malawi last month and is worried he might have malaria. On examination, a papular rash is noted around his feet and there is a palpable liver edge. Initial blood tests show a raised white cell count with an eosinophilia. What is the most likely diagnosis?

    A. Leishmaniasis
    B. Schistosomiasis
    C. African trypanosomiasis
    D. Malaria
    E. Influenza

27. Pale stools

A 35-year-old man presents to his GP with diarrhoea, abdominal pain and nausea. He says he his stools have been pale and he has felt persistently bloated. His symptoms started 6 weeks ago while on a surfing holiday in Peru. What is the most likely diagnosis?

    A. Coeliac disease
    B. Enterotoxigenic *E. coli* gastroenteritis
    C. Salmonella
    D. Giardia
    E. Cryptosporidiosis

28. Rash (4)

A 26-year-old Bangladeshi man presents to accident and emergency with a 1-week history of fever, headache, malaise and dry cough. He returned to the UK 2 weeks ago, having spent his summer in Bangladesh. On examination, his temperature is 39°C and a patchy maculopapular rash is seen over his trunk. On examination of the abdomen, there is splenomegaly. Blood tests reveal a low white cell count. What is the most likely diagnosis?

    A. Tetanus
    B. Malaria
    C. Typhoid
    D. Cholera
    E. Primary syphilis

29. Lockjaw

A 32-year-old man presents to accident and emergency with the inability to open his jaw, starting a few hours earlier. His wife mentions that he has 'had the flu' since returning from a weekend camping trip. What is the most likely diagnosis?

A. Tetanus
B. Dislocation of the temporomandibular joint
C. *Clostridium perfringens* infection
D. Influenza
E. *Clostridium difficile* infection

30. Sepsis

Following a colonic resection, a 72-year-old woman becomes unwell with acute confusion, pyrexia, tachycardia and hypotension. The patient has had a difficult postoperative period, which has included an admission to ITU for the management of a chest infection. Blood cultures are sent and grow methicillin-resistant *Staphylococcus aureus* (MRSA). The patient is placed in isolation and barrier nursing is implemented. What is the most appropriate management of this patient?

A. Manage conservatively
B. Start intravenous vancomycin
C. Start intravenous co-amoxiclav
D. Start intravenous co-amoxiclav and gentamicin
E. Start oral metronidazole

31. Heart murmur

A 90-year-old man presents to accident and emergency with a 2-week history of fevers, lethargy and night sweats. He has recently had crowns fitted at the dentists. He has a past medical history of hypertension, gout and type 2 diabetes mellitus. On examination his temperature is 39°C, his pulse is 120 bpm and splinter haemorrhages are seen in the nails. On auscultation of the heart a pansystolic murmur is audible. A diagnosis of endocarditis is suspected and blood cultures are taken. What organism is most likely to be grown?

A. *Staphlococcus aureus*
B. *Staphlococcus epidermidis*
C. *Actinobacillus*
D. *Enterococcus faecalis*
E. *Streptococcus viridans*

32. Itchy rash (2)

A 45-year-old man who lives in a homeless shelter presents to accident and emergency with an itchy rash. The itching is particularly bad at night. On examination, there is a papular rash between the web spaces of the fingers and toes, the palms of the hands and soles of the feet, the axilla and on the genitalia. What is the most likely diagnosis?

   A. Scabies
   B. Shingles
   C. Chicken pox
   D. Molluscum contagiosum
   E. Tinea cruris

33. Knee pain (1)

A 20-year-old man presents to accident and emergency with extreme pain in the right knee. On examination, his temperature is 38.5°C and the knee is hot and swollen. He is unable to move his knee due to pain. The joint is aspirated and blood cultures are taken. The patient is admitted and started on intravenous antibiotics. Gram staining of the joint aspirate shows gram-negative diplococci. What is the most likely responsible organism?

   A. *Chlamydia trachomatis*
   B. *Neisseriae gonnorrheae*
   C. *Haemophilus influenzae*
   D. *Streptococcus pneumoniae*
   E. *Streptococcus viridans*

34. Knee pain (2)

A 74-year-old man presents to accident and emergency with extreme pain in the left knee. On examination, his temperature is 39°C and the knee is swollen and hot. He is unable to move the joint due to pain. The joint is aspirated and the patient is admitted and started on intravenous antibiotics. What is the most likely causative organism?

   A. *Neisseriae gonorrheae*
   B. *Mycobacterium tuberculosis*
   C. *Neisseria meningitidis*
   D. *Staphylococcus aureus*
   E. *Haemophilus influenzae*

35. Shortness of breath

A 42-year-old man presents to accident and emergency with a 3-week history of shortness of breath, dry cough, fevers and malaise. He has presented as his exercise tolerance has deteriorated. He mentions that he has been HIV positive for ten years. On examination, there are fine crackles throughout both lung fields. Chest x-ray demonstrates bilateral perihilar interstitial shadowing. What is the most likely causative organism?

    A. *Pneumocystis jiroveci*
    B. Herpes simples virus type 1
    C. Herpes simplex virus type 2
    D. *Streptococcus pneumoniae*
    E. *Mycoplasma pneumoniae*

36. Dysphagia

A 42-year-old man presents to accident and emergency with a 3-week history of retrosternal discomfort after swallowing. He mentions that he has been unable to keep any food down at all. He has been HIV positive for ten years. He is admitted and endoscopy shows areas of ulceration throughout the oesophagus. What is the most likely causative organism?

    A. *Staphylococcus aureus*
    B. *Crytosporidium parvus*
    C. *Candida albicans*
    D. *Pneumocystis jiroveci*
    E. *Cryptococcus neoformans*

37. Skin lesions (2)

A 42-year-old man presents to his GP with 'blotches' over his legs. He has been HIV positive for ten years. On examination, there are multiple purple and brown papules over his legs and his gums. What is the most likely diagnosis?

    A. Malignant melanoma
    B. Squamous cell carcinoma
    C. Basal cell carcinoma
    D. Kaposi's sarcoma
    E. Toxoplasmosis

38. Skin lesions (3)

A 42-year-old man presents to his GP with 'blotches' over his legs. He has been HIV positive for ten years. On examination, there are multiple purple and brown papules over his legs and his gums. A diagnosis of Kaposi's sarcoma is suspected. What is the most likely causative organism?

    A. Herpes simplex virus type 1
    B. Herpes simplex virus type 2
    C. Human herpes virus type 3
    D. Human herpes virus type 8
    E. *Pneumocystis jiroveci*

39. Visual disturbance

A 42-year-old man presents to his GP complaining of deterioration in his vision in the right eye and the presence of floaters. The change in his vision has been causing him to suffer from headaches. He has been HIV positive for ten years. Fundoscopy reveals haemorrhages and exudates on the retina. What is the most likely diagnosis?

    A. Retinal detachment
    B. CMV retinitis
    C. Kaposi's sarcoma
    D. Optic atrophy
    E. Diabetic retinopathy

40. Confusion

A 42-year-old man presents to accident and emergency with a 1-day history of headache and fevers. He presents with his partner who says he has been becoming increasingly confused and disorientated. On examination, his temperature is 38.5°C. On cranial nerve examination there is a right-sided superior quadrantanopia. An urgent CT scan of the head is organized which shows multiple ring enhancing lesions. What is the most likely diagnosis?

    A. Toxoplasmosis
    B. Meningitis
    C. Cryptosporidiosis
    D. CMV encephalitis
    E. Histoplasmosis

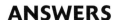

ANSWERS

Fever (1)

1 A   Malaria (A) should be considered as the most likely diagnosis of patients presenting with fever, having returned from malaria endemic areas. The most common presenting features are fever, malaise, headache, vomiting or diarrhoea. Tuberculosis (B) has a variable presentation, but most commonly presents with pulmonary symptoms such as cough, fever and sweats, malaise and weight loss. Tuberculosis is also an unlikely answer as the initial infection (primary tuberculosis) that may have been picked up during the trip is usually asymptomatic. Symptoms are usually manifestations of reactivation of primary tuberculosis (post-primary tuberculosis). Influenza (C) must be considered as a possible diagnosis – just because the patient has travelled to a malaria endemic area does not mean that they have not picked up flu! However, the travel history means that malaria is the more likely diagnosis, which requires investigation. Typhoid (D) presents with gastrointestinal symptoms, making this answer wrong. Finally, Dengue fever (E) is also transmitted by mosquitos and may present with abrupt onset fever. However, additional features include headache, facial flushing and retrobulbar pain. There may also be a generalized maculopapular rash. The absence of these features makes malaria the more likely diagnosis.

Fever (2)

2 C   The diagnosis of malaria is usually confirmed with thick and thin blood films (C). Note that a negative result does not rule out malaria and usually three negative blood films are required to exclude the diagnosis. Blood cultures (A) should be sent in the pyrexial patient, but are not used to confirm the diagnosis. Similarly, a full set of blood tests, including the full blood count (B), should be sent. Full blood count may show a low haemoglobin or platelet count. However, the diagnosis of malaria cannot be confirmed on full blood count alone. Ziehl–Nielson staining (D) is used to detect acid-fast bacilli in the investigation of tuberculosis. A Paul–Bunnell (E) test is used in the investigation of infectious mononucleosis.

Fever (3)

3 E   Falciparum malaria may develop into a potentially life-threatening disease if left untreated. Therefore, conservative management (A) is not the appropriate answer. Aciclovir (B) is a commonly used antiviral drug that is not used in the treatment of malaria. Widespread chloroquine (D) resistance means that this is not the first-line drug of choice for patient with falciparium malaria. Quinine (E) is used to treat falciparium malaria and can be given orally or intravenously. Omeprazole (C) is not used in the treatment of malaria.

Haemoptysis (1)

4 D The symptoms of fevers, night sweats and weight loss in an Indian male are characterisitic of post-primary pulmonary tuberculosis (D). Initial infection with *Mycobacterium tuberculosis* is known as primary tuberculosis (C) and is usually asymptomatic. The bacilli reaching the lung causes an initial reaction, resulting in the granulomatous lesions (with central caseating, necrotic material) walled in by surrounding epitheloid cells). These lesions may contain the tubercle bacilli, which can become reactivated later in life, usually caused by depression in host immunity, resulting in post-primary tuberculosis. Post-primary tuberculosis may manifest itself in a number of ways, the most common of which is pulmonary tuberculosis. Fever and night sweats are not a feature of sarcoidosis (A). Furthermore, the cough in sarcoid is usually dry and characteristic chest x-ray findings are bilateral hilar lymphadenopathy with pulmonary infitrates. Small cell carcinoma of the lung (B) should be considered in patients with haemoptysis and chest x-ray changes. However, the patient is a non-smoker, making this diagnosis less likely than tuberculosis. *Pneumocystis pneumonia* (E) is caused by *Pneumocystis jiroveci* and is seen in immunocompromised patients. While night sweats and fevers may occur, the cough in *Pneumocystis pneumoniae* is usually non-productive. In addition, chest x-ray usually shows widespread pulmonary infiltrates. Thus, this is the incorrect answer.

Cough

5 E The most common cause of a community-acquired pneumonia as described in this question is *Streptococcus pneumoniae* (E), making this the correct answer. Epidemics of pneumonia caused by *Mycoplasma pneumonia* (A) usually occur every 3–4 years and may present with generalized features such as headache, arthralgia and myalgia. A chest x-ray may show patchy consolidation through the lung fields. In addition, the clinical features of disease often do not usually correlate with the x-ray findings. *Klebsiella pneumoniae* (B) is relatively rare and usually occurs in elderly patients with other underlying co-morbidities. It results in a cavitating pneumonia in which patients present with a productive cough of purulent or blood-stained sputum. Pneumonia caused by *Staphylococcus aureus* (C) usually occurs following influenzal viral infection. Staphyloccocal peumonia may become life-threatening and must be treated aggressively and quickly. *Haemophilus influenza* (D) is frequently the cause of infective exacerbations of chronic obstructive pulmonary disease (COPD).

Diarrhoea (1)

6 B *Clostridium difficile* colitis is caused by the use of broad-spectrum antibiotics which eradicate the normal gut flora and result in colonization of the gut by *Clostridium difficile*. This extensive infection results in pseudomembranous colitis and patients will usually present with profuse watery diarrhoea. The treatment of this is with oral metronidazole (B). Intravenous co-amoxiclav (A) may cause pseudomembranous colitis due to *Clostridium difficile* infection and must be stopped if possible. The patient must be isolated and treated with oral rehydration solution (D) or intravenous fluids (C) but conservative measures alone are not sufficient. Prednisolone (E) is not used in the treatment of pseudomembranous colitis.

Diarrhoea (2)

7 A Cholera (A) is caused by *Vibrio cholerae*, transmitted by the faeco-oral route, and normally presents with a mild diarrhoea. However, some patients may present with sudden onset profuse watery diarrhoea, fever and vomiting. The diarrhoea is classically described as 'rice-water stools' and may result in significant dehydration. Typhoid (B) is caused by *Salmonella typhi*, spread by the faeco-oral route and may present with gradual onset fever, headache, malaise and either constipation or diarrhoea. The profuse rice-water diarrhoea described in this case is not a feature. In addition, a patient with typhoid may develop a maculopapular rash, known as rose spots over the trunk. Pseudomembranous colitis (C) is caused by *Clostridium difficile* colonization of the gut and is caused by use of broad-spectrum antibiotics. Shigella (D) usually presents with bloody diarrhoea, making this answer incorrect. Enterotoxigenic *E. coli* diarrhoea (E) is the most common cause of travellers' diarrhoea. However, the profuse watery diarrhoea described in this case makes cholera the most likely diagnosis.

Diarrhoea (3)

8 B The most appropriate management for patients with profuse diarrhoea due to cholera is rehydration with intravenous fluids (B). Rehydration with intravenous fluids is favoured here as the patient is tachycardic and shows signs of hypovolaemia. Oral rehydration solution (A) are favoured in developing countries and recommended by the WHO. Metronidazole (C) is not used in the treatment of cholera. However, ciprofloxacin is occasionally used. Codeine phosphate (D) and oral azithromycin (E) are not used in the treatment of profuse diarrhoea due to cholera.

Diarrhoea (4)

9 C Rotavirus (C) is an important cause of outbreaks of childhood diarrhoea and should be considered the most likely cause in this question. Enterotoxigenic *E. coli* (A) is the most common cause of travellers' diarrhoea. The outbreak of diarrhoea within the nursery makes this option unlikely. Salmonella (B) should be considered as a possible diagnosis. It is usually caused by eating contaminated foods, especially poultry. Salmonella may cause outbreaks of diarrhoea and vomiting when communal food is contaminated. However, the age group affected in this question makes rotavirus the more likely answer. Influenza (D) usually presents with fever, headache, myalgia and dry cough, making this answer incorrect. Shigella (E) usually presents with bloody diarrhoea, making this answer incorrect.

Rash (1)

10 C The case in this question is describing the presentation of chicken pox. This is caused by VZV infection (C). This is transmitted by droplet infection and presents with a prodromal illness of fever, headache and malaise and is followed by widespread eruption of a vesicular rash over the scalp, face, trunk and, to a lesser extent, the extremities. Epstein–Barr virus (A) causes infectious mononucleosis. Cytomegalovirus usually causes an opportunistic infection in an immunocompromised host (for example, transplant recipients on immunosuppression) which may resemble infectious mononucleosis. *Staphlococcus aureus* (D) is a commensal skin bacteria which can cause skin infections. However, it does not cause a widespread itchy vesicular rash. Herpes-simplex type 1 virus (E) causes cold sores and genital herpes.

Rash (2)

11 A The case in this question describes the presentation of a patient with shingles. This is caused by reactivation of VZV. The normal presentation of shingles is with a prodromal phase of tingling or pain, followed by an eruption of a painful, blistering rash in a dermatomal distribution. Complications of shingles include post-herpetic neuralgia (severe pain in the dermatomes affected after shingles) and ocular disease. Early in the disease, as in this case, oral aciclovir (A) is the most appropriate treatment as it may help shorten the course of the disease. High-dose intravenous acyclovir (B) is given to immunocompromised patients. Topical steroids (C) are not helpful in the management of shingles. Paracetamol (D) is an important analgesic for symptomatic relief of patients with shingles, but in early onset disease acyclovir should be given to try and reduce the course of the disease, making this the incorrect answer. Amitryptiline (E) is a useful drug for the management of post-herpetic neuralgia, but is not used for the management of shingles.

Painful rash

12 A The case in this question describes a patient presenting with genital herpes. This is caused by infection with herpes simplex virus type 1 or type 2. It is transmitted by skin to skin contact during sexual contact. Both of these viral subtypes can also cause cold sores. The treatment of genital herpes is with antivirals, such as acyclovir or ganciclovir. Oral acyclovir (A) is preferred, unless the patient is immunocompromised, when high-dose intravenous acyclovir (B) may be considered. Oral flucloxacillin (C) is not used in the treatment of genital herpes. Paracetamol (D) is likely to be an important analgesic in patients with genital herpes. However, it does not limit the extent of disease and should be used with an antiviral. Glyceryl trinitrate cream (E) is used in the treatment of anal fissures and not genital herpes.

Penile discharge

13 D Gonorrhoea (D) is caused by *Neisseria gonorrheae*. In men, this usually presents with a purulent urethral discharge and dysuria. Women are often asymptomatic but may present with vaginal discharge, pelvic pain, dysuria or intermenstrual bleeding. Chlamydia (A) is the most common sexually transmitted infection in the UK. It is often asymptomatic in both men and women. In symptomatic men, clinical features include urethral discharge and dysuria. This is similar to the features described in this question. However, the presence of large amounts of yellow-coloured penile discharge make gonorrhoea a more likely answer than chlamydia. Genital herpes (B) presents with the prodromal symptoms of fever and feeling generally unwell, followed by a sudden outbreak of a painful vesicular rash over the genitalia. Urethral discharge may occur, but the absence of a rash makes this answer incorrect. Cystitis (C) may cause discomfort on urinating and increased frequency but is unlikely to cause a purulent urethral discharge, making this answer incorrect. Syphilis (E) does not present with discomfort on urinating or a purulent urethral discharge.

Penile lesion (1)

14 D The presence of a painless, hard ulcer on the penis is describing the chancre of primary syphilis (D). Syphilis is caused by the spirochaete *Treponema pallidum*, which is transmitted through sexual contact or can be acquired trans-placentally. Primary syphilis occurs approximately 3 weeks after initial exposure to the pathogen, when a macule develops at the site of sexual contact. This ulcerates to form a hard, painless chancre, which may resolve spontaneously after a few weeks. Four to eight weeks following primary syphilis, secondary syphilis (E) may occur, which is characterized by general symptoms including lymphadenopathy, malaise, a generalized rash and other symptoms depending on which organ has been affected by infection. Tertiary syphilis may occur over two years from initial infection and is characterized by granulomas of the skin and bones. Neurosyphilis refers to infection of the central nervous system, which may occur at any point in the disease. Similarly, involvement of the cardiovascular system results in cardiovascular syphilis (which may result in aortic aneurysms of aortic regurgitation). Chancroid (A) is caused by *Haemophilus ducreyi* and is characterized by the formation of a soft genital ulcer. Genital herpes (B) presents as an abrupt onset, painful vesicular rash over the genitalia. Thus, this is the incorrect answer. Chlamydia (C) is usually asymptomatic and when clinical features are present it does not cause the formation of a hard painless chancre.

Penile lesion (2)

15 E This is a difficult question. Primary syphilis is treated with procaine penicillin (E). A shorter course can be used in the treatment of primary syphilis compared to the later stages of disease (for example 14 days instead of 28 days). If penicillin cannot be tolerated, doxycycline or tetracycline can be used. Co-amoxiclav (A) is not used in the treatment of syphilis. Aciclovir (B) is an antiviral that is not used in the treatment of syphilis. Azithromycin (C) is a macrolide antibiotic that has been used to treat syphilis in the past. It is also used to treat chancroid. However, the drug of choice in this patient is procaine penicillin, making azithromycin (C) the incorrect answer. Ciprofloxacin (D) is a quinolone antibiotic that is also used in the treatment of chancroid, but not in the treatment of primary syphilis.

Jaundice (1)

16 A Hepatitis A (A) is the most common type of viral hepatitis in the world. The hepatitis A virus is a picornovirus that is transmitted faeco-orally, usually due to the ingestion of contaminated water. The virus replicates in the liver and is excreted in the bile and then the faeces of infected individuals. Following infection, the viraemia causes the prodromal symptoms of fever, malaise, anorexia and nausea. Subsequently, jaundice may develop. As this happens, the spleen or liver may be palpable. The history of travel, the friends being affected and the clinical features should identify hepatitis A as the correct answer in this case. Gilbert's syndrome (D) is an inherited hyperbilirubinaemia that is completely asymptomatic and is normally detected as an incidental finding of a raised bilirubin with other blood results within the normal parameters. While the affected individuals in this question are brothers, the jaundice has been acquired, making Gilbert's syndrome the incorrect answer. Hepatitis B (B) is transmitted intravenously and is also sexually transmitted. In addition, it may also be transmitted vertically from mother to child. Clinical features may be similar to those seen in hepatitis A. In addition, extrahepatic features, such as rashes, arthralgia and glomerulonephritis, are more common. The outbreak of disease among three travellers makes hepatitis A the more likely option in this question. Hepatitis C (C) is transmitted by the intravenous route and is sexually transmitted. Acute infection is usually asymptomatic or mild, making this answer incorrect for this question. The majority of patients develop a chronic infection which predisposes to developing liver cirrhosis. The most common presenting features of malaria (E) are fevers, headache, vomiting or diarrhoea. While patients with malaria may develop jaundice and have a palpable liver, the absence of the other features of malaria, including pyrexia, make this answer incorrect.

Jaundice (2)

17 C Treatment of hepatitis A infection is with conservative management (C), using supportive measures where required. Hepatitis A usually has a self-limiting course and the majority of patients make a full recovery. A small minority of patients may develop fulminant hepatitis. Intravenous hydrocortisone (A) is not a treatment for hepatitis A. Pegylated interferon alpha plus ribavirin (B) is a treatment for hepatitis C. Acyclovir (D) is a guanosine analogue antiviral drug, but it is not used in the treatment of hepatitis A. Chloroquine (E) is an anti-malarial.

Sore throat

18 C This case describes the presentation of infectious mononucleosis (C) or glandular fever. This is caused by Epstein–Barr virus (EBV), spread by saliva or droplet infection. When acquired in the young, it is usually asymptomatic. However, infection in young adults can result in illness. Additional clinical features to those described in this case include splenomegaly, hepatitis and severe fatigue (particularly when the infection is chronic). Complications of illness include meningitis, encephalitis and Guillain–Barré syndrome. Toxoplasmosis (A) is caused by the protozoan *Toxoplasma gondii* and is usually acquired following the ingestion of poorly cooked meat. Most infections are asymptomatic but it can occasionally resemble infectious mononucleosis. Cytomegalovirus (CMV) infection (B) is acquired by blood-borne transmission, direct contact or organ transplantation. In the immunocompetent, primary infection is usually latent and there may be reactivation in times of immunocompromise. Clinical features include fever, pneumonitis, colitis, hepatitis, retinitis and CNS disease. In patients with AIDS, CMV most commonly causes retinitis. Streptococcal sore throat (D) is an important differential and may produce a sore throat similar to that seen in infectious mononucleosis. However, it will not produce the widespread lymphadenopathy described in this case. In addition, atypical mononuclear cells are not seen on blood film in patients with streptococcal sore throat. While influenza (E) can cause some of the non-specific symptoms in this case, such as fever and anorexia, it will not result in the presence of atypical lymphocytes on blood film, making this answer incorrect.

Neck stiffness

19 C This case is describing the presentation of a patient with bacterial meningitis. Typical features on presentation include signs of meningism, such as neck stiffness and photophobia, deceased consciousness and a non-blanching petechial rash over the trunk and lower limbs. The immediate management of this life-threatening condition is crucial knowledge as it will save lives, and drugs and doses are worth remembering. The best management is administration of 1.2 mg of IM or IV benzylpenicillin (C) and then immediate transfer to a hospital. Sending this patient home (B) is thus inappropriate. Ciprofloxacin (D) is a usually given to contacts of the patient as prophylaxis against infection, rather than in the treatment. Bloods (E), blood cultures and, if possible, a lumbar puncture are all necessary investigations, but the patient must be given the initial dose of antibiotic and then sent urgently to accident and emergency (A).

Facial swelling

20 B Mumps (B) is caused by a paramyxovirus and is transmitted by droplet infection or direct contact. Clinical features of mumps include fever, malaise, headache, lethargy and pain and swelling of the parotid glands. Parotid gland swelling may be unilateral or bilateral. Complications of disease include CNS involvement, causing a clinical meningitis, epididymo-orchitis, oophiritis, myocarditis, pancreatitis, mastitis and hepatitis. Measles (A) is also caused by a paramyxovirus and its clinical features include initial onset of fevers, cough, coryza and conjuncitivits. Koplik's spots, which are clustered grey lesions in the buccal mucosa adjacent to the second molar, may be seen and are pathognomonic of measles. Following the initial symptoms, there is development of a maculopapular rash over the face, which then spreads to the rest of the body, Therefore, measles is not the correct answer in this question. While influenza (C) may cause fevers and lethargy, it does not produce the parotid gland swelling described in this question, making it the wrong answer. Similarly, while fevers, lethargy and swollen erythematous tonsils may be seen in patients with infectious mononucleosis (D), parotid swelling is not a feature, making this answer wrong. Petrussis (E) is whooping cough and is caused by the gram-negative bacteria *Bordetella pertussis*. The absence of the paroxysms of coughing seen in whooping cough make this the incorrect answer.

Rash (3)

21 A Lyme disease (A) is caused by the spirochaete *Borrelia burgdorferi*. Infection is transmitted by ixodid ticks. Initial symptoms usually manifest around 10 days after the bite. Characteristically, there is a flu-like illness, as described in the case in this question, and an expanding skin rash, known as 'erythema chronicum migrans'. The second stage of the disease may occur some weeks later and cause neurological manifestations (such as encephalitis or neuropathies), arthritis or cardiac manifestations. Acute sarcoidosis (B) may present with erythema nodosum and arthritis. However, it does not present with erythema chronicum migrans or flu-like symptoms, making this answer incorrect. Brucellosis (C) or Malta fever may present with the flu-like symptoms described in this case. However, onset of symptoms is usually slower and infection may become chronic. In addition, erythema chronicum migrans is not seen in Brucellosis, making this answer wrong. Similarly, the description of this distinctive rash allows exclusion of syphilis (D) as the correct answer. Erythema ab igne (E) is a skin reaction that is caused by long-term exposure to heat (for example hot water bottles or heaters).

Haemoptysis (2)

22 D This is a straightforward question. The diagnosis of tuberculosis is confirmed on staining of sputum with Ziehl–Nielsen staining (D) for acid-fast bacilli. Tuberculin skin testing (A) is when the tuberculosis antigen is injected intradermally and the size of the reaction is measured 48–72 hours later. While this test indicates immunity to tuberculosis, it does not help confirm a diagnosis of the disease. Blood cultures (B) are not useful in the diagnosis of tuberculosis. Sputum cultures however, which are grown on Lowenstein–Jensen medium for up to 12 weeks, can confirm the diagnosis. This test has the added advantage that antibiotic sensitivity can also be determined. Chest x-ray (C) is highly useful and may demonstrate a cavitating lesion of pulmonary tuberculosis. However, a diagnosis on microscopy or culture is needed to confirm the x-ray findings. CTPA (E) is the investigation of choice in the diagnosis of pulmonary embolism.

Neck stiffness

23 E *Streptococcus pneumoniae* (A) and *Neisseria meningitidis* (C) account for 80 per cent of acute bacterial meningitis in adults. Meningitis caused by *Neisseria meningitidis* is called meningococcal meningitis. The presence of a non-blanching, petechial rash indicates that the meningitis is caused by *Neisseria meningitidis*. While VZV (D) can cause viral meningitis, the presence of the rash should indicate that this is not the correct answer. *Neisseria gonorrhoeae* (C) causes gonorrhoea while *Listeria monocytogenes* (B) is an important cause of neonatal meningitis.

Skin lesion (1)

24 A Leishmaniasis (A) is caused by the *Leishmania* protozoa, transmitted by sandflies, and is seen in areas of Africa, Europe, Asia, Central and South America. The case described in this question is of cutaneous leishmaniaisis.

In cutaneous leishmaniaisis, lesions develop at the bite site. These start as an itchy papule and develop into erythematous ulcers with raised edges. In visceral leishmaniasis, the protozoa spread from the cutaneous lesions, via the lymphatics to the reticuloendothelial system. Onset of symptoms may be insidious and features include fever, sweats, cough and arthralgia. The liver, spleen and lymph nodes are usually enlarged on physical examination. Mucocutaenous leishmaniasis occurs when primary cutaneous lesions spread to the mucosa of the nose, palate, pharynx or larynx. African typanosomiasis (B) is sleeping sickness and is caused by *Trypanosoma gambiense*. Herpes zoster (C) is shingles, which presents with a blistering rash across a well-demarcated dermatomal distribution. Schistosomiasis (D) is caused by water-borne fluke worms and does not result in the cutaneous lesions described in this question, making the answer incorrect. Cryptosporidiosis (E) is a parasitic disease that results in fever and watery diarrhoea.

Leishmaniasis

25 E Leishman–Donovan bodies (E) may be seen in bone marrow, spleen, lymph node or skin lesions in patients with leishmaniasis and confirms the disease. Leishmania is transmitted by the phlebotomine sandfly, making options (A) and (D) incorrect. Leishmania are not bacteria (B), they are protozoa. There are multiple *Leishmania* species found in different parts of the world that result in cutaneous, mucocutaneoous and visceral leishmaniasis. The clinical picture produced is dependent on the *Leishmania* species and the reaction of the host immune system. Visceral leishmaniasis is not a self-limiting condition (C) and, if left untreated, may result in pancytopenia which can be life threatening.

Itchy rash (1)

26 B Schistosomiasis (B) is caused by water-borne flukes. Snail vectors release cercariae into the water where they can penetrate the skin or mucous membranes of humans. An itchy papular rash (known as a swimmer's itch) may develop at the site of penetration. Once they have penetrated through the skin or the mucous membranes, the schistosomoules migrate to the liver. Approximately 3 weeks after infection, the host may develop fever, rash, myalgia, diarrhoea and there may be hepatosplenomegaly on examination (this reaction is termed Katayama fever). The flukes mature in the liver and then migrate to their final destination (either the mesenteric veins or the vesicular plexus). In their final positions, the flukes may result in a chronic infection with varying clinical features.

Leishmaniasis (B) is a parasitic infection transmitted via sand flies. While cutaneous leishmaniasis may present with skin signs and symptoms, the itchy papular rash seen in this case is not a feature. The fevers and palpable liver edge described in this case may be the initial features of visceral leishmaniasis, but onset tends be slower that what has been described in this case and take a longer time to be manifested from the initial infection. African trypanosomiasis (C) is sleeping sickness. Malaria might present with the fever, lethargy and myalgia described. This should be considered as a potential diagnosis, especially due to the travel history. However, the presence of the papular rash and eosinophilia mean that malaria (D) is the wrong answer. Similarly, influenza (E) does not result in an eosinophilia, making this answer incorrect.

Pale stools

27 D Giardia (D) is caused by the protozoa *Giardia intestinalis/lamblia*. It causes small intestinal disease with diarrhoea, abdominal discomfort and bloating. Stools may become pale and offensive and symptoms may persist. Diagnosis can be made from stool cultures, although a negative stool culture does not exclude giardia. Treatment is with a short course of metronidazole. Coeliac disease (A) is caused by inflammation of the jejunal mucosa and is characterized by gluten intolerance. While it can occur at any age, peak incidence is in infancy and in the fifth decade. The symptoms of coeliac disease may be similar to the symptoms in this question with abdominal discomfort, bloating, diarrhoea and pale stools. There may also be other features such as mouth ulcers and angular stomatitis. The travel history and the age of the patient mean that Giardia (D) is the more likely answer than coeliac disease (A). While enterotoxigenic *E. coli* gastroenteritis (B) and salmonella (C) both cause diarrhoea, the duration of symptoms mean that these answers are not the correct answers. Cryptosporidiosis (E) causes general malaise and watery diarrhoea, which normally improves after 10 days, making this answer unlikely.

Rash (4)

28 C The case in this question describes the presentation of a patient with typhoid (C). This is caused by infection with *Salmonella typhi*. The features in the question that should alert the diagnosis of typhoid are the patchy maculopapular rash (known as rose spots), which occur in approximately 40 per cent of cases, and the low white cell count, due to a leukopenia. The patient may initially be constipated and subsequently develop diarrhoea. Complications of disease include meningitis, pneumonia, osteomyelitis and intestinal perforation. Diagnosis of typhoid is confirmed on culture of blood, bone marrow, urine or stool. Tetanus (A) may initially present with fevers and malaise, but the rash on the trunk, splenomegaly and low white cell count are not features, making this answer incorrect. Malaria (B) should be considered in returning travellers with a pyrexia and thick and thin blood films sent. However, the maculopapular rash is not seen in malaria, thus making this answer incorrect. Cholera (D) presents with diarrhoea, which is occasionally profuse and watery. Primary syphilis (E) does not present with a fever, rash or splenomegaly making this answer incorrect.

Lockjaw

29 A Tetanus is caused by *Clostridium tetani* (A). This is a toxin-secreting organism which is usually found in the soil or metalwork. Infection occurs following contaminated wounds. Clinical features include fevers, malaise and headache followed by the classical features of trismus (lockjaw), risus sardomicus (characteristic facial expression), muscular spasms or autonomic dysfunction. Patients who present with wounds in which there is a suspicion of contamination should be vaccinated with human tetanus immunoglobulin. Dislocation of the temporomandibular joint (B) is unlikely due to the flu-like symptoms preceding the presentation and the absence of trauma. *Clostridium perfringens* (C) may cause gastroenteritis following ingestion of contaminated food or gas gangrene when wounds are infected. Influenza (D) does not cause trismus and *Clostridium difficile* (E) infection causes offensive diarrhoea and is related to the use of broad spectrum antibiotics.

Sepsis

30 B MRSA is a hospital-acquired infection which may colonize the skin, cause wound infections, pneumonias or septicaemia. The case in this question is describing sepsis as a result of MRSA. The most appropriate management of this patient is with isolation, barrier nursing and intravenous vancomycin (B). The patient is septic and thus conservative management (A) is inappropriate. Co-amoxiclav (C), gentamicin (D) and metronidazole (E) are not used in the treatment of MRSA. Isolation, barrier nursing, hand washing and removal of lines when possible are needed to prevent the spread of MRSA.

Heart murmur

31 E The most common organism causing endocarditis is *Streptoccus viridans* (E), which is thought to account for 30–50 per cent of cases, infection commonly occurs following dental procedures. *Staphlococcus aureus* (A) is a common cause of infective endocarditis and accounts for a greater proportion of cases among intravenous drug users and those with prosthetic heart valves. *Staphlococcus epidermidis* (B) can cause infective endocarditis and tends to cause a more indolent disease. *Actinobacillus* (C) is a gram-negative bacteria that is a relatively rare cause of endocarditis. *Enterococcus faecalis* (D) is fairly common cause of endocarditis but is less common that streptococcus viridans. It is important to note that sometimes, no cause of endocarditis is found.

Itchy rash (2)

32 A Scabies is caused by *Sarcoptes scabiei* (A). It presents with an itchy papular rash, which most commonly involves the web spaces of the fingers, on the palms of the hands and soles of the feet, in the axilla and genitalia. There might be visible skin burrows where the mite has tunnelled and this is a classic sign. Shingles (B) presents with a painful blistering rash over a dermatomal distribution, hence this is not the answer. Chicken pox (C) presents with a widespread itchy vesicular rash. Molluscum contagiosum (D) is caused by a pox virus and presents with multiple small papules. This can affect any part of the body and is spread by direct contact. It usually occurs in children or immunosuppressed adults. Tinea cruris (E) is ringworm of the groin, presenting as well-demarcated red plaques in the groin.

Knee pain (1)

33 B The case in this question describes a patient presenting with septic arthritis. The most common cause of septic arthritis in young fit adults is gonococcal arthritis. The results of the Gram stain should also identify *Neisseriae gonnorrheae* (B) as the correct answer. *Chlamydia trachomatis* (A) may cause reactive arthritis and is a gram-negative bacteria. However, it does not cause septic arthritis and the Gram stain finding of diplococci means that this is the incorrect answer. *Haemophilus influenzae* (C) is a gram-negative bacteria that causes septic arthritis in children. *Streptococcus pneumoniae* (D) is a gram-positive bacteria that commonly causes pneumonia. It is possible for this bacteria to cause septic arthritis. However, the result of the Gram stain and the age of the patient make the answer incorrect in this question. *Streptococcus viridans* (E) is a gram-positive bacteria that is commonly responsible for infective endocarditis.

Knee pain (2)

34 D Like the previous question, this case is describing a patient with septic arthritis. However, this is an older patient. In this category of patients, *Staphlococcus aureus* (D) is the most likely causative organism. As mentioned in the previous question, *Neisseriae gonorrheae* (A) is the most common causative organism of septic arthritis in young fit adults. Therefore, the age of the patient in this case makes this option incorrect. A small proportion of patients with tuberculosis develop septic arthritis. The absence of any features of tuberculosis makes *Mycobacterium tuberculosis* (B) an unlikely option. *Neisseria meningitidis* (C) causes meningococcal septicaemia. These patients may also develop septic arthritis. The absence of features of septic arthritis make this answer incorrect. *Haemophilus influenzae* (E) causes septic arthritis in children. Therefore, the age of the patient makes this option incorrect.

Shortness of breath

35 A *Pneumocystis jiroveci* (A), formerly known as *Pneumocystis carinii*, is a fungal infection that is the most common life-threatening opportunistic infection for people with AIDS. It presents with dry cough, exertional dyspnoea, fever and malaise. Chest x-ray may be normal or show bilateral perihilar interstitial shadowing. On CT scan of the chest, there might be a characteristic ground-glass appearance. Herpes simplex virus type 1 (B) and type 2 (C) cause oral and genital ulcers. *Streptococcus pneumoniae* (D) is the most common cause of pneumonia, but the clinical signs of exertional dyspnoea and dry cough in a patient with HIV make *Pneumocystis jiroveci* far more likely in this question. *Mycoplasma pneumoniae* (E) is a cause of atypical pneumonia, which presents with dry cough, fever and malaise. The patient subgroup, presence of fine crepitations in both lung fields and the x-ray findings make this option incorrect.

Dysphagia

36 C *Candida albicans* (C) is a fungal infection that may colonize the oesophagus of patients with HIV, causing dysphagia and retrosternal discomfort. It is treated with fluconazole or ketoconazole. However, resistance to these organisms is becoming increasingly common. *Staphylococcus aureus* (A) does not colonize the oesophagus and causes ulceration in patients with HIV. *Crytosporidium parvum* (B) is a protozoal infection that presents with abdominal pain, nausea or vomiting and profuse watery diarrhoea. *Pneumocystis jiroveci* (D) causes pneumocystis pneumonia in HIV patients. *Cryptococcus neoformans* (E) causes meningitis in patients with HIV; these patients present with fever, headache and drowsiness. *Cryptococcus neoformans* may then be identified from the cerebrospinal fluid obtained at lumbar puncture.

Skin lesions (2)

37 D Kaposi sarcoma lesions are characteristically well-defined pigmented papules. Lesions may also have surrounding soft tissue swelling and, in patients with HIV, they often occur in the mouth. Within the HIV population, Kaposi's sarcoma has a predisposition for homosexual men and tends to be more aggressive. Kaposi's sarcoma may also involve the gastrointestinal tract and the respiratory system. This visceral Kaposi's sarcoma has a worse prognosis than disease just confined to the skin. Malignant melanoma (A) and basal cell carcinoma (C) are not associated with HIV, making this answer incorrect. Squamous cell carcinoma (B), however, is associated with HIV, but presents with ulcerated lesions with raised edges. Toxoplasmosis (E) is caused by *Toxoplasma gondii* and normally presents with cerebral abscesses or encephalitis in patients with HIV.

Skin lesions (3)

38 D Human herpes virus type 8 (D) is associated with Kaposi's sarcoma. Kaposi's sarcoma is derived from vascular endothelial cells and fibrous tissue. Herpes simplex virus type 1 (A) and herpes simplex virus type 2 (B) cause oral and genital ulcers. Human herpes virus type 3 (C) is also known as VZV and causes chicken pox and shingles. It is important to note that the herpes viruses occur more frequently and with a greater severity in patients who are HIV positive. *Pneumocystis jiroveci* (E) causes pneumocystis pneumonia in patients with HIV.

Visual disturbance

39 B Cytomegalovirus can cause varying pathology in patients with HIV including retinitis, colitis, oesophagitis and pneumonitis. CMV retinitis (B) causes varying symptoms, depending on which part of the retina is involved. The common presenting features include loss of visual acuity, floaters, headache and eye pain. If the macular is involved, there may be complete loss of vision. The characteristic appearance on fundoscopy is the presence of haemorrhages and exudates, described as a 'pizza-pie' appearance. Treatment of CMV retinitis should be started as soon as possible to prevent the infection from spreading and compromising the vision. Retinal detachment (A) should be considered in patients who give a history of floaters. However, the appearance on fundoscopy is characteristic of CMV retinitis, thus making retinal detachment (A) the incorrect answer. Kaposi's sarcoma (C) does not involve the retina, but there may be lesions around the eye. Optic atrophy (D) presents with decreased visual acuity, but pale optic disks are seen on fundoscopy. There is no history to suggest that this patient has diabetes, thus making diabetic retinopathy (E) the incorrect answer.

Confusion

40 A Toxoplasmosis (A) is caused by the protozoa *Toxoplasmosis gondii*. In patients with HIV, it may present with encephalitis. Clinical features include fever, headache confusion and convulsions. As in this case, there may be focal neurological signs on examination. The multiple ring enhancing lesions are the characteristic CT finding. Meningitis (B) may present with a high fever, headache and confusion. However, the focal neurological signs and the presence of multiple ring-enhancing lesions on CT make this answer incorrect. Cryptosporidiosis (C) may affect HIV patients and presents with abdominal pain, nausea and vomiting and profuse diarrhoea. While CMV encephalitis (D) may produce the clinical features described in this question, the CT finding of the multiple ring enhancing lesions makes this answer incorrect. Histoplasmosis (E) may affect HIV patients and presents with respiratory symptoms.

SECTION 12:
EMERGENCIES

Questions

QUESTIONS

1. Epigastric pain

A 43-year-old woman presents to accident and emergency with epigastric pain that started 4 hours ago. The woman describes the pain as being sharp and radiating to her back. She feels nauseous but has not vomited and is fully alert and orientated. The patient responds well to IV fluids and analgesia. Biochemical blood results show:

Bilirubin	8 μmol/L
ALT	38 IU/L
AST	34 IU/L
ALP	421 IU/L
Amylase	1850 U/L

The most appropriate investigation would be:

   A. Abdominal ultrasound (US) scan
   B. Computed tomography (CT) scan
   C. Erect chest x-ray
   D. Endoscopic retrograde cholangiopancreatography (ERCP)
   E. Magnetic resonance imaging (MRI) scan

2. Aspirin overdose

A 28-year-old woman is rushed to accident and emergency in a confused state. Her partner reports seeing the patient vomiting and breathing very rapidly before falling ill, at which point he called the ambulance. Empty aspirin packets were found close to the patient, the partner estimates it has been approximately 45 minutes since the patient may have ingested the pills. The most appropriate first-line management would be:

   A. Haemodialysis
   B. Activated charcoal
   C. IV sodium bicarbonate
   D. Gastric lavage
   E. Intravenous fluids and electrolytes

3. Gum discoloration

A 43-year-old man presents with profuse vomiting, abdominal pain and a faint metallic taste in the mouth. The patient is mildly jaundiced on examination with faint green discoloration of the gums. The patient denies taking any recreational drugs, but mentions he has been away on sabbatical in rural India. The most likely diagnosis is:

    A. Copper poisoning
    B. Magnesium poisoning
    C. Iron toxicity
    D. Liver failure
    E. Organophosphate poisoning

4. Confusion (1)

A 16-year-old boy presents to accident and emergency in a confused state. He appears pale, sweaty and has a heart rate of 110 bpm and temperature of 37°C. Respiratory examination reveals good air entry and a respiratory rate of 12. He is accompanied by a group of friends who admit they had been drinking alcohol earlier and smoking marijuana. They deny he has any medical problems apart from mild asthma and deny ingesting any other recreational substances. Urine dipstick is negative for any significant findings. His blood glucose is 2.1 mmol/L. The most likely cause of the patient's symptoms is:

    A. Diabetic ketoacidosis
    B. Ethanol toxicity
    C. Ecstasy ingestion
    D. Asthma attack
    E. Cannabis toxicity

5. Unconscious man

A 22-year-old unconscious man is brought into accident and emergency. He was found lying alone on the street by passers-by who called the ambulance and the crew mention seeing needles on the floor. The patient's Glasgow Coma Scale is 12, he has a respiratory rate of 10 and blood pressure of 97/65 mmHg. During your examination you notice pinpoint pupils. The most appropriate treatment is:

    A. Mechanical ventilation
    B. IV naloxone
    C. IV naloxazone
    D. IV naltrexone
    E. Methadone

6. Acute headache

An 18-year-old woman presents to her GP. She appears anxious and explains she has been revising for her exams but suffered an acute severe headache this morning which left her unable to work and she has not felt well ever since. She denies any recent travelling, fever or neck stiffness. She appears tearful but otherwise well, with no signs following a neurological examination. The most likely diagnosis is:

    A. Tension headache
    B. Migraine
    C. Subarachnoid haemorrhage
    D. Meningitis
    E. Space-occupying lesion in the brain

7. Breathing difficulty

A 26-year-old man with a past medical history of asthma presents to accident and emergency with difficulty breathing. He has a respiratory rate of 35 bpm, heart rate 120 bpm and difficulty in answering questions. On auscultation, a polyphonic wheeze is heard and SpO_2 is 93 per cent. The patient is unable to perform a peak expiratory flow rate (PEFR). The most appropriate treatment is:

    A. Nebulized adrenaline
    B. IV magnesium sulphate
    C. 100 per cent oxygen
    D. Salbutamol nebulizer
    E. Oral prednisolone

8. Chest pain (1)

A 65-year-old Asian man with type 2 diabetes complains of central chest pain which he describes as severe and crushing in nature. On appearance, the patient appears anxious, sweaty and has difficulty breathing. The most appropriate first-line treatment is:

    A. β-blocker
    B. Glyceryl trinitrate (GTN) sublingual spray
    C. Non-steroidal anti-inflammatory drug (NSAID)
    D. Aspirin
    E. Oxygen therapy

9. Shortness of breath (1)

A 74-year-old man with a known history of chronic obstructive pulmonary disease (COPD) presents with a 3-day history of worsening shortness of breath, wheeze, non-purulent cough and fever. He appears unwell and the following blood results were obtained:

WCC	13.8×10^9/L
CRP	39.2 mg/L
PO_2	49 mmHg
PCO_2	33.2 mmHg
SaO_2	95 per cent

The most appropriate treatment is:

A. Oxygen therapy
B. Antibiotic treatment
C. Physiotherapy
D. Short-acting bronchodilator therapy
E. Intravenous theophylline

10. Chest pain (2)

A 54-year-old known hypertensive male presented with a 3-day history of shortness of breath. The patient reported feeling unwell with a sharp pain in the left side of the chest and loss of appetite. His clinical findings included a heart rate of 117 bpm, blood pressure of 97/85 mmHg, temperature 37.2°C and a respiratory rate of 22 bpm. Respiratory examination showed reduced air entry and hyper-resonance on percussion. The most likely diagnosis is:

A. Tension pneumothorax
B. Pneumonia
C. Pleural effusion
D. Aortic dissection
E. Pulmonary embolism

11. Postoperative chest pain

A 59-year-old obese woman underwent a coronary artery stent procedure. She is a well-controlled type 2 diabetic. The operation was successful. However, after 1 week during recovery, the patient complained of severe chest pain and shortness of breath. Her heart rate was 115 bpm and blood pressure 107/89 mHg. Following resuscitation of the airway, breathing and circulation, an electrocardiogram (ECG) showed sinus tachycardia and right axis deviation. The most appropriate treatment is:

    A. Warfarin
    B. Intravenous adrenaline
    C. Alteplase
    D. Salbutamol
    E. Intravenous heparin

12. Malaena

A 47-year-old man presents to accident and emergency with a 3-day history of melaena. The patient appears pale, has a heart rate of 110 bbpm and blood pressure of 105/71 mmHg. The patient reports suffering a sprained ankle 1 week previously and has been using NSAIDs to control his symptoms. The most likely diagnosis is:

    A. Duodenal ulcer
    B. Gastric ulcer
    C. Colon cancer
    D. Rectal varices
    E. Diverticular disease

13. Shortness of breath (2)

A 69-year-old woman presents to accident and emergency in a distressed state. She is extremely breathless and an audible wheeze can be heard, frothy clear sputum is produced each time she coughs. A gallop rhythm and widespread wheezes and crackles are heard on auscultation. The most likely diagnosis is:

    A. Acute asthma attack
    B. Emphysema
    C. Pneumonia
    D. Pulmonary oedema
    E. COPD

14. Malaise

A 19-year-old woman complains of general malaise and lethargy. She has recently started university after a gap year in the Western Cape of South Africa and is now returning home to visit her parents. She felt feverish with a headache which has become considerably worse by the afternoon with nausea and vomiting. Supine flexion of the patient's neck causes unassisted knee flexion. The most likely diagnosis is:

A. Subarachnoid haemorrhage
B. Encephalitis
C. Bacterial meningitis
D. Epstein–Barr virus (EBV)
E. Malaria

15. Seizures (1)

A 17-year-old male is brought unconscious to accident and emergency. His friends report they were at a nightclub while celebrating his birthday, they deny having any alcohol or recreational drugs. The club has strobe light effects and while these were on he suffered a seizure. The friends called an ambulance and while waiting the patient suffered another seizure shortly after the first, he was not conscious during any of the attacks. The most appropriate treatment is:

A. Intravenous lorazepam
B. Rectal diazepam
C. Intravenous thiamine
D. Intravenous midazolam
E. Intravenous thiopental

16. Diffuse abdominal pain

A 20-year-old woman presents with a 3-day history of diffuse acute abdominal pain. The patient reports feeling generally unwell earlier during the week with a strange sensation in her mouth. She denies any recent travel history or sexual activity. On examination, skin turgor is reduced and a fruity odour can be smelt. The most likely diagnosis is:

A. Pancreatitis
B. Diabetic ketoacidosis
C. Acute porphyria
D. Liver failure
E. Maple syrup urine disease

17. Confusion (2)

A 75-year-old woman presents with confusion to accident and emergency, she was brought in by her neighbours who found her outside her house in her nightclothes during the middle of the day. She appears oedematous in appearance, particularly of her neck. The patient's hand is visibly shaking and while coughing a rust-coloured sputum is produced. Blood tests reveal a mild hyponatraemia while blood pressure is 110/82. The most likely diagnosis is:

A. Sepsis
B. Pneumonia
C. Myxoedema coma
D. Lung cancer
E. Schmidt's syndrome

18. Collapse

A 52-year-old man presents to accident and emergency after collapsing at home. He appears pale on appearance with cold extremities. Blood pressure is 97/73 mmHg, heart rate 110 bpm, temperature 36.9°C and an ECG shows normal findings. Blood culture and urine culture are negative for any findings. He reports returning from a weekend break in Wales, but forgot to take his medication for Crohn's disease with him. The most likely diagnosis is:

A. Addisonian crisis
B. Sepsis
C. Myocardial infarction
D. Abdominal aneurysm rupture
E. Nelson's syndrome

19. Haemoptysis

A 44-year-old woman is brought to accident and emergency after becoming ill at the airport after a flight from Australia. She presents with mild pain that causes her to catch her breath and has been coughing blood-stained sputum. On examination, her respiratory rate is 25, heart rate 100 bpm and blood pressure is 130/85 mmHg. The most appropriate management is:

A. D-dimers
B. Chest x-ray
C. Start heparin therapy
D. Start warfarin
E. CT pulmonary angiography

20. Fever

A 27-year-old woman visits her GP complaining of a fever. She returned from India almost 2 weeks ago and had felt unwell but attributed this to jet lag. After suffering from a fever she rested for 2 days and on recovering returned to work as an accountant. After another 2 days she now reports waking up at night again with a high fever, feeling drowsy and confused. On presentation she appears unwell, pale and sweaty. The most likely diagnosis is:

    A. *Plasmodium falciparum*
    B. *Plasmodium vivax*
    C. *Plasmodium malariae*
    D. *Plasmodium ovale*
    E. *Plasmodium knowlesi*

21. Headaches (1)

A 35-year-old man complains of a three-month history of intermittent excruciating headaches. They are very variable and occur from once a month to three times a week. The headaches are associated with extreme anxiety and sweating. On examination, the patient's blood pressure is 152/95 mmHg and during palpation of the abdomen the patient's skin flushes red. The most likely diagnosis is:

    A. Cluster headache
    B. Phaeochromocytoma
    C. Subarachnoid haemorrhage
    D. Migraine
    E. Temporal arteritis

22. Chest pain (3)

A 47-year-old obese Asian man complains of a sharp pain on the left side of his chest with difficulty breathing. The pain started a few hours ago and does not radiate anywhere, the patient also reports feeling increasingly short of breath and became extremely anxious when he started coughing blood-stained sputum. He states he has been flying all week on business trips and is getting late for his next flight. The most likely diagnosis is:

    A. Myocardial infarction
    B. Muscular injury
    C. Pneumothorax
    D. Pulmonary embolism
    E. Pericarditis

23. Confusion (3)

A 53-year-old severely distressed and confused woman presents to accident and emergency with her husband. A collateral history reveals she has been suffering increasingly severe tremors, sweating and weight loss during the week. Since yesterday she has started to suffer from palpitations and increasing confusion. Blood pressure is 157/93 mmHg and there is an irregularly irregular pulse. The most likely diagnosis is:

- A. Phaeochromocytoma
- B. Carcinoid tumour
- C. Thyroid crisis
- D. Addisonian crisis
- E. Serotonin syndrome

24. Central chest pain

A 57-year-old man complains of a two-month history of chest pain which has recently become more severe. The patient describes the pain as a tightness occurring in the centre of the chest which he most often notices when reaching the top of the stairs. The pain usually recedes after a short rest. In the last 2 weeks he has noticed the pain is more severe and, unless he is sitting down or sleeping, is present all the time. The most likely diagnosis is:

- A. Classical angina
- B. Crescendo angina
- C. Decubitus angina
- D. Prinzmetal angina
- E. Nocturnal angina

25. Headache (2)

A 57-year-old woman complains of a headache and weakness on the right side of her body. The headache is normally worst first thing in the morning and is particularly painful on her left hand side. The weakness has occurred very gradually over several weeks and is most noticeable when lifting objects. On examination, her temperature is 38.5°C, she has recently had a left ear infection which is not causing any pain now. The most likely diagnosis is:

- A. Cerebral abscess
- B. Otitis media
- C. Subdural haemorrhage
- D. Mollaret's meningitis
- E. Cerebellar abscess

26. Chest pain (4)

A 42-year-old man presents with a 2-day history of severe chest pain. The patient reports a sudden ripping sensation at the front of the chest that occasionally radiates to the back. The patient has tried paracetamol and ibuprofen to alleviate the pain, but has had no success. The patient suffers from poorly controlled hypertension and at the last GP appointment his blood pressure was 167/95 mmHg. The most definitive investigation is:

A. ECG
B. Chest x-ray
C. MRI scan
D. Transoesophageal echo
E. CT scan with contrast

27. Muscle weakness

A 53-year-old woman with hypertension presents with muscle weakness and painful cramping. She admits some confusion with her new medication spironolactone after a recent dosage change, and may have taken more than the new prescribed dose. On examination, the patient appears well, an ECG shows absent p waves and widened QRS complexes. The most appropriate treatment is:

A. Intravenous fluids only
B. Intravenous 10 per cent calcium gluconate
C. Nebulized salbutamol
D. Intravenous insulin and dextrose
E. Intravenous insulin alone

28. Dyspnoea

A 17-year-old boy is rushed to accident and emergency after breathing difficulties in a restaurant. The parents report the patient feeling unwell after eating a cake containing nuts. The patient has swollen lips and tongue and an audible wheeze is heard. The most appropriate first-line treatment is:

A. 0.05 mg intravenous adrenaline
B. 100 mg intravenous hydrocortisone
C. 20 mg intravenous chlorphenamine
D. 0.5 mg intramuscular adrenaline
E. 0.3 mg intramuscular adrenaline

29. Confusion (4)

A 51-year-old Caucasian male with poorly controlled hypertension presents to accident and emergency with confusion, nausea and vomiting. His daughter visits him weekly and called the ambulance on finding him in this state at home. Blood pressure measurement shows 200/140 mmHg. The most appropriate management is:

    A. Thiazide diuretic
    B. Angiotension II receptor antagonist
    C. Calcium channel blocker
    D. ACE inhibitor
    E. Beta blocker

30. Leg pain

A 67-year-old woman suffered a fracture to her hip during a fall and undergoes a successful hip replacement. After 2 weeks, the patient complains of pain in her right leg, particularly on movement. On examination, the leg is swollen below the knee, erythematous and tender on palpation. The most appropriate management is:

    A. Unfractionated heparin
    B. Low weight molecular heparin
    C. Warfarin
    D. Early ambulation
    E. Thrombolytic therapy

31. Seizure (2)

A 29-year-old woman is brought to accident and emergency after suffering from a seizure at work witnessed by a colleague. She reports the patient has been unwell for the past week with headaches and nasal congestion, but refused any sick leave. The patient has a temperature of 38.3°C, a swollen bulging eye and an ipsilateral gaze palsy. The most likely diagnosis is:

    A. Cavernous sinus thrombosis
    B. Giant cell arteritis
    C. Duane syndrome
    D. Cerebral abscess
    E. Meningitis

32. Confusion (5)

A 30-year-old man is brought to accident and emergency by his wife in a confused state. After an argument at home, the wife had left the patient and on returning found him unconscious. She suspects he may have made a suicide attempt but had not thought to look for any pills or bottles close to the patient. While waiting to be seen, the patient suffers a seizure. On recovery, an examination shows the patient's temperature is 39°C, pulse is irregular, respiratory rate is 20 and the patient's pupils are dilated. An ECG recording reveals tachycardia and widened QRS complexes, while a blood gas is normal. The most likely substance ingested is:

    A. Carbamazepine
    B. Gabapentin
    C. Aspirin
    D. Sodium valproate
    E. Amitryptiline

33. Petechial rash

A 49-year-old man is assaulted by a gang and is brought into accident and emergency. After resuscitation, he regains consciousness with a Glasgow Coma Scale (GCS) of 15. He has suffered multiple fractures of the left leg and left arm but remains stable. While in the intensive care unit, he becomes agitated and complains of difficulty breathing which does not improve despite high flow oxygen. You notice a widespread petechial rash. The most likely diagnosis is:

    A. Cardiac tamponade
    B. Fat embolism
    C. Pulmonary embolism
    D. Disseminated intravascular coagulation
    E. Pulmonary infarction

34. Chest pain (5)

A 65-year-old man presents with a 25-minute history of severe chest pain that he describes as 'gripping' in nature. The pain does not radiate anywhere and is the most severe pain the patient has experienced. The patient is sweaty and anxious in appearance, tachycardic and has a normal blood pressure. An ECG shows hyperacute T-waves and serum creatinine kinase levels are not raised. The patient has a history of peptic ulcer disease but is otherwise healthy. The most likely diagnosis is:

    A. Prinzemetal angina
    B. Gastro-oesophageal reflux disease (GORD)
    C. Tension pneumothorax
    D. Myocardial infarction
    E. Oesophageal rupture

35. Headache (3)

A 19-year-old woman presents with an acute episode of feeling unwell. While in the middle of moving to a new house, she experienced an extremely severe pain near the back of her head. She denies any recent travelling, fever or neck stiffness. The most definitive investigation is:

    A. Lumbar puncture
    B. Blood culture
    C. CT scan
    D. Fundoscopy
    E. MRI scan

ANSWERS

Epigastric pain

1 A   This patient's history and biochemical results indicate acute pancreatitis, possibly due to biliary tract obstruction such as gallstones indicated by the elevated alkaline phosphatase. An abdominal ultrasound scan (A) is the optimal investigation for gallstones and can reveal pancreatic swelling from pancreatitis. A CT scan (B) is important to investigate pancreatic necrosis, although this usually occurs in severe or recurrent attacks, it is also useful in differentiating between pancreatic carcinoma and chronic pancreatitis. Once a diagnosis has been made, a CT scan is appropriate to determine the next step in management. An MRI scan (E) is more often used in chronic pancreatitis sufferers as often more detailed information can be acquired, such as changes in an already diseased pancreas. Rarely, in other gastrointestinal disorders, e.g. perforated peptic ulcer disease, the serum amylase can be elevated enough (>600) to overlap with pancreatitis. For this reason, an erect chest x-ray (C) can help exclude such causes of pain and amylase elevation. An endoscopic retrograde cholangiopancreatography (ERCP) (D) is often used in emergency situations, e.g. stone impaction in the common bile duct causing worsening symptoms of liver and pancreas.

Aspirin overdose

2 E   In patients who have taken a suspected aspirin overdose, the metabolic pathways to consider include the breakdown of aspirin to salicylic acid by the action of hydrolases which are especially prevalent in the liver. Saturation of these enzymes, as occurs in overdose, causes an increase in the plasma salicylate concentration with systemic consequences, for example renal excretion of bicarbonate creating a metabolic acidosis while respiratory centres are stimulated causing hyperventilation. In all patients first-line therapy must include fluid resuscitation (E) in order to correct dehydration or electrolyte derangement. This is likely to result due to the respiratory alkalosis and metabolic acidosis that occurs in aspirin overdose. Activated charcoal (B) and gastric lavage (D) should also be considered within 1 hour of patients ingesting tablets. Dependent on patient compliance, lavage tends to be used in more serious cases, and then only if the airway is definitively protected, in order to slow absorption. There is, however, no evidence that this improves clinical outcome. In moderate poisoning where salicylate concentration reaches 500–700 mg/L, sodium bicarbonate infusion (C) should be given to create an alkaline urine which increases excretion via the kidney. Sodium bicarbonate first line would aggravate existing hypokalaemia and so this must be corrected first. Haemodialysis (A) is reserved for patients with severe poisoning with plasma salicylate concentration exceeding 700 mg/L, such patients are usually in a coma with severe metabolic acidosis.

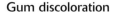

Gum discoloration

3 A   Copper poisoning (A) most often occurs due to ingestion of copper salt-contaminated food products. In India, copper sulphate is used in fertilizer and fungicides and is the most common cause of copper poisoning. The majority of ingested copper accumulates within the liver and is eliminated through the bile. Poisoning features include profuse emesis, diarrhoea, abdominal discomfort and a metallic taste in the oral cavity. In more serious cases, haemolysis and hepatorenal failure can occur, causing death. Treatment is usually with D-penicillamine which acts as a chelator. Magnesium (B) toxicity most often occurs in patients with renal failure, clinical features include narcosis, muscle weakness and hyporeflexia. Calcium gluconate is usually given for cardioprotection. A substantial amount of iron (C) is required before toxicity features present and usually this occurs in patients undergoing regular blood transfusions. Features include black or grey vomitus and gastrointestinal disturbance including pain and diarrhoea. In more severe cases metabolic acidosis, haematemesis and shock can occur. Liver failure (D) is acutely life-threatening in fulminant disease whereby encephalopathy symptoms develop within 2 weeks alongside severe liver function impairment. Patients are most often jaundiced, confused, disorientated and have atrophied livers. Organophosphate poisoning (E) most commonly involves insecticides and in the developing world is a common cause of organophosphorus contamination. Acetylcholinesterase inhibition results from organophosphate exposure causing sympathetic activation with anxiety, sweating, emesis and miosis. In life-threatening situations, respiratory failure can develop requiring atropine injection.

Confusion (1)

4 B   Ethanol intoxication (B) sequelae are usually dependent on the blood alcohol concentration. Alcohol acts primarily as a depressant and in high concentrations can cause renal failure, hypothermia and respiratory depression. In children, more commonly than adults, severe hypoglycaemia refractory to glucagon can occur alongside intoxication. This is due to gluconeogenesis blockage which is the case in this patient, treatment involves glucose infusion. Diabetic ketoacidosis (A) usually occurs in precipitous insulin secretion failure, patients suffer from metabolic acidosis due to ketone production which would be detected alongside glucose in the urine. Ecstasy ingestion (C) results in symptoms of euphoria with patients feeling energetic and foregoing any desire to sleep or eat. Patients often exhibit hyperthermia, tachycardia and hypertension. In more severe cases, patients can develop delusions and become agitated, which are not features here. An asthma attack (D) would result in tachypnoea, poor air entry and polyphonic auscultatory sounds. In an emergency, a silent chest would be present. Cannabis (E) is usually smoked and causes initial euphoria, altered sensations and tachycardia. Naive users can suffer acute psychosis but do not suffer hypoglycaemia as a direct result of use.

Unconscious man

5 B This patient is most likely suffering from an opiate overdose which is treated by an opiate antagonist such as naloxone (B). The characteristic features of opiate use include pinpoint pupils, respiratory depression and a comatose state. Methadone (E) is a partial opioid antagonist and, although useful in weaning patients off drugs such as heroin, it would only act to exacerbate the patient's symptoms, especially in this case given its relatively long half-life. Since the patient is able to maintain a respiratory effort, mechanical ventilation (A) would not be necessary. IV naltrexone (D) is another opioid antagonist which has a longer half-life than naloxone and so is less often used in an emergency situation and more for long-term dependency control. Naloxazone (C) is an irreversible opioid receptor antagonist and so is not appropriate in an emergency situation since this requires short-term reversal so that more controlled weaning can be started.

Acute headache

6 C A subarachnoid haemorrhage (SAH) (C) is the result of sudden arterial bleeding into the subarachnoid space and has a characteristic presentation in patients as a sudden, extremely severe headache that typically, but not exclusively, occurs in the occipital region. Vulnerable areas that bleeding may occur include between the posterior communicating and internal carotid artery, between the anterior communicating and anterior cerebral artery and also at the bifurcation of the middle cerebral artery. Other features associated with a SAH include nausea, vomiting and in severe cases a confused state or even coma. A tension headache (A) is often precipitated by periods of stress and typically presents as a tight constriction around the circumference of the head but can also manifest as a diffuse throbbing or pulsing sensation. Such headaches are benign in nature and usually dissipate with reassurance and rest. An exploration of depressive symptoms should always be conducted as it is a common co-morbidity. A migraine (B) can be broad in presentation and often presents similarly in nature to tension headaches or hemicranially. However, they are also associated with premonatory prodromal auras that can be varied in presentation, such as visual disturbances, transient neurological sensations such as paraesthesia or simply as nausea. Meningitis (D) often presents with the characteristic triad of fever, headache and neck stiffness. Sensitivity to light, nausea and vomiting are often associated with these symptoms which are not present in this patient. A space-occupying lesion in the brain (E) will present, most likely dependent on the structures that it impinges upon. This most often occurs in one of the following three mechanisms: local destruction of brain structure, secondary to the effects of raised intracranial pressure (look for Kernig's sign and Brudzinski's sign) and lastly generalized or partial seizures.

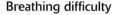

Breathing difficulty

7 C   The British Thoracic Society guidelines identify clinical signs of severe asthma as including exhaustion, cyanosis, silent chest and hypotension while measurements include peak expiratory flow (PEF) <33 per cent of predicted flow, SpO_2 <92 per cent, PaO_2 <8 kPa and a normal $PaCO_2$ (4.6–6.0 kPa). An acute attack is defined by any one the following criteria: PEF 33–50 per cent, respiratory rate ≥25/min, heart rate ≥110/min or inability to complete sentences. In this patient, the diagnosis best fits an episode of acute asthma with hypoxaemia for which the optimal management is oxygen (C) in order to maintain an SpO_2 between 94 and 98 per cent and combat hypoxaemia. β_2 agonist bronchodilators (D), such as salbutamol, constitute second-line therapy in the presence of hypoxaemia. In acute asthma with normal oxygen levels, high dose inhaled bronchodilators are first-line therapy as they act efficiently to reduce bronchospasm, there is no advantage in giving nebulized adrenaline (A) which acts as a non-selective β_2 agonist when compared to salbutamol or terbutaline. High-dose steroid (E) therapy follows oxygen and bronchodilator interventions and may be given orally or parenterally dependent on the patient's ability to swallow. IV magnesium sulphate (B) has bronchodilatory effects also and is considered only if there is no response to inhaled bronchodilators or in life-threatening asthma.

Chest pain (1)

8 B   In an acute presentation of suspected acute coronary syndrome, pain relief through a glyceryl trinitrate (GTN) spray (B) or intravenous opioids should be given to relieve the patient's symptoms. This allows them to be more cooperative during history taking as well as interventions. NSAIDs (C) do not provide adequate pain relief and are not appropriate. Following pain relief, a loading dose of 300 mg aspirin (D) should be given unless the patient is allergic to it. Oxygen therapy (E) should not be given routinely unless oxygen saturation falls below 94 per cent. Once patients are stable, β-blockers (A) are given for the relief of on-going chest pain.

Shortness of breath

9 D   This patient is suffering an exacerbation of pre-existing COPD and management should follow a step-wise approach. Increased frequency of bronchodilator use (D) is first-line therapy to stabilize the patient and provide acute relief of symptoms. Following a short-acting bronchodilator, oxygen therapy (A) is considered only to maintain SaO_2 within an appropriate target range for the patient, since the patient is not hypoxaemic it is not required here. The guidelines for oxygen delivery in acute exacerbations of COPD are currently being reviewed. IV theophyllines (E) are considered following poor response to bronchodilator therapy.

Physiotherapy (C) is useful in clearing sputum once symptomatic relief has been provided. Antibiotics (B) are considered if there are clinical signs of pneumonia or if the patient has purulent sputum, however, this does not precede airway stabilization.

Chest pain (2)

10 A A tension pneumothorax (A) is a medical emergency and is characterized by the occupation of gas within the pleural cavity in between the chest wall and lung, through a one-way valve, such that air enters the lung but cannot escape. This results in a number of dangerous complications including mediastinal shift away from the site of the pneumothorax including heart and associated vessels, collapse of the lung on the affected side and compression of the opposite lung. Patients appear clinically unwell and associated signs include a progressive hypoxic and hypercapnoeic state, tachycardia, late hypotension and hyper-resonance on chest percussion which does not occur in answers (B) to (E). A chest x-ray is helpful in confirming the clinical signs, a needle thoracostomy provides emergency treatment until a chest drain can be inserted for more definitive management. Pneumonia (B) is the inflammation of the lung tissue most often due to a bacterial infection. Patients typically present with fever, cough, pleuritic pain and purulent sputum. Clinical signs include that of lung consolidation with dullness on percussion. A pleural effusion (C) is excess fluid that surrounds the lung due to a number of causes, such as heart failure and liver failure. The excess fluid can impair lung expansion and typically patients have a stony dullness to percussion. An aortic dissection (D) is often precipitated by hypertension causing a tear into the arterial intima, this is expanded by blood penetration and can involve the aortic arch or descending thoracic aorta. Patients complain of a severe 'tearing' pain that begins in the chest and radiates to the back. A pulmonary embolism (E) is a dislodged thrombus which usually originates in the venous system and travels to the pulmonary vasculature. Symptoms typically include abrupt shortness of breath and as further lung damage and infarction ensues, haemoptysis and pleuritic chest pain can occur.

Postoperative chest pain

11 E This patient most likely has a pulmonary embolism which occurs following the migration of a thrombus from the venous vasculature or less commonly from the right side of the heart into the pulmonary vasculature where it eventually causes pulmonary infarction. Risk factors for venous thromboembolism include major surgical procedures, pregnancy, malignancy and hypertension among others. In the absence of dyspnoea and/or tachypnoea, a pulmonary embolism is less likely. Treatment in a suspected pulmonary embolism is with heparin (E) which is then followed by warfarin (A). Unfractionated heparin is given intravenously and low molecular weight heparin is given subcutaneously. Warfarin is not started first without heparin cover because the risk of clotting becomes elevated. Warfarin inhibits clotting factors II, VII, IX, X which promote coagulation and protein C and S which are anticoagulant. However, protein C and S disappear first, leaving the blood in a procoagulant state. Alteplase (C) is reserved for use in stable patients with a confirmed massive pulmonary embolism. Salbutamol (D) is β_2 agonist that would aid air entry but would not stabilize the patient's cardiovascular system. Adrenaline (B) does not feature in suspected pulmonary embolism management.

Malaena

12 B This patient has most likely suffered a gastric ulcer bleed (B), the action of NSAIDs such as aspirin causes a reduction of mucosal prostaglandins by inhibiting the cyclo-oxygenase pathway. This leads to increased damage to the gastric mucosa from increased gastric acid exposure causing pain and in severe cases severe bleeding. Although duodenal ulcer perforation (A) occurs more commonly than gastric ulcers, this incidence is now decreasing due to pharmacological action against *Helicobacter pylori*. The use of NSAIDs more commonly causes gastric ulceration, otherwise duodenal ulcers share the same risk factors as gastric ulcers. Colon cancer (C) is often accompanied by a distinct set of symptoms that include changes in regular bowel movements, changes in frequency and consistency of stool, abdominal masses and rectal bleeding. Symptoms of malignancy, such as unexplained weight loss, should always raise suspicions of a malignancy, which is not a feature in this case. Rectal varices (D) can produce painless bleeding, however they tend to occur in older patients and are not associated with analgesia use and so are less likely in this case. Diverticular disease (E) is most often asymptomatic in most patients unless complicated by diverticulitis. Symptoms most often arise in the left iliac fossa with changes in normal bowel habits and intermittent pain.

Shortness of breath

13 D Pulmonary oedema (D) is the accumulation of fluid within the lung, most often occurring due to cardiac failure leading to hydrostatic backpressure of fluid into the lung or direct lung injury. The excess fluid causes impaired gaseous exchange presenting as shortness of breath with frothy sputum often being produced. The presence of a gallop rhythm in this case most likely signifies heart failure. A patient with an acute asthma attack (A) can present similarly to this case of pulmonary oedema. However, on auscultation, reduced breath sounds, polyphonic wheeze and the presence of frothy sputum is not a common feature in pulmonary oedema. Emphysema (B) is a progressive lung disease characterized by destruction of small lung tissue, air becomes trapped causing shortness of breath and lung expansion. Such patients often have less sputum and suffer weight loss. Pneumonia (C) infection commonly presents with fever, pleuritic chest pain and a dry cough or rust-coloured sputum. In COPD (E), there is a common association with smoking and patients usually present with a cough which tends to be worse in the morning, shortness of breath and small volumes of colourless sputum, unless there is an underlying infection.

Malaise

14 C Bacterial meningitis (C) is often defined by the important triad of fever, headache and neck stiffness. Nausea, vomiting, acute malaise, severe headache, irritability and photophobia are also commonly associated features. These symptoms can progress within minutes and mild symptoms can be deceiving. A subarachnoid haemorrhage (A) is due to sudden arterial bleeding into the subarachnoid space and characteristically presents with a sudden, extremely severe headache. Other features associated with a SAH include nausea, vomiting and in severe cases a confused state or even coma. An encephalitis (B) describes an acute inflammation of the brain and can be similar to meningitis with symptoms of headache and fever. More prominent in this condition, however, are progressive drowsiness, confusion and in severe disease neurological problems such as seizures and hallucinations. EBV (D) often occurs in individuals under five years of age and is often asymptomatic. In older patients symptoms are more severe with fever, headache, lethargy and a painful throat and is otherwise known as infectious mononucleosis. Prominent in disease is the presentation of neck lymphadenopathy and splenomegaly. Malaria (E) typically causes a tertian or quartan fever shortly after infection and is associated with rigors and night sweats. Malaria is endemic in the northern and eastern parts of South Africa with low risk in the western and southern-most areas.

Seizures (1)

15 B This patient is suffering from status epilepticus, a medical emergency that causes continuous, prolonged seizures while the patient is unconscious with significant mortality occurring in those affected. Prior to resuscitation, first-line management is to give rectal diazepam pre-hospital arrival (B). Intravenous thiamine (C) is given during resuscitation if alcohol abuse or malnutrition is suspected. Once the patient is resuscitated in hospital the next antiepileptic therapy should be intravenous lorazepam (A). Only in refractory status epilepticus should alternatives such as thiopental (E) be used. Intravenous midazolam (D) is optimal for controlling refractory status epilepticus in children.

Diffuse abdominal pain

16 B This patient is most likely suffering from diabetic ketoacidosis (B) whereby insulin deficiency causes a state of uncontrolled metabolism as the body perceives low energy stores. Increased glycogen breakdown from the liver and reduced muscle uptake of glucose causes hyperglycaemia and excess ketones. The hyperglycaemia results in an osmotic diuresis and dehydration which in severe cases can cause renal hypoperfusion. Excess ketones cause a metabolic acidosis and are often discernible as excreted acetones in exhaled breath as a sweet odour. The resultant nausea and vomiting further the degree of dehydration and electrolyte loss. Pancreatitis (A) is most often characterized by severe pain in the epigastric or umbilical region of the abdomen with radiation towards the back. Nausea and vomiting can cause dehydration but ketone production is not a feature in an acute presentation. Acute porphyria (C) occurs due to errors of inborn metabolism with a broad range of potential manifestations which are loosely divided into neurovisceral and photosensitive. Diffuse abdominal pain is a common feature with precipitants such as stress or alcohol intake, but there is no uncontrolled catabolic state causing excess ketones or hyperglycaemia. Although liver failure (D) can also result in a musty sweet odour, this patient is very young with none of the other peripheral stigmata of liver disease such as gynaecomastia, jaundice and abdominal distension, among others. Maple syrup urine disease (E) is a metabolic abnormality that affects branched chain amino acids resulting in a toxic accumulation of amino acids such as valine and leucine. The disorder primarily affects infants and young children with characteristically sweet smelling urine similar to the odour from maple syrup.

Confusion (2)

17 C A myxoedema coma (C) is a medical emergency that results due to the progression of hypothyroidism, typically in elderly females. There are a number of factors that can exacerbate pre-existing hypothyroidism into a state of myxoedema. Patients can present with severe symptoms of hypothyroidism including hypothermia, hyponatraemia, weight gain, confusion and heart failure. The absence of coma does not negate a diagnosis. Although rust-coloured sputum is strongly suggestive of pneumonia (B), this is likely to be the precipitant that has caused the underlying diagnosis of myxoedema with signs of heart failure, hyponatraemia and confusion. Sepsis (A) is unlikely in this patient despite signs of infection. Blood pressure is well maintained. Patients often present with a bounding pulse and warm peripheries due to carbon dioxide retention, other features can include fever and rigors. Lung cancer (D) most commonly presents with features of malignancy such as significant weight loss over a short period of time, coughing and blood stained sputum. Paraneoplastic syndromes can emerge producing strange symptoms such as hyponatraemia secondary to anti-diuretic hormone.

However, this does not account for other features such as heart failure, poor tolerance to environmental temperature and confusion in the presence of mild hyponatraemia. Schmidt's syndrome (E) is otherwise known as polyglandular autoimmune syndrome type II and is part of the immunoendocrinopathy syndromes. It consists of Addison's disease and is most commonly associated with autoimmune thyroid disease and type 1 diabetes. Other diseases can include hypogonadism and myasthenia gravis.

Collapse

18 A This patient is suffering from an acute addisonian crisis (A). The adrenal cortex secretes three steroid based hormones: glucocorticoids (cortisol), mineralocorticoids (aldosterone) and the sex steroids. In primary adrenocortical insufficiency, the abnormality lies at the level of the adrenals which become refractory to the action of increasing adrenocorticotroph hormone (ACTH). In this case, the patient is suffering from secondary adrenocortical insufficiency whereby the use of exogenous steroids, such as in Crohn's disease, causes suppression of the hypothalamic–pituitary–adrenal axis. Long-term use of steroids must be properly managed and never stopped abruptly as this can cause an adrenal crisis whereby the sudden increase in ACTH may exceed the adrenal glands ability to respond in an acute setting. Other precipitants, such as acute stress or infection, can also cause an adrenal crisis and steroid doses should be increased during such periods. Symptoms of crisis can include shock, nausea, vomiting, hypothermia and abdominal pain. A massive adrenal haemorrhage can be caused by a severe stressor such as sepsis (B) or myocardial infarction (C). In sepsis, a precipitating organism in blood culture or urine culture is likely to have been identified and in most cases a high fever is present. Signs of a myocardial infarction are likely to have been seen on ECG, as well as symptoms such as chest pain. An abdominal aneurysm rupture (D) causes catastrophic bleeding and usually occurs in males ≥60 years of age and is accompanied by excruciating pain in the lower back or flanks. Nelson's syndrome (E) encompasses the presentation following a therapeutic bilateral adrenelectomy, most often conducted in children. An ACTH-secreting adenoma arises in the pituitary causing loss of pituitary function and local mass effects, such as vision impairment and hyperpigmentation of the skin due to melanocyte stimulating hormone (MSH), a breakdown product of pro-opiomelanocortin (POMC) which produces ACTH and MSH.

Haemoptysis

19 A This patient is possibly suffering from a pulmonary embolism (PE), risk factors for which include major surgical procedures, pregnancy, malignancy and hypertension among others (see Wells score). Dyspnoea, tachypnoea, pleuritic chest pain and haemoptysis are suggestive of a pulmonary embolism. Although D-dimers (A) are not routine screening tests, a negative result strongly negates a PE and are suitable in this patient where there is no clear diagnosis of PE. In massive PE, they should not be used. Such patients present with collapse, unexplained hypoxia, engorged neck veins and commonly with a right ventricular gallop. If D-dimers are positive, low molecular weight heparin (C) should then be started and a chest x-ray (B) should be considered. If there are signs of a PE on x-ray, a CT pulmonary angiogram (E) is then used to confirm a PE after which warfarin is started once confirmed (D).

Fever

20 A Human malaria is caused most often by one of four species of plasmodium which include *P. falciparum*, *P. vivax*, *P. ovale* and *P. malariae*. Transmission occurs through the bite of the female anopheline mosquito. The incidence of malaria is strongly affected by the appropriate environmental temperature which influences the temperature-dependent development of the parasite in the mosquito gut. Sporozoites, the infective stage of the plasmodium, accumulate in the salivary glands of the mosquito and enter the bloodstream when a human is bitten. Rapid uptake occurs in the liver whereby the sporozoites undergo rapid multiplication as merozoites. *P. vivax* and *P. ovale* often remain dormant in the liver as hypnozoites reactivating at a later date. The other infected hepatocyte cells rupture releasing merozoites into the bloodstream where they are taken up by erythrocyte cells. The merozoites again undergo cyclic multiplication transforming from merozoites to trophozoites to schizonts and then back to mature merozoites. At this stage, the erythrocytes rupture releasing new merozoites to infect fresh erythrocytes. This follows a tertian cycle (48 hours) in *P. falciparum*, *P. vivax* and *P. ovale,* while *P. falciparum* follows a quartan cycle (72 hours), although this more often occurs in more long-standing disease. In *P. vivax* (B) or *P. ovale* (D), infection symptoms tend to be relatively mild, with a slower progression of anaemia and recovery within 6 weeks. However, hypnozoites may reactivate years after initial infection. *P. malariae* (C) is similarly mild in progression but is much more chronic and can last for years. *P. falciparum* (A) infection is distinguishable by its high parasitaemia which can cause mental state changes while elevated cytokines can cause end stage organ damage. *P. knowlesi* (E) is a new malarial infection in humans and can cause severe malarial symptoms. Its asexual cycle lasts around 24 hours with a typical fever following a quotidian/daily cycle.

Headaches (1)

21 B A phaeochromocytoma (B) is a rare malignancy of the sympathetic nervous system. In 90 per cent the tumour occurs in the adrenal gland. In the majority of cases both adrenaline and noradrenaline are produced, although in larger tumours and those arising in the sympathetic chain solely noradrenaline is produced. Clinical features are secondary to the action of excess catecholamine release, which is usually at random. Symptoms include hypertension, sweating, panic attacks, tremor and flushing among many others. Over time, a severe burden is placed on end organs, particularly the cardiovascular system. A cluster headache (A) is a neurovascular abnormality due to unclear mechanisms possibly involving histamine. Patients suffer severe headaches often localized unilaterally to the periorbital area and temple. Pain can last from a few minutes to a few hours with associated lacrimation on the side of the headache, nasal congestion and eye-lid oedema. Diagnosis requires five separate episodes of headache occurring every other day or eight attacks in one day. A subarachnoid haemorrhage (C) is the result of sudden arterial bleeding into the subarachnoid space and characteristically presents as a sudden, extremely severe headache, often called a thunderclap headache. Other features associated with an SAH include nausea, vomiting and in severe cases a confused state or even coma. A migraine (D) defines a recurrent headache that often occurs with premonatory prodromal auras involving visual, gastrointestinal or neurological symptoms, such as paraesthesia, nausea and irritability. Hypertension is not usually an associated feature. Temporal arteritis (E) or giant cell arteritis is an inflammatory granulomatous disease affecting the large cerebral arteries. There is often a strong association with polymyalgia rheumatica. Patients in virtually all cases are over 50 years old, symptoms include severe headaches, scalp and skull tenderness and in severe cases temporary or permanent loss of vision in one eye due to ophthalmic artery involvement can occur.

Chest pain (3)

22 D A pulmonary embolism (D) occurs due to the migration of a dislodged thrombus, usually originating in the venous system and travelling to the pulmonary vasculature. Symptoms typically include abrupt shortness of breath and, as further lung damage and infarction ensues, haemoptysis and pleuritic chest pain occur. Abnormalities in Virchow's triad increase the risk of thromboembolism, namely changes in vessel wall, blood coagulation and in this case blood stasis compounded by the patient's body habitus and long-haul flights which makes pulmonary embolism the most likely answer. A myocardial infarction (A) can have a varied manifestation but classically presents with severe crushing chest pain that is relieved with the action of opiate analgesia. Pain can originate in the centre of the chest, but may radiate to the jaw, arm or even epigastric area, while the patient can appear pale, anxious and sweaty. Atypical features can include shortness of breath and syncope. A muscular injury (B) can be mistaken for a more sinister diagnosis but is characteristically recognized by pain precipitated by movement and also reports of an event causing injury or strain. A pneumothorax (C) is due to the presence of air within the pleural space and can occur due to a myriad of reasons, often in tall young men a spontaneous pneumothorax can occur. In older patients, COPD is often the cause of pleural rupture leading to air escaping into the pleural space. Patients usually present with abrupt pleuritic pain affecting the side of the pneumothorax with progressive difficulty in breathing, pallor and tachycardia. A tension pneumothorax is a medical emergency; in both scenarios there is no association with long haul flights and haemoptysis. Pericarditis (E) is inflammation of the pericardial sac around the heart; patients experience sharp often exquisite pleuritic pain exacerbated by movement such as breathing, coughing and lying down.

Confusion (3)

23 C This patient is most likely suffering from a thyroid storm or crisis (C), a medical emergency that results from complication of hyperthyroidism. Patients present with tachycardia, agitation, palpitation and symptoms of heart failure among others. Precipitants, such as infection, can cause hyperthyroidism to progress towards crisis. Management is tailored towards cardiovascular protection and inhibiting further thyroid hormone production. A phaeochromocytoma (A) is a malignancy of the sympathetic tract and most commonly affects the adrenals. Symptoms tend to be intermittent following excess catecholamine release rather than progressive, and headaches and flushing are more prominent compared to weight loss and confusion. Carcinoid tumour (B) consists of enterochromaffin cells from the small intestine and can secrete vasoactive hormones such as serotonin and histamine. Patients present with flushing, abdominal pain and diarrhoea. An addisonian crisis (D) can be due to a number of stresses such as sepsis, cardiac failure, etc. Symptoms include acute shock, nausea, vomiting, hypothermia and abdominal pain. Blood pressure tends to fall and atrial fibrillation is not an associated feature. Serotonin syndrome (E) is an iatrogenic disorder that is characterized by the triad of autonomic, cognitive and neuromuscular derangements. Symptoms can include confusion, muscular spasms, hyperpyrexia, diarrhoea and tachycardia. The syndrome is precipitated shortly after use of serotonin-based medications such as selective serotonin reuptake inhibitors (SSRIs). Progressive symptoms, atrial fibrillation and weight loss do not usually occur.

Central chest pain

24 B Angina can present in a number of different manifestations. In most patients chest pain is central but can radiate to the jaw or either arm. Breathlessness can be associated and the severity of the pain can range from mild to severe. Crescendo/unstable angina (B) becomes progressively worse and can be symptomatic even at rest. Classical or exertional angina (A) is exacerbated by physical stressors such as exercise, in cold temperature or increased emotional states. Once the stressor is removed, such as with rest, the angina tends to fade rapidly. In most patients, there is a threshold of exercise past which angina pain is precipitated. Decubitus angina (C) is precipitated by changing from a vertical to supine position, most often due to left ventricular impairment. Variant or Prinzmetal angina (D) describes pain that occurs randomly and without a discernible stressor, the patient is usually at rest. The pain occurs due to coronary artery spasm. Nocturnal angina (E) occurs while the patient is asleep and often wakens them. Critical coronary artery disease and vasospasm are believed to be the cause.

Headache (2)

25 A This patient most likely has a cerebral abscess (A), infection into the brain most commonly occurs secondary to another area of infection such as mastoiditis or the paranasal sinuses. Infective organisms tend to be streptococci and staphylococci. A cerebral abscess has four recognized stages of symptoms: stage 1 is early cerebritis lasting less than 5 days, and is initial abscess formation with little local tissue destruction; stage 2 is late cerebritis with a more focal site of infection and necrotic core and lasts less than 14 days; stage 3 is early capsule formation with a reduction in space-occupying effects due to reduction in oedema and formation of a thickened capsule; stage 4 is a late capsule formation and can last for months with a well-defined area of inflammatory debris and necrosis. Symptoms produced include altered cognitive processes, headache, seizures, vomiting, hemiparesis and cranial nerve palsy. Simple otitis media (B) would account for signs of infection such as discharge or fever but more likely is the passage of infection to the brain causing an abscess which explains the neurological symptoms. Mollaret's meningitis (D) is a self-limiting occurrence of meningitis that occurs over years with no bacterial cause. Symptoms include recurrent meningism, headaches and fever with a symptom-free period lasting up to several months. A subdural haemorrhage (C) is the accumulation of venous blood within the subdural space, most often due to a head injury. The occurrence of symptoms following the trauma can range from days to months depending on the degree and rapidity of bleeding. Symptoms include headaches, increasing drowsiness and confusion. Hemiparesism, stupor and coma can also occur. Fever and signs of infection are not usually associated. A cerebellar abscess (E) tends to manifest much more acutely compared to a cerebral abscess with symptoms occurring over hours and days; hydrocephalus also often occurs.

Chest pain (4)

26 E An aortic dissection is often precipitated by hypertension, allowing blood expansion into the arterial intima. The aortic arch or descending thoracic aorta is most commonly involved. Patients complain of a severe 'tearing' pain in the chest which can radiate to the back. There are a number of investigations that may show signs of an aortic dissection. A CT scan with contrast (E) has a sensitivity and specificity close to 100 per cent for diagnosis and can also provide vital information about location and complications distal to the abnormality. A transoesophageal echo (D) has high sensitivity and specificity, but has now largely been replaced by CT scans which are less invasive and more accessible. An MRI scan (C) has similar sensitivity and specificity, to CT scanning and is ideal in patients with renal damage; it is, however, more difficult to conduct in unstable patients. A chest x-ray (B) and ECG (A) may show signs suggestive of an aortic dissection but do not have high enough sensitivity or specificity when compared to other modalities. On chest x-ray, signs may include a widened mediastinum and irregular aortic contours, while on ECG signs may mimic findings of an acute ischaemia. ST segments may be elevated or depressed depending on the location of the dissection.

Muscle weakness

27 B Spironolactone is a potassium-sparing diuretic that acts as an aldosterone antagonist as well as having anti-androgen effects. Common side effects include gynaecomastia in males and risk of hyperkalaemia. Elevated potassium levels can be dangerous due to cardiac abnormalities such as absent P waves, widening of the QRS complexes and peaked T waves. Other symptoms include muscle weakness or painful cramping, paraesthesia and neurological derangement. Severe hyperkalaemia can be asymptomatic and patients are at risk of sudden cardiac death. Management of hyperkalaemia is initially centred around cardiac protection. Slow intravenous 10 per cent calcium gluconate infusion (B) does not lower potassium levels but acts to inhibit cardiac membrane depolarization and so this is first-line therapy. Intravenous insulin and dextrose (D) should follow calcium gluconate infusion. The insulin drives potassium back into cells while dextrose prevents hypoglycaemia. Nebulized salbutamol (C) also acts to lower potassium levels but acts in 30 minutes and so should follow insulin and dextrose infusion. Intravenous fluid (A) and sodium bicarbonate should be infused to correct any metabolic acidosis and to correct fluid deficits following interventions to protect the heart and lower serum potassium. Intravenous insulin (E) should never be infused alone as this puts the patient at risk of developing hypoglycaemia which would be compounded if the patient is also dehydrated.

Dyspnoea

28 D In this patient suffering from a suspected anaphylactic reaction following resuscitation of the airway, breathing and circulation intramuscular adrenaline must be given (0.5–1.0 mL of 1:1000 dilution) (D) in an adult and children above the age of 12. In children between 6 and 12 years, 0.3 mg of intramuscular adrenaline (E) is appropriate. Intravenous adrenaline (A) should only be given by experienced specialists and is rarely considered due to potential cardiac risks. Twenty milligrams intravenous chlorphenamine (C) and 100 mg of intravenous hydrocortisone (B) is only given after adrenaline therapy and fluid challenges.

Confusion (4)

29 D Uncontrolled hypertension presents many risks to the patient and should be dealt with swiftly using appropriate pharmacological intervention. This patient has most likely suffered a cerebrovascular haemorrhage due to uncontrolled hypertension. Patients with blood pressure ≥160/100 or ≥140/90 mmHg with cardiovascular risk factors should receive drug therapy. If they are younger than 55 years and not of African-Caribbean descent, first-line therapy is an oral ACE inhibitor (D). If patients are more than 55 years of age or of African-Caribbean descent a calcium channel blocker (C) or thiazide diuretic (A) should be considered. Angiotension II receptor antagonists (B) should follow in patients intolerant to ACE inhibitors. Beta blockers (E) are no longer preferred as routine first-line therapy for hypertension.

Leg pain

30 B This patient is suffering from deep vein thrombosis, most likely from postoperative venous stasis. There is a risk of embolization of a thrombus to the lung vasculature causing death. Low molecular weight heparin (B) is the best initial therapy compared to unfractionated heparin (A) since they have greater efficacy, require no monitoring and put patients at less risk of bleeding. If low molecular weight heparin is not readily available, then unfractionated heparin may be used. Warfarin (C) follows heparin therapy and is continued once the international normalized ratio enters an appropriate range (approximately 2.5) after which heparin is stopped. Warfarin is not started first with no heparin cover because the risk of clotting becomes elevated. Warfarin inhibits clotting factors II, VII, IX, X which promote coagulation and protein C and S which are anticoagulant. However, protein C and S disappear first leaving the blood in a procoagulant state. Heparin cover is therefore required. Once patients have been fully anticoagulated, ambulation (D) is advised with compression stockings; until then bed rest is advised. Thrombolytic therapy (E) is not currently advised and is reserved for patients with significant deep vein thrombi.

Seizure (2)

31 A This patient is suffering from a cavernous sinus thrombosis (A). The cavernous sinuses are irregular cavities at the base of the skull lying either side of the sella turcica. Blood enters from multiple directions into the cavernous sinus including the facial veins, sphenoid and middle cerebral veins. Any infection of the face may therefore enter the nose or tonsils and spread into the cavernous sinus with disastrous consequences. The third, fourth and sixth cranial nerves are in close proximity while the ophthalmic and maxillary divisions of the trigeminal nerve are also adjacent to the sinus wall. A cavernous sinus thrombosis therefore presents with an assortment of headache, orbital pain, eye swelling and cranial nerve palsies affecting III, IV, VI and part of V. A giant cell arteritis (B) is an inflammatory granulomatous disease which typically affects the large cerebral arteries. Symptoms can include severe headaches, scalp and skull tenderness. In severe cases temporary or permanent loss of vision in one eye can occur due to ophthalmic artery involvement. Patients tend to be over 50 years of age which makes it unlikely in this case. Duane syndrome (C) is a congenital syndrome that limits orbital movements, such as abduction and adduction. A cerebral abscess (D) most commonly produces symptoms of early to late cerebritis in this patient who has been symptomatic for one week. Symptoms such as headache, seizures, vomiting and cranial nerve palsy typically occur insidiously after weeks or months as the abscess grows. Meningitis (E) is characterized by the triad of fever, headache and neck stiffness (Kernig's sign). Sensitivity to light, nausea and vomiting are often associated with these symptoms which are not present in this patient. Cranial nerve symptoms are also unusual.

Confusion (5)

32 E This patient has most likely ingested excess tricyclic antidepressants such as amitryptiline (E). Toxicity results in elevated anticholinergic effects such as pupil dilation, skin flushing, seizures, hypotension and muscle twitching. Cardiac complications typically include prolonged QRS complexes and tachyarrhythmia. Aspirin (C) breaks down into salicylic acid by the action of hydrolases, mostly by the liver. In an overdose, elevated plasma salicylate levels cause several systemic effects: most importantly, renal impairment causing a metabolic acidosis, while respiratory centres are stimulated causing hyperventilation. Carbamazepine (A) is an anticonvulsant and in overdose can cause a dry mouth, convulsions, opthalmopathy, pupil dilation and hallucinations. Muscle twitching is not a usual feature. Gabapentin (B) is a GABA agonist, and in excess causes malaise, slurring of speech and gastrointestinal abnormalities. Sodium valproate (D) is often characterized in excess by drowsiness, respiratory depression and seizures. The patient's respiratory movements have not been affected.

Petechial rash

33 B A fat embolism (B) is the most likely cause of the patient's acute symptoms although the pathophysiology of this disease has not been fully elucidated. Suggestions include the escape of adipose fat cells into the circulation within 1–3 days after trauma of the long bones. The fat globules break down into free fatty acids which then cause local toxic effects all over the body. This supports the occurrence of petechiae, mental state changes and dyspnoea, which is the characteristic triad in fat embolism. A cardiac tamponade (A) would most likely occur soon after trauma and include features such as muffled heart sounds, hypotension and raised jugular venous pressure. Disseminated intravascular coagulation (D) is an uncommon complication during recovery and patients do not normally suffer severe breathlessness. A pulmonary infarction (E) can result in severe dyspnoea but is characteristically the result of longer periods of recovery rather than an acute presentation. A pulmonary embolism (C) can also cause abrupt shortness of breath, haemoptysis and pleuritic chest pain. Petechiae, however, are not a common associated feature.

Chest pain (5)

34 D The patient's clinical presentation with substernal chest pain and ECG changes are strongly suggestive of a myocardial infarction (D). Hyperacute T waves are seen in early ECG changes followed by ST elevation, T wave inversion and then Q waves. Creatinine kinase is not an accurate measure of cardiac damage as they can take several hours to increase, troponins are now more commonly used. Prinzmetal angina (A) is pain that occurs at random and usually when the patient is at rest. The pain is likely due to coronary artery spasm and is not associated with hyperacute T waves on ECG. Gastroesophageal reflux disease (B) can be mistaken for myocardial infarction though the pain is often described as burning more often than gripping and usually occurs for several days rather than abruptly. There are no associated abnormal ECG changes. A tension pneumothorax (C) usually causes pleuritic chest pain and difficulty breathing is a more predominant feature. Such patients can decompensate extremely quickly. An oesophageal rupture (E) can cause pain of a similar site and magnitude as a myocardial infarction, however it is associated with severe retching and vomiting and not T-wave changes on ECG.

Headache (3)

35 C An unenhanced CT scan (C) as soon as possible is the investigation of choice in a patient with a suspected subarachnoid haemorrhage. Over time, signs of a haemorrhage can fade so that a normal scan report occurs. Blood is much easier to see on a CT than on an MRI (E). Blood is white on a CT scan. If a CT scan report is negative for any findings despite clinical symptoms, a lumbar puncture (A) should be offered. A subarachnoid haemorrhage is reabsorbed within 10 days and so may not appear on a CT scan if it is delayed. Hours after haemorrhage the CSF becomes yellow (xanthochromic) due to bilirubin and this is strongly indicative of a subarachnoid haemorrhage. A blood culture (B) would not be appropriate as the patient does not have any features of meningism or infection. Fundoscopy (D) may support cerebral changes, such as papilloedema, due to raised intracranial pressure which would negate a lumbar puncture, however, since a CT scan is first-line investigation it is not appropriate in this case.

SECTION 13:
PRACTICE EXAM

QUESTIONS

1. Cerebral abscess

A 17-year-old boy suffered a generalized seizure at school and is brought to accident and emergency by ambulance. His teachers report he was well during the day but has suffered from repetitive ear infections and despite taking antibiotics during the week still suffered from headaches and ear discharge. On examination, he appears well but complains of headache, his temperature is 39°C and he is neurologically intact. A CT scan confirms a cerebral abscess and rapid culture tests confirm streptococcal infection. The most appropriate management is:

    A. Cefuroxime alone
    B. Cefuroxime and metronidazole
    C. Flucloxacillin alone
    D. Flucloxacillin and cefuroxime
    E. Surgical decompression

2. Hypothalamic–adrenal axis

A 55-year-old woman presented with truncal obesity, easy bruising, a dorsal fat pad and depression. She denies any headaches, weight loss or any other abnormalities. An ultrasound scan showed bilateral adrenal atrophy. The most likely cause is:

    A. Exogenous steroid use
    B. Pituitary dependent Cushing's disease
    C. Ectopic adrenocorticotroph hormone (ACTH) production
    D. Adrenal malignancy
    E. 21-Hydroxylase deficiency

3. Management of cold sores

Which of the following treatment options would be the most appropriate for the management of a cold sore?

    A. Oral acyclovir
    B. Topical acyclovir
    C. Oral amoxicillin
    D. Topical fusidic acid
    E. Topical ketonconazole

4. Onycholysis

Onycholysis is described as separation of the nail from the nail bed which usually starts from the distal and/or lateral attachment and moves proximally. Which of the following is not a cause of onycholysis?

    A. Psoralens
    B. Psoriasis
    C. Thyrotoxicosis
    D. Streptococcal pneumonia
    E. Trauma

5. Peutz–Jeghers syndrome

You see a 21-year-old woman on your ward round who has been admitted for further investigation for longstanding iron deficiency anaemia. You are told by your registrar that colonoscopy revealed multiple hamartomatous polyps suggestive of Peutz–Jeghers syndrome. From the list below, which one of the following is the most likely mode of inheritance of Peutz–Jeghers syndrome:

    A. Autosomal recessive
    B. Autosomal dominant
    C. X-linked dominant
    D. Polygenic
    E. None of the above

6. Chest pain

A 35-year-old woman complains of a sharp central chest that is acutely exacerbated each time she moves, breathes in or lies flat. The pain tends to stay in the centre of the chest but occasionally moves towards her neck and shoulders. The pain is relieved by sitting forward. The patient does not drink alcohol, is not diabetic and does not smoke. A pericardial rub is heard on auscultation. The most appropriate diagnostic investigation is:

    A. CT calcium score
    B. ECG
    C. Serum amylase
    D. Chest x-ray
    E. Echocardiography

7. Dilated cardiomyopathy

A 45-year-old man with a strong family history of dilated cardiomyopathy presents with peripheral oedema, finger clubbing, jugular venous distension and pulmonary rales. A gallop rhythm is heard on auscultation. Which investigation would not be useful in dilated cardiomyopathy?

    A. Chest x-ray
    B. ECG
    C. Biopsy
    D. Echocardiogram
    E. Cardiac MR

8. Inflammatory bowel disease

Which of the following extra-intestinal signs is not seen in ulcerative colitis:

    A. Finger clubbing
    B. Erythema nodosum
    C. Iritis
    D. Sacroiliitis
    E. Granuloma annulare

9. Haemoptysis (1)

A 66-year-old woman presents to your clinic with a 1-week history of haemoptysis. Which of the following from the list of answers below is not a cause of haemoptysis?

    A. Pulmonary tuberculosis
    B. Bronchiectasis
    C. Aspergilloma
    D. Wegener's granulomatosis
    E. Asthma

10. Extrapulmonary manifestations of sarcoidosis

A 60-year-old man presents to you with some signs and symptoms which may be associated with pulmonary sarcoidoisis which was diagnosed nine months ago. From the list below which of the following is not an extrapulmonary manifestation of sarcoidosis?

    A. Splenomegaly
    B. Anterior uveitis
    C. Erythema marginatum
    D. Hepatic granuloma infiltration
    E. Bilateral parotitis and swelling

11. Laboratory investigations (1)

Before the start of a ward round you asked to check the blood results of patients on the general medicine ward round. A new patient has the following results:

Prothrombin time	Normal
Partial thromboplastin time	Prolonged
Bleeding time	Normal
Platelet count	Normal

What is the most likely diagnosis?

    A. Bernard Soulier syndrome
    B. Glanzmann's thrombasthenia
    C. Disseminated intravascular coagulation
    D. Haemophilia
    E. Liver disease

12. Diarrhoea (1)

A 76-year-old man has a 4-day history of profuse watery diarrhoea coupled with abdominal pain. He was seen by his GP 2 weeks ago and started on oral amoxicillin for a lower respiratory tract infection. Stool sample analysis reveals *Clostridium difficile* enterotoxin. His observations are within normal range and the patient is apyrexial. Which of the following is the most appropriate treatment for this patient's condition?

    A. Oral vancomycin
    B. Oral metronidazole
    C. Intravenous metronidazole
    D. Oral ciprofloxacin
    E. No antibiotic treatment required

13. Papilloedema

A 50-year-old woman is brought to accident and emergency by her son who has become increasingly worried about her confused state. Her son states she suffers from chronic hypertension but is poorly compliant with medication and has become increasingly confused over the past week and complaining of hallucinations. On examination, the patient's Glasgow Coma Scale (GCS) is 14, blood pressure is 210/120 mmHg, pulse is 112/min and there is papilloedema on fundoscopy. The most likely diagnosis is:

    A. Subdural haemorrhage
    B. Hypertensive encephalopathy
    C. Lacunar infarction
    D. Vascular dementia
    E. Phaeochromocytoma

14. Ischaemic stroke

A 38-year-old woman with a history of classical migraine is admitted with a right hemisphere ischaemic stroke. She has optimal blood pressure and a very favourable lipid profile, and duplex scanning of the carotids shows total absence of atheromatous plaque. Echocardiography, however, reveals an abnormality which may be relevant. Which of the following is it likely to be?

    A. Ventricular septal defect
    B. Tricuspid incompetence
    C. Left ventricular hypertrophy
    D. Patent foramen ovale (PFO)
    E. Dilate left atrium

15. Glycated haemoglobin

A 50-year-old man is diagnosed with type 2 diabetes and you advise an improved diet alongside exercise. You mention monitoring the patient's HbA1c levels until the glucose becomes more stable. What is the most appropriate HbA1c target?

    A. 6.5 per cent
    B. 6.2 per cent
    C. 6.3 per cent
    D. The patient should select an appropriate achievable target
    E. 6.0 per cent

16. Breathlessness

A 24-year-old woman presents with increasing breathlessness on exertion, which has been developing over several months. There are no abnormal physical signs on examination. On the ECG, there is right axis deviation and an R wave in V1, with peaked P waves. Chest x-ray showed prominent hilar vessels with sparse vasculature peripherally in the lungs. Doppler echocardiography revealed a pulmonary artery pressure of 60 mmHg and primary pulmonary hypertension was diagnosed. Which of the following medications would not be appropriate in managing this patient?

    A. Sildenafil
    B. Bosentan
    C. Warfarin
    D. Prostacyclin
    E. Doxazosin

17. Jaundice

You are told that a patient has been admitted to accident and emergency with jaundice and right upper quadrant pain. What levels of plasma bilirubin would this patient have in order for jaundice to be clinically visible:

    A. >30 µmol/L
    B. >25 µmol/L
    C. >35 µmol/L
    D. >15 µmol/L
    E. >20 µmol/L

18. Abdominal pain

A 64-year-old man presents with a 2-day history of abdominal pain which he describes as constant, dull and around his umbilicus and occasionally migrating to his groin. He has a body mass index (BMI) of 27 and a past medical history of poorly controlled hypertension. Abdominal examination reveals a pulsatile and expansile mass just below the umbilicus. The most appropriate screening investigation is:

    A. Abdominal ultrasound
    B. Abdominal x-ray
    C. Computed tomography (CT) scan of the abdomen
    D. Abdominal magnetic resonance imaging (MRI) scan
    E. Angiography

19. Fever (1)

An 18-year-old man presents with a 3-day history of fever, vomiting and headaches on waking in the morning. He has recently started at university and denies taking any illicit substances prior to or during his time at university. He has tried paracetamol but they have not helped. He decided to see a doctor when his neck became painful and stiff to move. On further examination, a non-blanching petechial rash is discovered. The most appropriate management is:

    A. Intravenous ceftriaxone
    B. Fundoscopy
    C. Lumbar puncture
    D. Intravenous cephalexin
    E. Blood culture

20. Erythroderma

Erythroderma is described as a chronic inflammatory skin condition characterized by scaling affecting greater than 50 per cent of the total body. Which one of the following cutaneous malignancies would you expect erythroderma to be associated with?

    A. T-cell lymphoma
    B. Squamous cell carcinoma (SCC)
    C. Basal cell carcinoma (BCC)
    D. Malignant melanoma
    E. Kaposi's sarcoma

21. Knee pain

A 71-year old woman presents to accident and emergency with pain in the right knee. This has been ongoing for the past five months but she is now finding it difficult to walk. Pain is usually worse after exertion. On examination, the right knee is swollen. There is a reduced range of active movement and palpable crepitus. What are the most likely findings on x-ray?

    A. Increased joint space, subchondral sclerosis, bone cysts and osteophytes
    B. Increased joint space, soft tissue swelling and peri-articular osteopenia
    C. Normal x-ray
    D. Reduced joint space, subchondral sclerosis, bone cysts and osteophytes
    E. Reduced joint space, soft tissue swelling and peri-articular osteopenia

22. Anterior myocardial infarction

A 64-year-old man suffers an anterior myocardial infarction. A few hours later, his pulse rate is noted to be 46/minute and his blood pressure 94/59 mm Hg. He is short of breath and has slight central chest pain. The monitor showed sinus bradycardia. What would be your choice of management?

    A. Insertion of temporary pacing wire
    B. Intravenous isoprenaline
    C. Intravenous atropine
    D. Intravenous adrenaline
    E. Oral salbutamol

23. Heart failure

A 60-year-old man presents to his GP with gradually increasing fatigue and some exertional dyspnoea. Blood pressure is 118/74 mmHg and pulse rate is 81/minute. There are no abnormal physical findings and on echocardiography the ejection fraction is 0.47. However, the clinical impression remains one of early heart failure. Which of the following circulating biomarkers would lend support to that conclusion?

A. Atrial natriuretic peptide
B. Brain natriuretic peptide
C. Endothelin
D. Noradrenaline
E. Adrenomedullin

24. Skin hyperpigmentation

Which of the following conditions from the list below is not associated with cutaneous hyperpigmentation?

A. Hypopituitarism
B. Pregnancy
C. Addison's disease
D. Cushing's syndrome
E. Nelson's syndrome

25. Prosthetic valve endocarditis

A 50-year-old man with type 2 diabetes undergoes a prosthetic aortic valve replacement after suffering from congestive heart failure due to native valve endocarditis. Following the operation, he presents with fever, janeway lesions, splinter haemorrhages and night sweats. The most definitive investigation for prosthetic valve endocarditis is:

A. Auscultation
B. Transthoracic echocardiography
C. Transoesophageal echocardiography
D. Chest x-ray
E. ECG

26. Arterial blood gas interpretation

You are informed that one of your ward patients has been breathless over the last hour and has been quite anxious since her relatives left after visiting. The patient is a 67-year-old woman who was admitted 6 days ago for a left basal pneumonia which has responded well with intravenous antibiotics. Her past medical history includes dementia and hypertension. You are asked by your registrar to interpret the patient's arterial blood gas (ABG) measurements taken during her tachypnoea: pH 7.49 kPa, PO_2 14.1, PCO_2 3.1 kPa, HCO_3 24. From the list of answers below, choose the most appropriate ABG interpretation:

    A. Metabolic alkalosis
    B. Respiratory alkalosis
    C. Type 1 respiratory failure
    D. Respiratory acidosis
    E. None of the above

27. Hypertension

A 41-year-old woman with type 2 diabetes attends a hypertension clinic. She has been doing well on metformin and has maintained good glycaemic control alongside dietary changes and regular physical exercise. She has been meeting her HbA1c targets consistently. However, her blood pressure has been poorly controlled despite lifestyle changes and is currently 157/97 mmHg. The most appropriate first-line therapy is:

    A. Diuretics
    B. Angiotensin II receptor blocker
    C. Calcium channel blocker
    D. β-blocker
    E. Angiotensin-converting enzyme (ACE) inhibitor

28. Seizure (1)

A 46-year-old woman with atrial fibrillation is seen in clinic following an episode of syncope while shopping. She has a family history of epilepsy and a past medical history of breast cancer. She remembers feeling dizzy for a couple of seconds then waking up on the floor. What is the most useful step in management?

    A. Lying–standing blood pressure
    B. A collateral history
    C. An ECG
    D. An MRI brain
    E. A CT head

29. Malignant melanoma

A 36-year-old man has been diagnosed with superficial spreading malignant melanoma. Which one of the following factors will determine the patient's prognosis?

    A. Size of the lesion
    B. Shape of the lesion
    C. Thickness of the lesion
    D. Colour of the lesion
    E. Patient age

30. Chest signs

A 55-year-old man who has been smoking 20 cigarettes a day for the last 30 years has been diagnosed with a right-sided pleural effusion following admission with a week's history of shortness of breath. From the list below, select the most likely findings that one would ascertain during examination of the chest wall:

    A. Decreased air entry coupled increased vocal fremitus and resonant percussion on the right side of the chest
    B. Normal air entry coupled decreased vocal fremitus and resonant percussion on the right side of the chest
    C. Normal air entry coupled increased vocal fremitus and dull percussion on the right side of the chest
    D. Decreased air entry coupled decreased vocal fremitus and dull percussion on the side of the chest
    E. None of the above

31. Diabetes in pregnancy

A 34-year-old diabetic woman attends your hypertension clinic to discuss her blood pressure control. She is currently following lifestyle advice and has started to lose weight and maintain good glycaemic control. Her blood pressure was 155/93 mmHg at her last clinic appointment and is now 150/90 mmHg. She informs you she has recently become pregnant, which was planned, and intends to keep the baby. The most appropriate first-line therapy is:

    A. ACE-inhibitor
    B. Angiotensin II receptor blocker
    C. Calcium channel blocker
    D. Diuretics
    E. β-blocker

32. Severity of pneumonia

You are told by your registrar that a 66-year-old woman from a residential home has been admitted with a right mid-zone community-acquired pneumonia. She is very drowsy and her CURB-65 score is 4. On admission, the patient's oxygen saturations are 91–92 per cent on room air, respiratory rate of 20, temperature of 37.7°C, PO_2 7.1 kPa and PCO_2 4.7 kPa. Her oxygen saturations have improved to 95 per cent on 15 L O_2 via a non-rebreather oxygen mask. From the list below, which is the most appropriate management plan for this patient?

    A.   Oral antibiotics and alert the ITU SpR
    B.   Intravenous antibiotics and transfer to respiratory ward
    C.   Intravenous antibiotics and alert the ITU SpR
    D.   Oral antibiotics and transfer to the respiratory ward
    E.   Alert ITU SpR

33. Hepatocellular carcinoma

You see a 57-year-old man who has been diagnosed with hepatocellular carcinoma (HCC). You are asked about risk factors in HCC by your consultant. Which of the following is not a known predisposing factor for developing hepatocellular carcinoma?

    A.   Hepatitis B virus
    B.   Liver cirrhosis
    C.   Hepatitis C virus
    D.   Hepatitis A virus
    E.   Aflatoxin

34. Diarrhoea (2)

A 69-year-old man, who is recovering from an emergency laparotomy for a ruptured duodenal ulcer, develops profuse offensive diarrhoea. His postoperative course has been complicated by chest infections and he has just been stepped down onto the main wards from the intensive care unit. Stool cultures have revealed C. *difficile* toxin. What is the most appropriate treatment?

    A.   Oral metronidazole
    B.   Intravenous fluids
    C.   Intravenous hydrocortisone
    D.   Oral aciclovir
    E.   Oral co-amoxiclav

35. Blood groups

A child with blood type AB rhesus positive requires a blood transfusion Which of the following blood types would be suitable?

    A. AB rhesus negative
    B. A rhesus positive
    C. B rhesus positive
    D. O rhesus positive
    E. All of the above

36. Confusion (1)

A 69-year-old man presents with confusion. His wife reports he has become increasingly depressed and confused in the last month. Prior to this, he had been complaining of pain in his right arm and abdomen but he refused to visit his GP. The patient has brisk reflexes, reduced skin turgor, sunken eyes and an x-ray of his right arm shows lytic lesions. The most appropriate management is:

    A. Calcitonin
    B. Non-steroidal anti-inflammatory drugs (NSAIDs)
    C. Intravenous bisphosphonates
    D. Stem cell transplant
    E. Intravenous saline

37. Palpitations

An 18-year-old woman is referred with the complaint of recurrent palpitations lasting 2–3 hours and terminating as abruptly as they started. She is otherwise well and finds the episodes uncomfortable but not especially distressing. Examination is entirely normal between attacks. The electrocardiogram (ECG) shows a PR interval of 0.1 seconds and slow upstrokes in the R waves of several leads. What is the most likely diagnosis?

    A. Sinus tachycardia
    B. Acute anxiety
    C. Lown–Ganong–Levine syndrome
    D. Wolff–Parkinson–White syndrome
    E. Nodal tachycardia

38. Seizure (2)

A 23-year-old woman is brought into accident and emergency after collapsing at her office. She admits having been stressed and had stayed up all night preparing for a presentation she gave this morning. She describes sitting at her desk and seeing multicoloured circles of light in her right visual field then waking in the ambulance with an oxygen mask on. She feels tired, achy and confused. Her colleague who witnessed the event tells of his fright as he saw her collapse and start jerking both arms and legs. What best describes her seizure?

A. Tonic–clonic seizure
B. Generalized seizure
C. Grand mal seizure
D. Simple partial seizure with secondary generalization
E. Pseudoseizure

39. Marfans' syndrome

You are asked to examine a 16-year-old boy with suspected Marfans' syndrome. The patient is tall and thin limbed with long slender fingers, you notice a pectus excavatum of the chest and on examination of the mouth a high arched palate is visible. Which of the following is not included in the cardiovascular criteria for Marfans?

A. Aortic dissection
B. Aortic dilatation
C. Mitral valve prolapse
D. Mitral valve regurgitation
E. Mitral valve calcification

40. Thrombocytopenia

A 12-year-old patient complains of easy bruising and nose bleeds, small ecchymoses can be seen on the patient's skin. The patient reports feeling ill in the last week with mild fever and a sore throat. The nose bleeds are not prolonged and stop soon after pressure is applied. A blood test shows a mild thrombocytopenia. The most likely diagnosis is:

A. Immune thrombocytopenic purpura
B. Aplastic anaemia
C. Bernard Soulier syndrome
D. Glanzmann's thrombasthenia
E. Thrombotic thrombocytopenic purpura

41. Stroke complications

An 88-year-old woman who lives in a nursing home has a past medical history of hypertension, diabetes and ischaemic stroke resulting in left-sided hemiplegia. She suffers from frequent urinary tract infections. Her drug history includes aspirin, simvastatin, insulin and lisinopril. She presents with an ulcer on her left heel. Her HbA1c = 6.1 per cent. Her BM is 8.9, blood pressure is 112/87, heart rate 62. She seems comfortable at rest. Her lungs are clear and her abdomen is soft and non-tender. There is a 2×2 cm ulcer on her left heel. Her right foot is normal. What is the most likely cause of her ulcer?

    A. Decubitus ulcer
    B. Venous insufficiency
    C. Hyperglycaemia
    D. Arterial insufficiency
    E. Bacterial infection

42. Diabetes treatment

A type 2 diabetic patient has been taking metformin with good effect for the last four months. He has started to lose weight and maintained good glucose control. In the last two months, however, the patient has been persistently hyperglycaemic despite increased metformin dosage and HbA1c targets have not been achieved. The most appropriate management is:

    A. Thiazolidinedione
    B. Insulin
    C. Sulfonylurea
    D. Increase metformin dose
    E. Exenatide

43. Pyrexia

A 59-year-old man, who has completed five cycles of chemotherapy for metastatic colorectal carcinoma, presents to accident and emergency complaining of feeling generally unwell. On examination, he is pyrexial at 38.9°C and there are crepitations in the right lung base. What is the most urgent investigation?

    A. Full blood count
    B. Chest x-ray
    C. Urine microscopy, culture and sensitivity
    D. Blood cultures
    E. CT abdomen

44. Fever (2)

A 30-year-old man presents to accident and emergency with a 5-day history of fevers, sweats and lethargy. On further questioning, he mentions that he has just returned from a 6 week trip to Tanzania. On examination his temperature is 40°C. What is the most likely diagnosis?

A. Influenza
B. Malaria
C. Typhoid
D. Infectious mononucelosis
E. Cholera

45. Haemoptysis (2)

A 39-year-old Indian man presents to accident and emergency with a 6-week history of haemoptysis, night sweats and weight loss. Chest x-ray reveals some shadowing in the left upper zone. What is the most appropriate diagnostic investigation?

A. Blood cultures
B. Full blood count
C. CT chest
D. Ziehl–Nielsen sputum staining
E. Tuberculin skin testing

46. Atrial myxoma

A 44-year-old man presents with non-specific symptoms of fever, shortness of breath and syncope. Blood tests show a raised erythrocyte sedimentation rate (ESR) and a transoesophageal echo shows an atrial myxoma. What is characteristically heard on auscultation in atrial myxoma?

A. End-diastolic murmur
B. Loud first heart sound
C. Fourth heart sound
D. Pansystolic murmur
E. Loud third heart sound

47. Diarrhoea (3)

A four-year-old girl presents to her GP, with her mother, with a 2-day history of fevers and diarrhoea. Her mother has contacted her nursery, who have informed her that several of the other children have been off sick with the same problem. What is the most likely causative organism?

A. Rotavirus
B. Salmonella
C. Enterotoxigenic *Escherichia coli*
D. Influenza
E. Varicella zoster virus

48. Headache (1)

A 28-year-old junior doctor has been complaining of a headache for the last 6 hours. It started gradually, intensifying slowly and involving the entire cranium but over the last hour she has noticed that turning her head is uncomfortable. She feels generally unwell and prefers to lie in a dark room. Her boyfriend has noticed that she seems irritable. On examination, heart rate is 110, blood pressure is 89/60. She is flushed and has warm extremities. She exhibits photophobia and there is neck stiffness. Close examination of her skin reveals no rashes. Kernig's sign is negative. What is the most important next step in management?

    A. Carry out a lumbar puncture
    B. Check for papilloedema
    C. Administer cefotaxime
    D. Request a CT
    E. Perform blood cultures

49. Heavy legs

A 52-year-old woman who has recently finished a course of chemotherapy for metastatic adenocarcinoma of the lung presents to accident and emergency following a fall at home. She mentions that her legs have been feeling heavy for 2 days. On examination there is reduced power through the lower limbs. Her lower limb reflexes are brisk and she has upgoing plantars. On examination of the abdomen, there is a palpable bladder. There is a sensory level below L1. What is the most important diagnostic investigation?

    A. MRI lumbar spine
    B. MRI whole spine
    C. CT thorax, abdomen, pelvis
    D. Positron emission tomography (PET) scan
    E. Bone scan

50. Confusion (2)

A 66-year-old man presents to accident and emergency in a confused state accompanied by his wife. She states that the patient has become increasingly obtunded in the last 3 days and has not opened his bowels for the same period of time. She mentions he has been suffering from multiple myeloma, but is otherwise healthy. On examination, the patient has brisk tendon reflexes, dry mucosal membranes, reduced skin turgor and the eyes appear sunken. The most appropriate management is:

    A. Intravenous fluids and diuretics
    B. Diuretics alone
    C. Intravenous calcitonin
    D. Psychiatric referral
    E. Intravenous fluid resuscitation

51. Sore throat

An 18-year-old woman presents to accident and emergency with a 5-day history of fevers, malaise and severe sore throat. On examination, she has a temperature of 40°C and her tonsils are inflamed with visible palatal petechiae. In addition, her cervical lymph nodes are palpable. A full blood count shows a raised lymphocyte count. What is the most likely diagnosis?

    A. Influenza
    B. Streptococcal sore throat
    C. Infectious mononucleosis
    D. Malaria
    E. Mumps

52. Back pain

A 45-year-old man presents to accident and emergency with back pain. He works as a builder and the pain started after he had moved a cement mixer. On presentation, he is in considerable distress and unable to walk. He has not passed urine or opened his bowels since the incident. On peripheral neurological examination of the lower limbs, power is reduced throughout due to the pain. Sensation is preserved except for around the perineum. On digital rectal exam, there is poor anal tone. What is the most likely diagnosis?

    A. Spinal cord compression
    B. Cauda equina syndrome
    C. Nerve root compression
    D. Bony injury
    E. Muscular strain

53. Headache (2)

A 75-year-old woman presents to accident and emergency with severe left-sided headache. She also mentions that the vision in her left eye is blurred. She has previously been fit and well but has been feeling increasing worn down in the last few months with aching, weak shoulders and legs. On examination, the left side of her scalp is painful to touch. Blood tests reveal a raised ESR. What is the most appropriate immediate management?

    A. Discharge with advice to use paracetamol
    B. Intravenous hydrocortisone
    C. Oral prednisolone
    D. Arrange urgent CT head
    E. Opthalmology opinion

54. Creutzfeldt–Jakob disease

A 45-year-old man is admitted with ataxia and myoconus on a background of increasing confusion and personality change. What is the most likely cause of his illness?

    A. Sporadic
    B. Familial
    C. Bovine meat
    D. Iatrogenic
    E. Canibalism

55. Laboratory investigations (2)

A seven-year-old girl is brought to accident and emergency by her mother because of a nose bleed that keeps on bleeding despite pressure and ice-packs. Petechiae and ecchymoses can be seen on examination and the mother reports the child has recently recovered from a throat infection. You suspect the patient is suffering from immune thrombocytopenic purpura and organize tests to measure platelets (Plt), bleeding time (BT), prothrombin time (PT) and partial thromboplastin time (PTT). Which of the following is the most appropriate result?

    A. PT: prolonged; PTT: prolonged; BT: prolonged; Plt: decreased
    B. PT: normal; PTT: normal; BT: prolonged; Plt: decreased
    C. PT: normal; PTT: normal; BT: prolonged; Plt: normal
    D. PT: normal; PTT: prolonged; BT: prolonged; Plt: normal
    E. PT: normal; PTT: prolonged; BT: normal; Plt: normal

56. Metatarsophalangeal joint pain

A 60-year-old man presents to accident and emergency with sudden onset pain in the right metatarsophalangeal joint. He is unable to walk without a stick. On further questioning, the patient reports experiencing two similar episodes in the past. Blood tests reveal a raised urate. What is the most appropriate treatment?

    A. NSAIDs
    B. Intra-articular steroid injection
    C. Methotrexate
    D. Allopurinol
    E. Paracetamol and bed rest

57. Haematuria (1)

A 17-year-old anxious Chinese boy presents to clinic with a 1-day history of haematuria. He first noticed the abnormality after a rugby match. His blood pressure is 123/75 mmHg. There is nothing of note on examination and the patient denies any recent illness or on-going medical problems. Urine dipstick confirms the presence of blood and protein. The most likely diagnosis is:

- A. Urinary tract infection
- B. Nephrotic syndrome
- C. IgA nephropathy
- D. Renal cell cancer
- E. Bladder cancer

58. Painful hands

A 39-year-old woman presents to her GP with a 3-month history of pain in the hands. She mentions that her hands have been particularly stiff in the mornings after waking up. On examination of the hands, there is pain on palpation of the proximal interphalangeal joints and metacarpophalangeal joints. What is the most likely diagnosis?

- A. Osteoarthritis
- B. Septic arthritis
- C. Rheumatoid arthritis
- D. Reactive arthritis
- E. Gout

59. Hypertension in chronic kidney disease

A 45-year-old diabetic man is diagnosed with chronic kidney disease and attends a hypertension clinic to discuss the optimal target for blood pressure control. The best systolic blood pressure target is:

- A. <120 mmHg
- B. 120–130 mmHg
- C. 130–140 mmHg
- D. 140–150 mmHg
- E. 150–160 mmHg

60. Flank pain

A 45-year-old man presents with a 1-day history of severe, excruciating pain in his right flank, vomiting and fever. He describes the pain as 'needle-like' and it moves towards his groin. He has tried diclofenac which has had little effect. When passing urine, the pain increased and his urine was blood-tinged. He denies any other symptoms or medical problems. The patient's temperature is 38°C and a CT scan shows a renal staghorn calculus. The most appropriate treatment is:

A. Shock wave lithotripsy
B. Ureteroscopy
C. Percutaneous nephrolithotomy
D. Open surgery
E. Conservative management, allow stone to pass

61. Per vaginam bleeding

A 30-year-old woman, who is 8 weeks pregnant, presents to accident and emergency with PV bleeding and crampy abdominal pain. She has a past medical history of a right-sided deep vein thrombosis and two previous miscarriages. She is sent to the early pregnancy assessment unit, where ultrasound confirms miscarriage. What is the most likely underlying diagnosis?

A. Rheumatoid arthritis
B. Anti-phospholipid syndrome
C. Sjögren's syndrome
D. Discoid lupus
E. Systemic lupus erythematosus (SLE)

62. Painful knee

A 21-year-old man presents to accident and emergency with a hot, swollen, painful right knee and feeling generally unwell. On examination, his temperature is 38.5°C and he is unable to weight bear. He cannot move his right knee joint due to the pain. A diagnosis of septic arthritis is suspected and the joint is aspirated. What organism is most likely to be seen on the Gram stain of the joint aspirate.

A. *Neisseria meningitidis*
B. *Haemophilus influenzae*
C. *Staphylococcus aureus*
D. *Streptococcus pneumoniae*
E. *Neisseria gonorrheae*

63. Haematuria (2)

A 40-year-old man patient presents with visible haematuria. He denies any other symptoms such as fever or pain, and suffers from no other medical problems. He does not smoke or drink alcohol and denies any illicit substance abuse. The most appropriate management is:

    A. Repeat urine dipstick
    B. Cystoscopy
    C. Record blood pressure
    D. Record albumin:creatinine ratio
    E. Urine microscopy, culture and sensitivity

64. Haemoptysis (3)

A 44-year-old man presents with a 3-day history of haemoptysis. He has suffered from a chronic cough in the last three months, but has only recently noticed blood in the sputum. He denies any medical problems and does not drink or smoke. A urine dipstick is positive for haematuria and proteinuria and inspiratory crackles are ausculated over both lung bases. Blood results confirm the presence of anti-glomerular basement membrane antibodies and blood pressure is 125/86 mmHg. The most likely diagnosis is:

    A. Goodpasture's syndrome
    B. Wegener's granulomatosis
    C. Primary biliary cirrhosis
    D. Pernicious anaemia
    E. Post-streptococcal glomerulonephritis

65. Skin rash

A 26-year-old woman presents with an erythematous, palpable rash present on her feet, thighs, palms and soles. The rash is not itchy or painful. She mentions a dull pain in her elbows and knees whenever she moves. A full blood count is normal and a urine dipstick is positive for haematuria. The most likely diagnosis is:

    A. Post-streptococcal glomerulonephritis
    B. Goodpasture's syndrome
    C. Wegener's granulomatosis
    D. Meningococcal septicaemia
    E. Henoch–Schönlein purpura

ANSWERS

Cerebral abscess

1 B   A cerebral abscess is one the most dangerous complications that can result from infections affecting the face and any of the routes that allow infection into the brain, such as sinusitis and otitis media. Patients can complain of fever, headaches and seizures among other presentations. In stable patients, pharmacological therapy is dependent on the suspected organism. For streptococcal and anaerobic infections, intravenous cefuroxime and metronidazole (B) are required. Staphylococcal infections require intravenous flucloxacillin with cefuroxime (D). In general, staphylococcal infections are more common in abscesses. Cefuroxime (A) and flucloxacillin (C) alone are not adequate treatments. Surgical decompression (E) is required in patients who are unstable or have remained refractory to antibiotic therapy.

Hypothalamic–adrenal axis

2 A   Exogenous steroid use (A) causes a negative feedback response whereby pituitary ACTH production is halted, adrenal stimulation also stops causing bilateral atrophy. In pituitary-dependent Cushing's disease (B), ACTH is produced in excess which would cause bilateral adrenal hypertrophy. An ectopic malignancy (C) producing ACTH would similarly cause adrenal hypertrophy. An adrenal malignancy (D) such as an adenoma in one adrenal gland would suppress ACTH production causing atrophy in the normal adrenal gland, while the adrenal malignancy would remain normal or hypertrophied from malignant growth. 21-hydroxylase deficiency (E) would cause an increase in ACTH production from the pituitary also causing adrenal hyperplasia.

Management of cold sores

3 B   Topical acyclovir is the recommended first-line treatment of cold sores caused by Herpes simplex virus.

Onycholysis

4 D   Psoralens (A), psoriasis (B), thyrotoxicosis (C), trauma (E), porphyria and tetracyclines are all known causes of onycholysis. Streptococcal pneumonia (D) is not known to cause onycholysis.

Peutz–Jeghers syndrome

5 B   Peutz–Jeghers syndrome is an autosomal dominant disease characterized by peri-oral (and mucosal) pigmentation and development of hamartomatous polyps within the gastrointestinal (GI) tract. Patients usually present with a positive family history, deeply pigmented lesions on the lips and buccal mucosa, abdominal pain (secondary to obstruction or intussception), iron-deficiency anaemia, rectal prolapse, precocious puberty. Investigations include iron studies, faecal occult blood (may reveal GI bleeding), endoscopy and genetic analysis. Patients are usually referred for genetic analysis/counselling and surgical excision of polyps may be required. Colonoscopy/flexible sigmoidoscopy is recommended from the age of 18 years at three-yearly intervals and upper GI endoscopy is recommended from the age of 25 years at three-yearly intervals. Complications include: (1) High risk of colorectal, pancreatic, gastro-oesophageal and small bowel cancers – risk increases with age; (2) GI bleeding; (3) Intussusception; (4) Rectal prolapse.

Chest pain

6 B This patient is suffering from an acute episode of pericarditis, the change of symptoms with sitting position, lack of cardiovascular risk factors and pericardial rub deviate away from other differentials such as pleurisy and angina. The ECG (B) is diagnostic in pericardial disease with classic saddle-shaped ST elevation indicating pericarditis. The ECG usually undergoes changes over time, beginning with ST elevation that evolves into T-wave flattening and then normalization. A CT calcium score (A) is used in the prediction of coronary artery disease risk and is not appropriate here. Serum amylase (C) may be useful if investigating pancreatitis. A chest x-ray (D) may be useful if exploring differentials such as a pneumothorax, but alongside echocardiography (E) is not useful for diagnosing pericarditis.

Dilated cardiomyopathy

7 C Although familial dilated cardiomyopathy is associated with a number of cytoskeletal abnormalities, such as actin, troponin T and beta myosin heavy chain, a cardiac biopsy (C) is not indicated unless the patient is referred to specialist care centres. A chest x-ray (A) is useful in showing generalized enlargement of the heart. An ECG (B) may show ST segment changes while an echocardiogram (D) can reveal the presence of left or right ventricle dilatation. A cardiac MR (E) is useful in exploring the presence of a cardiac thrombus in dilated cardiomyopathy (DCM).

Inflammatory bowel disease

8 E Answers (A–D) are all known extraintestinal signs of ulcerative colitis. Granuloma annulare is a benign chronic skin condition characterized by dermal papules and annular plaques. It has been associated with non-insulin dependent diabetes mellitus, but is primarily idiopathic. The papules can occur anywhere on the body and usually resolve in a few months without treatment being required.

Haemoptysis (1)

9 E Pulmonary tuberculosis (A), Bronchiectasis (B), Aspergilloma (C) and Wegener's granulomatosis (D) cause haemoptysis. Other causes include:

- bronchogenic carcinoma;
- pulmonary abscess;
- farmer's lung;
- pulmonary embolus;
- Goodpasture's syndrome.

Asthma (E) does not result in patients presenting with haemoptysis.

Extrapulmonary manifestations of sarcoidosis

10 C Apart from answer (C), all the above answers are documented extrapulmonary manifestations of sarcoidosis. Erythema marginatum (C) is described as the presence of pink annular macules which appear on the trunk and primarily on the extensor surfaces of the skin. It is usually associated with acute rheumatic fever and forms part of one of the major conditions that are mentioned in the Jones criteria. Erythema nodosum (which are tender red circular nodules usually present on the shins bilaterally but can appear anywhere on the body) along with lupus pernio and subcutaneous nodules are the known documented cutaneous manifestations of sarcoidosis.

Laboratory investigations (1)

11 D Haemophilia (D) A (factor VIII dysfunction) and B (factor IX dysfunction) present similarly with neonatal bleeding during birth, soft tissue haemorrhage as young children, gum bleeding and, in older children and adults, haematomas and haemarthroses. Since factor VII is preserved as well as platelets, only the partial thromboplastin time is affected. Bernard Soulier syndrome (A) causes prolonged bleeding time alongside decreased platelet numbers. Glanzmann's thrombasthenia (B) causes prolonged bleeding time, disseminated intravascular coagulation (C) causes prolonged prothrombin time, partial thromboplastin time, bleeding time and with reduced platelets. Liver disease (E) (end-stage) causes a similar derangement of prothrombin time, partial thromboplastin time, bleeding time and platelets to disseminated intravascular coagulation (DIC).

Diarrhoea (1)

12 B The treatment of *C. difficile* diarrhoea is with antibiotics. The antibiotic of choice is oral metronidazole. Oral metronidazole (B) is preferred over its intravenous form (C) due to relatively increased efficacy; enhanced gut lumen concentrations are achieved via oral administration. Vancomycin (A) is usually reserved for patients who are either allergic to metronidazole or with *C. difficile* diarrhoea resistant to metronidazole. Ciprofloxacin (D) is not usually used to treat *C. difficile* diarrhoea.

Papilloedema

13 B This patient is suffering from a hypertensive encephalopathy (B), the elevated blood pressure compromises the integrity of the blood–brain barrier causing increased cerebral perfusion leading to cerebral oedema. Patients may present with a broad range of symptoms which include vomiting, headaches, confusion, visual disturbances and eventually coma if left untreated. Multiple acute infarctions can cause papilloedema to develop and this also compounds the patient's confused state. A lacunar infarction (C) is often associated with hypertension and is often asymptomatic. Symptomatic patients often exhibit the effects of minor strokes such as abrupt dysarthria, pure sensory or motor loss. Papilloedema is not a commonly associated feature. Vascular dementia (D) can occur due to the accumulation of several small lacunar infarctions or from a few large infarctions. Patients usually exhibit cerebral decline, pseudobulbar palsy and abnormal gait. Papilloedema is again not a commonly associated feature. A subdural haemorrhage (A) can exhibit symptoms from days to months depending on the degree and rapidity of bleeding which is often traceable to a precipitant such as a fall or blow to the head, which is not present in this case. Symptoms include headaches, increasing drowsiness and confusion. A phaeochromocytoma (E) is a rare malignancy of the sympathetic nervous system, clinical features are secondary to the action of excess catecholamine release, which is usually at random rather than a constant feature and include sweating, panic attacks, tremor and flushing.

Ischaemic stroke

14 D Although the prevalence of patent foramen ovale (PFO) in the general population is about 5 per cent, it is several-fold higher in patients with stroke, especially where there is no other likely cause. There are thought to be emboli originating in the venous circulation. The association between migraine and PFO is more controversial and the mechanisms are certainly unclear, but evidence in favour of it is increasing.

Glycated haemoglobin

15 D The recent NICE guidelines recommend that when setting a target glycated haemoglobin the patient should be involved in deciding their target HbA1c which can be above the recommended level of 6.5 per cent (A). Patients are encouraged to maintain their target levels, however this is discouraged if side effects such as hypoglycaemia cause a significant impairment of quality of life. Highly intensive management with HbA1c levels between 6.0 and 6.5 per cent are discouraged.

Breathlessness

16 E   Doxazosin (E) is a selective α_1-receptor blocker which is used in systemic but not pulmonary hypertension. Sildenafil (A), a phosphodiesterase-5 inhibitor which increases cyclic guanosine monophosphate (GMP) levels in pulmonary vessels, is frequently combined with bosentan (B), an endothelin receptor antagonist (there are several other drugs available in each class). Prostacyclin (D) has to be given intravenously, unlike the previously mentioned drugs, and has both vasodilator and anti-platelet properties, while anti-coagulation (C) is usually recommended to prevent thrombosis aggravating the increased pulmonary resistance. Calcium channel blockers are also frequently used.

Jaundice

17 C   Jaundice, also known as icterus, refers to yellow pigmentation of the skin, sclerae and mucosa due to raised plasma bilirubin, usually visible at >35 μmol/L. Jaundice can be category\ed according to: (1) The site of the problem: pre-hepatic (e.g. haemolysis, physiological in neonates, dyserythropoesis, glucuronyl transferase deficency), hepatic (e.g. viral hepatitis, CMV, Epstein–Barr virus (EBV), drug induced, alcoholic hepatitis, cirrhosis) and post-hepatic (e.g. gallstones in the common bile duct, pancreatic cancer, cholangiocarcinoma, primary biliary cirrhosis); or (2) The type of circulating bilirubin (conjugated or unconjugated).

Abdominal pain

18 A   This patient is suffering from a suspected abdominal aortic aneurysm (AAA), these most commonly occur infrarenally and predominantly affect males. There is close association with atherosclerosis and genetic abnormalities such as Marfan's and Ehlers–Danlos syndrome. Although most aneurysms are asymptomatic, patients can present with renal colic-like symptoms, diverticular-like pain, umbilical pain and groin pain. A pusatile and expansile mass is strongly indicative of an abdominal aneurysm. In order to screen for an AAA an abdominal ultrasound scan (A) is the least invasive and safest screening investigation. In obese patients, it can be difficult to differentiate the entire aortic structure. An abdominal x-ray (B) would not be able to provide enough detail of the abdominal aorta to determine an aneurysm. An abdominal CT scan (C) provides the most accurate visualization of an AAA, especially with contrast, however due to the availability of resources and invasiveness it is not appropriate as a first-line screening investigation. An abdominal

MRI scan (D) is comparable to a CT scan if enhanced with contrast material, however, patients are unlikely to remain motionless during scanning and the modality is not as reliable when compared to CT and US scanning. Angiography (E) is an invasive procedure and the true size of the aneurysm cannot always be ascertained and so this modality is more appropriate when preparing the patient for surgical intervention.

Fever (1)

19 A This patient is likely to be suffering from meningococcal septicaemia and has the classic symptoms of fever, headache, non-blanching rash and neck stiffness alongside his new environment at university. Once meningitis is suspected, rapid management is required to prevent precipitation. The British Infection Society splits management dependent on whether the patient has predominantly septicaemic symptoms, as in this patient, or meningitic symptoms. In septicaemia, immediate antiobiotics must be started and this is usually IV ceftriaxone (A) or cefotaxime. Intravenous cephalexin (D) is not appropriate to provide enough safe cover. In suspected bacterial meningitis a lumbar puncture (C) is appropriate if there are no signs of raised intracranial pressure (ICP). Senior advice must always be sought and if there are any suspicions of raised ICP the critical care team should be called. A blood culture (E) in either pathway would take too long by which the patient may decompensate without any other treatment or intervention Fundoscopy (B) would be useful in a patient with suspected meningitis to assess for raised ICP which would negate a lumbar puncture, however this patient is suffering from septicaemic symptoms and so this is not appropriate.

Erythroderma

20 A Cutaneous T-cell lymphomas (A) have been known to be associated with the development of erythroderma. SCC (B), BCC (C), malignant melanoma (D) and Kaposi's sarcoma (E) have not been known to be associated with erythroderma.

Knee pain

21 D The case in this question is describing a patient with osteoarthritis. Reduced joint space, subchondral sclerosis, bone cysts and osteophytes (D) are the radiographical features of osteoarthritis. Reduced joint space, soft tissue swelling and peri-articular osteopenia (E) are the radiographical features of rheumatoid arthritis. It is likely that the woman in this case will have x-ray changes, thus making normal x-ray (C) an incorrect option. However, it is important to note that the radiographical changes of osteoarthritis may not correlate with the clinical features. The joint space in osteoarthritis is reduced, making options (A) and (B) incorrect.

Anterior myocardial infarction

22 C Transient vagal activation resulting in sinus bradycardia is common after myocardial infarction and may be symptomatic, as in this case, with hypotension and probably reduced cardiac output. It usually responds to one or more doses of atropine (C). Pacing (A) is unnecessary unless heart block is also present, while stimulant drugs (B, D and E) are not only ineffective in this situation but also dangerous, as they increase the risk of ventricular arrhythmias.

Heart failure

23 B Brain natriuretic peptide (B) is considered to have the greatest power as a diagnostic biomarker of the given answer options. In established heart failure, high levels of endothelin (C) and noradernaline (D) in particular are associated with poor prognosis. All of the given answers, including atrial natriuretic peptide (A) and adrenomedullin (E), may be increased in heart failure.

Skin hyperpigmentation

24 A Answers (B–E) are all associated with cutaneous hyperpigmentation. Hypopituitarism (A), however, leads to decreased hormone levels of pituitary melanotrophic hormones leading to generalized (hypopigmentation) pale yellow-tinged skin (with associated skin atrophy and loss of hair in androgenic-dependent areas).

Prosthetic valve endocarditis

25 C Transoesophageal echocardiography (C) is the investigation of choice since it provides high resolution images, as well as the option of alternative views. Simple auscultation (A) is appropriate to detect the structural breakdown of the valve. Transthoracic echocardiography (B) is the initial investigation and is ideal as it is non-invasive, however, definitive investigation is made difficult by the scattering of US signals the mechanical valve. A chest x-ray (D) and ECG (E) would be useful for detecting gross anomalies to heart function such as failure, but are not sensitive enough to detect vegetative damage.

Arterial blood gas interpretation

26 B Assessing the pH, with the normal range being between 7.35 and 7.45, this patient is suffering from an alkalosis. The PCO_2 level is below 4.7 kPa and is occurring as a result of the patient hyperventilating. Lastly, the bicarbonate level is within normal range (22–26) indicating that the alkalosis is resulting from a respiratory problem rather than a metabolic one. Tying in all these findings, the patient is suffering from an acute respiratory alkalosis (B) secondary to anxiety. Some other causes include central respiratory depression and other CNS disorders (e.g. drug-induced opiates, sedatives, CNS trauma, cervical cord lesion, etc.), muscle disorders (e.g. Guillain–Barré syndrome, myasthenia gravis), lung/chest wall defects (e.g. trauma, pneumothorax, diaphragmatic paralysis) and airway disorders (e.g. laryngospasms, upper airway obstruction).

Hypertension

27 E In type 2 diabetics blood pressure is monitored monthly if above 150/90 mmHg, bimonthly if above 140/80 mmHg and bimonthly if blood pressure is above 130/80 mmHg with renal, ophthalmic or cerebrovascular pathology. First-line therapy in type 2 diabetes patients with hypertension and no other abnormalities are ACE inhibitors (E) due to good blood pressure control and their renal and ophthalmic protective effects. An angiotensin II receptor antagonist (B) may be used if there is intolerance to an ACE inhibitor. Second-line therapy should be a calcium channel blocker (C) or a diuretic (A) if blood pressure remains high despite ACE inhibitor or angiotensin II blocker therapy. If this also fails to provide adequate control, α-blocker or β-blocker (D) therapy is used.

Seizure (1)

28 B The most important management step for any episode of loss of consciousness is to obtain a full history (B), including details before, during and after the event. Elicit the events just before the collapse including the activity, position (e.g. sitting versus standing), associated symptoms such as aura or palpitations and whether there were any witnesses. The patient should be able to describe events after they awake, including any post-ictal symptoms such as confusion or sleepiness. The patient will not know what happened while they were unconscious, although sometimes this can be inferred if they noticed incontinence, a sore tongue/muscles or bruising. A collateral history from a witness is key in determining the duration of the event, any colour changes or movements. The history often makes the diagnosis, investigations confirm it. Lying-standing blood pressure (A) is helpful in orthostatic hypotension, an ECG (C) or echo for cardiogenic causes, brain imaging (D and E) may detect structural abnormalities responsible for an epileptic focus.

Malignant melanoma

29 C The thickness of the lesion (C), which is known as the Breslow thickness (measured in millimetres), will determine the patient's five-year survival rate. The Breslow thickness can only be determined once an excision biopsy of the lesion is performed. Lesion shape (B), size (A), colour (D) and patient age (E) do not form part of ascertaining the prognosis in patients with malignant melanoma.

Chest signs

30 D On examination of the chest wall, one would typically find the following signs in a patient with a right-sided pleural effusion:

- Decreased air entry on the affected side

- Decreased vocal fremitus (which occurs as a result of decreased conduction of sound waves through liquid media)

- Dullness ('stony') on percussion on the affected side

Therefore (D) is the correct answer.

Diabetes in pregnancy

31 C A calcium channel blocker (C) is first-line therapy in a female who intends to/or has become pregnant, as well as in patients who are of African-Caribbean descent (with an ACE inhibitor). In a normal patient following lifestyle therapy ACE inhibitors (A) are first line, calcium channel blockers (C) are second line followed by a combination of diuretics (D) and calcium channel blockers. β-blockers (E) are used if despite the aforementioned therapy target blood pressure is not met. If there are any contraindications or poor compliance with ACE inhibitors, angiotensin II receptor blockers (B) are used instead.

Severity of pneumonia

32 C This patient has a CURB-65 score of 4. The BTS guidelines state that a CURB-65 score between 3 and 5 indicates severe pneumonia and requires hospitalization with the possibility of escalation to ITU. In this question, the patient has developed a secondary type-1 respiratory failure. Despite having 15 L of oxygen, her oxygen saturations have not vastly improved. This patient will therefore require review by the ITU team with the possibility of mechanical ventilation. In addition, severe pneumoniae are not usually treated with oral antibiotics; intravenous antibiotics are indicated due to quicker onset of action.

Hepatocellular carcinoma

33 D Chronic hepatitis B (A) and C (C) infections, liver cirrhosis (B) and aflatoxin (E) (a carcinogen from the mould *Aspergillus flavus*) are all known predisposing factors for developing hepatocellular carcinoma. Chronic inflammatory changes results in hepatocyte damage and mutation in the cellular reparation machinery. Hepatitis A (D) does not usually lead to chronic infection and thus is not deemed to be a predisposing factor to hepatocellular carcinoma.

Diarrhoea (2)

34 A *Clostridium difficile* colitis is a hospital-acquired infection that is caused by the use of broad-spectrum antibiotics. The use of these antibiotics causes eradication of normal gut flora and subsequent colonization of the gut by *C. difficile*. Patients may present with profuse, offensive diarrhoea. This is treated with a course of oral metronidazole (A). Intravenous fluids (B) may be required if the diarrhoea has resulted in significant dehydration. However, management with fluids alone does not eradicate the bacteria. Intravenous hydrocortisone (C) is not a treatment for *C. difficile* colitis. Oral acyclovir (D) is an anti-viral agent that is not useful in the treatment of *C. difficile* colitis. Oral co-amoxiclav (E) is a broad-spectrum antibiotic that may result in *C. difficile* colitis. Therefore, this is the incorrect answer.

Blood groups

35 E In a patient with blood type AB rhesus positive, they have no antibodies against blood groups A, B or O and only have rhesus antibodies. Since they cannot become sensitized they may receive blood from any of the given options (A), (B), (C) or (D).

Confusion (1)

36 E This patient is most likely suffering from hypercalcaemia due to an underlying condition of untreated multiple myeloma. Patients therefore suffer from symptoms that include dehydration, depression, bone and abdominal pain and increased risk of renal stones. Although the underlying disease is multiple myeloma, the patient must first be stabilized against the effects of hypercalcaemia. Intravenous saline (E) over several days stabilizes the patient and replaces any lost fluid volume. Calcitonin (A) has a short duration of action and is not particularly effective in lowering calcium levels and would not help with the patient's fluid loss. Intravenous bisphosphonates (C) are appropriate once the patient has been stabilized and is not dehydrated, especially important in a patient with myeloma to stem the excess serum calcium levels. Stem cell transplantation (D) would be aimed at trying to improve the patient's prognosis but would not be suitable or safe in an unstable patient. NSAIDs (B) would be helpful in alleviating the patient's pain, however, due to the production of Bence–Jones proteins they should be avoided as they might precipitate renal failure.

Palpitations

37 D Wolff–Parkinson–White syndrome (D) is due to an accessory bundle called the bundle of Kent, which provides a conducting pathway from the atria to the ventricles bypassing the AV node. Lown–Ganong–Levine syndrome (C) is similar but the PR interval is normal and not shortened as it is here. There is nothing to suggest anxiety (B) and although sinus tachycardia (A) can coexist with this arrhythmia, at other times the description of the episodes is not very typical. In the absence of the characteristic ECG findings, nodal tachycardia (E) would certainly be a possibility.

Seizure (2)

38 D This woman and her witness give a good description of a simple partial seizure (focal visual symptoms) which generalized into a tonic–clonic seizure (D). It is unlikely to be a pseudoseizure (E) (psychogenic non-epileptic seizure) and patients must be investigated with telemetry before being given this diagnosis. Insufficient sleep and stress can trigger seizures. The witness gives a good description of tonic–clonic seizures (A) which are a type of generalized seizure (B). Other types of generalized seizures include absence, tonic and atonic. The old name for tonic–clonic seizures is grand mal (C) (petit mal are now known as absence seizures). They may be primary or secondary. In this case there is secondary generalization as the patient describes an aura herald. Auras serve patients as warning signs and are in fact simple partial seizures (focal symptoms with preservation of consciousness). This helps localize the focus of the seizure, in this case the left occipital lobe, which then went on to generalize. Remember: auras are simple partial seizures.

Marfans' syndrome

39 D Marfans' syndrome is a connective tissue disorder inherited in an autosomal dominant fashion, although with several characteristic features there are no pathognomonic signs (for the full cardinal features list, see the Berlin criteria and Ghent critera). The following are the major and minor criteria for Marfans' syndrome: ascending aorta dissection (A) and ascending aorta dilatation (B), with or without regurgitation. Minor criteria include mitral valve calcification (E) in patients younger than 40, mitral valve prolapse (C), with or without the presence of mitral regurgitation (D), which therefore does not qualify as a criteria in Marfans' syndrome.

Thrombocytopenia

40 A An immune thrombocytopenic purpura (ITP) (A) is caused by anti-platelet antibodies from the spleen against antigens such as glycoprotein IIb-IIIa, an acute ITP can occur in children following a viral infection and is usually self-limited. Aplastic anaemia (B) causes a pancytopenia, Bernard Soulier syndrome (C) is an autosomal recessive disorder due to a deficiency in glycoprotein Ib characterized by prolonged bleeding time and reduced platelets but not related to infections. Glanzmann's thrombasthenia (D) is another autosomal recessive disorder due to a deficiency in glycoprotein

IIb-IIIa causing defective platelet aggregation. Patients have prolonged bleeding times but normal numbers of platelets. Thrombotic thrombocytopenic purpura (TTP) (E) is characterized by fever, thrombocytopenia, renal failure and neurological symptoms, which are not present in this case.

Stroke complications

41 A This woman is unable to move her left side secondary to ischaemic stroke. Hemiplegia means 'paralysis' as opposed to hemiparesis which is 'weakness'. She has developed a pressure sore or decubitus ulcer (A) as she is unable to move her leg, resulting in decreased perfusion from the weight of her own body resulting in ischaemia and breakdown of tissue. Good nursing care is important. Venous ulcers (B) typically affect the gator area, especially the medial maleolus. Nothing to suggest venous insufficiency is mentioned, such as varicose veins or previous deep vein thrombosis (DVT), shallow, irregular ulcers with surrounding skin changes (lipodermatosclerosis). She certainly has risk factors for arterial insufficiency (D). These typically 'punched-out' ulcers also have a predilection for the heel or between the toes, however you would expect reduced or absent leg pulses and perhaps a history of claudication. Bed sores better fit the history in this case. Diabetic ulcers (C) typically occur at the base of the first metatarsal head as a result of neuropathy causing decreased sensation and pressure ulcers. The neuropathy is typically symmetrical and you would expect bilateral sensory loss. There is nothing to suggest active bacterial infection (E).

Diabetes treatment

42 C Although metformin is a good first-line drug in overweight type 2 diabetics with poor glucose control, adjuncts are often needed. Metformin dosage should be titrated in the first few weeks of therapy to avoid the risk of gastrointestinal symptoms; however further increases should be avoided (D). The next step after metformin therapy is metformin and sulphonylurea, the latter has superior glucose-lowering ability and should be used as first-line treatment in overweight or obese patients with poor glucose control. Insulin secretagogues (C) (these include sulphonylureas and rapid-acting insulin secretagogues such as nateglinide and repaglinide) are particularly effective in controlling HbA1$_c$ levels and improve cardiovascular outcomes. Patients unable to maintain or achieve adequate glucose control may use sulphonylureas as second-line therapy and are only contraindicated if hypoglycaemia is a common problem for which thiazolidinedione (A) is used as a replacement. Insulin therapy (B) is only considered if, after metformin and sulphonylurea therapy, the patient's HbA1c remains above 7.5 per cent. Exenatide (E) can be used at this point as an alternative if weight is a particular problem.

Pyrexia

43 A Patients who become pyrexial while receiving chemotherapy must be managed with the diagnosis of neutropenic sepsis in mind. This is an oncological emergency. An urgent full blood count (A) is thus required to see if the patient is neutropenic ($<1.0 \times 10^9$ mmol/L). In this situation, blood tests and blood cultures (D) should be sent immediately and empirical broad spectrum antibiotic therapy commenced straight after, in accordance with local hospital guidelines. The antibiotic regimen can then be altered depending on the results. Following this, the source of sepsis can be sought using a chest x-ray (B) and urine microscopy, culture and sensitivity (C). Patients who are being treated for neutropenic sepsis should be kept in a side room and barrier nursing should be maintained.

Fever (2)

44 B Malaria (B) should be considered as the most likely diagnosis of a patient presenting with fevers, having travelled to a malaria endemic area. Patients usually present with fever, malaise, headache, vomiting or diarrhoea. This patient should have thick and thin blood films sent off, in addition to a full set of blood tests to confirm the diagnosis of malaria. Influenza (A) is a possible differential diagnosis. However, the travel history should identify malaria as the most likely differential. Typhoid (C) usually presents with gastrointestinal symptoms. Infectious mononucleosis (D) would present with fevers, sweats and malaise. However, in addition, there is likely to be a sore throat. Examination would reveal inflamed tonsils and widespread lymphadenopathy in addition to splenomegaly and hepatomegaly. Cholera (E) presents with profuse watery diarrhoea.

Haemoptysis (2)

45 D The case in this question should raise the suspicion of tuberculosis. The investigation of choice to confirm the diagnosis is Ziehl–Nielsen sputum staining (D) for acid fast bacilli. Blood cultures (A) should be sent if the patient is pyrexial on presentation, but are not useful in the diagnosis of tuberculosis. A CT chest (C) is not used in the diagnosis of tuberculosis. Tuberculin skin testing (E) is used to check immunity to tuberculosis and not to confirm the diagnosis. The diagnosis of tuberculosis can also be confirmed with sputum cultures, which are taken and grown in Lowenstein–Jensen medium for up to 12 weeks. A full blood count (B) would not provide any definitive information leading to a diagnosis here.

Atrial myxoma

46 E In atrial myxoma a characteristic loud third heart sound (E) or 'tumour plop' is heard along with a mid-diastolic murmur. An end-diastolic murmur (A) typically occurs in mitral or tricuspid stenosis, while a pansystolic murmur (D) typically occurs in mitral regurgitation and ventral septal defects. A loud first heart sound (B) is associated with mitral stenosis and Wolff–Parkinson–White syndrome. A fourth heart sound (C) tends to occur due to ventricular hypertrophy, which can be due to a number of causes such as chronic hypertension, aortic stenosis and congestive heart failure.

Diarrhoea (3)

47 A Rotavirus (A) is an important cause of outbreaks of childhood diarrhoea and should be considered as the most likely answer in this question. Salmonella (B) may cause outbreaks of gastroenteritis when food (commonly poultry) is contaminated. The age group of the affected individual and the absence of an obvious contaminated food source makes salmonella less likely than rotavirus. Enterotoxigenic *E. coli* (C) is the most common cause of travellers' diarrhoea. The absence of a travel history makes this an unlikely option in this case. Influenza (D) does not usually cause gastroenteritis. Rather, this presents with fever, headache, myalgia and dry cough. Therefore, it is the incorrect answer. Varicella zoster virus (E) is the cause of chicken pox and shingles, not gastroenteritis.

Headache (1)

48 C This is a medical emergency. The patient is hypotensive and tachycardic. She is in shock and needs immediate resuscitation with fluids and urgent administration of IV antibiotics (C) to treat her septicaemia. Blood cultures (E) and a lumbar puncture (LP) (A) should be performed, but should not delay treatment. Papilloedema (B) may be present if there is raised intracranial pressure and this should always be checked for before performing a lumbar puncture as there is a risk of herniation. In these cases, patients should have brain imaging prior to LP if indicated. A CT scan (D) is important and useful, but takes time to obtain and should not delay treatment.

Heavy legs

49 B The presence of upper motor neuron signs and a sensory level in the lower limbs must raise the suspicion of spinal cord compression. This is an oncological emergency and prompt action is required. It is important to note that often in acute cord compression, lower motor neuron signs may be seen below the level of the compression. The investigation of choice is MRI whole spine (B). While the findings on examination suggest that the cord compression is within the lumbar spine, MRI lumbar spine (A) is not the correct answer as metastatic lesions in the rest of the vertebral column may be present and influence treatment options. CT thorax, abdomen and pelvis (C), PET scan (D) and bone scan (E) are very useful investigations for the staging of cancers but are not used to identify spinal cord compression. Initial management of cord compression should be administration of dexamethasone and then contacting clinical oncology and neurosurgical teams to discuss treatment with either spinal radiotherapy or surgical decompression.

Confusion (2)

50 E This patient is suffering from hypercalcaemia secondary to multiple myeloma, a malignancy of plasma cells in the bone marrow. Monoclonal antibodies and/or light chains are released producing detectable serum M-proteins and urinary Bence–Jones protein, respectively. The impact of this is a hypercoagulative state, anaemia or pancytopenia, hypercalcaemia and an ESR that may or may not be raised. The acute management of hypercalcaemia is centred around eliminating the excess calcium via the urine and providing fluid support. Intravenous fluid (E) is therefore the most appropriate management. Intravenous fluids diuretic (A) does not address the electrolyte imbalance since diuretics have a small influence even after fluids are given. The most important treatment in hypercalcaemia is intravenous saline. Furosemide is occasionally added but this is to allow more saline to be given to older patients but runs the risk of hypokalaemia. Diuretics alone (B) are potentially lethal since they would exacerbate the dehydration. Intravenous calcitonin (C) would act to reduce calcium levels, however it is too slow and not as effective as fluid rehydration and diuresis. Although the confusion can make communicating with patients difficult, worrying clinical signs and collateral history should not be dismissed (D). In a patient with a history of multiple myeloma, hypercalcaemia is a common complication and further delay can be fatal.

Sore throat

51 C Infectious mononucleosis (C) is caused by Epstein–Barr virus infection and is characterized by fever, sore throat and anorexia. On examination, there may be widespread lymphadenophathy and hepatomegaly or splenomegaly. The tonsils usually appear inflamed and erythematous. The diagnosis can be confirmed with a blood film showing the presence of atypical mononuclear cells or a Paul Bunnell test. Influenza (A) should be considered as a differential in patients that present with this clinical picture. However, it is unusual for the tonsils to be so inflamed and for the cervical lymph nodes to be palpable. Therefore, influenza is not as likely as infectious mononucleosis. Streptococcal sore throat (B) may present with sore throat and fever. However, a lymphocytosis would not be seen on full blood count, making this answer incorrect. There is no history of travel mentioned. Therefore, malaria (D) is an unlikely answer. Finally, mumps (E) presents with fever, malaise and swelling of the parotid glands. There is no swelling of the parotid glands in this case. In addition, the swollen tonsils with palatal petechiae mean mumps is an unlikely answer.

Back pain

52 B Back pain is a very common problem in accident and emergency departments. The clinical features described in the case in this question of inability to open bowels, inability to urinate, reduced tone of digital rectal exam and a saddle anaesthesia, indicate that the patient has prolapsed a disc into the cauda equina **(B)** producing compression of the sacral nerves. Spinal cord compression **(A)** is not the correct answer, as clinical features would include a sensory level (i.e. a dermatomal level below which sensation is reduced) and upper motor neuron signs below the level of the compression (although it is important to note that in the acute injury, there may initially be lower motor neuron signs) A nerve root compression **(C)** would affect one particular nerve root and result in pain shooting down the leg and decreased sensation in that dermatome. Bony injury **(D)** and muscular strain **(E)** are incorrect answers due to the neurological signs.

Headache (2)

53 C The case in this question is describing a patient presenting with temporal arteritis or giant cell arteritis. This is a large vessel vasculitis that is associated with polymyalgia rheumatica. The temporal headache, which is exacerbated on palpation over the temporal area of the scalp, are the clinical features of disease. Vasculitis involvement of the ophthalmic arteries may result in irreversible loss of vision. The most appropriate treatment here is to start the patient on high dose oral prednisolone **(C)**. This is especially important in this case as the patient is describing visual loss. The patient must then be followed up with a temporal artery biopsy within the next 3–4 days to confirm the diagnosis. Paracetamol alone **(A)** may provide some symptomatic relief but will not alter the underlying vasculitic process, thus loss of vision may occur. Intravenous hydrocortisone **(B)** is not required, as the patient can have the steroid treatment as prednisolone orally. A CT head **(D)** is not useful as the underlying vasculitic process cannot be visualized. Opthalmology opinion **(E)** can be sought but the most important immediate management is to give the oral steroids.

Creutzfeldt–Jakob disease

54 A This patient has Creutzfeld–Jacob disease (CJD) or spongiform encephalitis. The most common cause is sporadic **(A)**. CJD is interesting as the causative agent is a simple protein (not a virus or bacteria, like other infectious diseases). The incidence is tiny – one in a million per year. Although there has been a large scare in transmission of this disease, especially the variant form, most cases of this very rare disease occur spontaneously in a person without any risk factors. Hereditary transmission **(B)** is the second most common cause with a clear genetic component. Blood transfusion, corneal transplant or surgery with contaminated instruments or human pituitary hormone replacement therapy have all been implicated in iatrogenic CJD

(D), but the actual risk of this is very low. Cannibalism (E) is the classic example of transmission. This type of CJD, Kuru, was seen in the Fore tribe of Papua New Guinea where in burial ceremonies, the women would eat the deceased's brain and be exposed to the prion protein. Men who traditionally did not eat the brain as part of the ceremony were spared. The profile of CJD was greatly raised with the mad cow disease scandal. The worry here was that humans were contracting the disease from contaminated meat, which meant that the causative prion had crossed the species barrier. This, coupled to the high exposure of the population to meat and the long (around ten years) incubation time, led to speculation of a future pandemic. This has not materialized and the number of cases of variant CJD is extremely small, albeit tragic.

Laboratory investigations (2)

55 B In immune thrombocytopenia a reduced number of platelets causes an increased bleeding, as is evident in this patient (B). Result (A) reflects disseminated intravascular coagulation, result (C) reflects the effect of aspirin, result (D) reflects Von Willebrand's disease and result (E) reflects haemophilia.

Metatarsophalangeal joint pain

56 A The case in this question is describing a patient presenting with acute gout. The most common presentation of acute gout is inflammation of the first metatarsophalangeal joint. The treatment of acute gout episodes is with an NSAID (A). Patients should also initiate conservative measures to reduce urate levels. These include weight loss and avoiding excess alcohol. Intra-articular steroid injection (B) can be given in some cases of acute gout, for example when NSAIDs are contraindicated. However, the first-line therapy is treatment with NSAIDs to control the local inflammation. Methotrexate (C) is a disease-modifying anti-rheumatic drug (DMARD) that is used in the treatment of rheumatoid arthritis. It is not however, used in the treatment of acute gout. Allopurinol must not be started during the acute attack of gout as it may worsen symptoms. This can be started after a few weeks to prevent further attacks. While paracetamol and bed rest may provide some symptomatic relief, the use of an NSAID is needed to control the acute inflammatory response.

Haematuria (1)

57 C The most common cause of idiopathic haematuria, particularly in Asia, is IgA nephropathy (C) which usually presents following a streptococcal throat infection or strenuous exercise. Mild proteinuria is also an associated feature. A urinary tract infection (A) is unlikely in painless haematuria and would most likely be associated with urinary symptoms such as urinary frequency, dysuria and the presence of leukocytes and nitrates detectable in the urine. The nephrotic syndrome (B) typically includes proteinuria, low serum albumin and oedema, which is not present in this case. Renal cell carcinoma (D) is usually associated with flank pain and an abdominal or flank mass which is again not present in this patient. Bladder malignancy (E) is a common and worrying cause of painless haematuria, however patient demographics typically describe patients above the age of 50 years with risk factors, such as smoking and exposure to chemicals, present in rubber, industrial dyes, etc.

Painful hands

58 C Rheumatoid arthritis (C) is a chronic, systemic inflammatory disease, which produces a symmetrical, deforming polyarthritis. It normally presents with pain in the small joints of the hands and feet, which is worse in the mornings. As the disease progresses, the affected joints can become deformed. Osteoarthrtis (A) affects the large weight-bearing joints and the joints of the hands. In the hands, the distal interphalangeal joints are affected more than the proximal interphalangeal joints in osteoarthritis. In addition, pain is characteristically worse at the end of the day. Septic arthritis (B) usually presents as an acutely inflamed, warm joint. There may also be systemic features. Therefore, this is the incorrect option in this question. Reactive arthritis (E) usually presents as an asymmetrical lower limb arthritis. Gout (E) normally presents as a monoarthritis, although it can present as a polyarthritis. It most commonly affects the first metatarsophalangeal joint.

Hypertension in chronic kidney disease

59 B Patients with chronic kidney disease must carefully maintain their blood pressure to avoid increasing their risk of co-morbidity. In patients with diabetes and chronic kidney disease, NICE guidelines recommend a systolic blood pressure in the target range of 120–129 mmHg (B) and diastolic blood pressure below 80 mmHg. Systolic blood pressure <120 mmHg (A) is associated with an increased risk of mortality, stroke and heart failure, 130–140 mmHg (C) is associated with end-stage renal disease, while 140–160 mmHg (D) and (E) is associated with end-stage renal failure and death.

Flank pain

60 C There are a number of factors that indicate urgent intervention, they include signs of an infection alongside urinary tract obstruction, pain refractory to analgesia and/or vomiting, signs of renal failure and bilateral renal calculi. Conservative management (E) is therefore not appropriate. Percutaneous nephrolithotomy (C) uses a nephroscope with a lithotripsy or laser device attached. All fragments can be removed using suction or grasping devices and this is the ideal treatment in large, complex stones in the kidney. Open surgery (D), although the first-line therapy in the past, has now been replaced by interventions that are effective and less invasive. Shock wave lithotripsy (A) utilizes shock waves in a focused manner to fragment stones, they are ideal in simple renal calculi. Ureteroscopy (B) introduces an endoscope that allows the passage of instruments that may be used for stone fragmentation. It is ideal for treating patients who are morbidly obese or pregnant.

Per vaginam bleeding

61 B Anti-phospholipid syndrome (B) is recurrent miscarriages and venous or arterial thrombosis. This patient should have an autoantibody screen sent. The presence of anti-cardiolipin antibodies would confirm the diagnosis. Rheumatoid arthritis (A) is a chronic, symmetrical deforming polyarthritis that is not associated with recurrent miscarriage and venous/arterial thrombosis. Sjögren's disease (C) occurs due to fibrosis of the exocrine glands and presents with decreased tear production and salivation and parotid gland swelling. Discoid lupus (D) is a variant of SLE where skin manifestations are the only feature. SLE (E) is a multisystem inflammatory disorder where clinical manifestations are variable and occur due to underlying vasculitis. SLE can be associated with anti-phospholipid syndrome. However, the absence of any clinical features of SLE in this case means that primary anti-phopsholipid syndrome is the most likely diagnosis.

Painful knee

62 E This case describes the presentation of a patient with septic arthritis. In young fit adults, the most common cause of this is *Neisseria gonorrhea* (E). The most common cause overall is *Staphylococcus aureus* (C). The age group of this patient means that this answer is less likely than *N. gonorrheae* (E). Patients with meningococcal septicaemia due to infection with *N. meningitidis* (A) may develop septic arthritis. The absence of any features of septic arthritis make this an unlikely diagnosis in this case. *Haeophilus influenzae* (B) causes septic arthritis in children. *Streptococci* may cause septic arthritis but the age range of this patient makes this a less likely option than *N. gonorrheae*.

Haematuria (2)

63 E The protocol for visible and non-visible haematuria starts with identifying transient causes such as a urinary tract infection, hence urinary microscopy, culture and sensitivity is the most appropriate management (E). Once this has been excluded in non-visible haematuria, a repeat urine dipstick (A) should be performed. If this is still positive then blood pressure (C) and albumin:creatinine ratio (D) should be recorded. The albumin:creatinine ratio is helpful in quantifying the degree of proteinuria, especially in diabetic patients. If these factors are abnormal

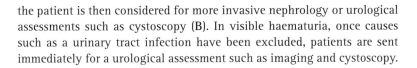

the patient is then considered for more invasive nephrology or urological assessments such as cystoscopy (B). In visible haematuria, once causes such as a urinary tract infection have been excluded, patients are sent immediately for a urological assessment such as imaging and cystoscopy.

Haemoptysis (3)

64 A The presentation of haematuria and haemoptysis raises the clinical suspicion of Goodpasture's syndrome (A) for which anti-glomerular basement membrane antibodies are pathognomonic. The antibodies, usually IgG, attack both the alveolar and basement membranes. Primary biliary cirrhosis is usually associated with anti-mitochondrial antibodies (C). Wegener's granulomatosis (B) is most commonly associated with anti-neutrophilic cytoplasmic antibodies. Pernicious anaemia (D) clinically presents with features of anaemia, such as pallor, malaise and shortness of breath, and is most commonly associated with anti-parietal antibodies. Post-streptococcal glomerulonephritis (E) is usually associated with haematuria and hypertension following a streptococcal infection, which leads to an acute nephritis due to antibody cross-reactivity. There is no associated alveolar damage.

Skin rash

65 E Henoch–Schönlein pupura (E) is a systemic autoimmmune disorder causing small vessel vasculitides. It is characterized by the deposition of IgA causing purpura especially prevalent on the legs, arthralgia, abdominal pain, vomiting and haematuria. Many patients suffer from a prodromal upper respiratory tract illness and anti-streptolysin O (ASO) titres can be raised. In most patients, the disease is self-limiting and responds well to steroids. A post-streptococcal glomerulonephritis (A) is associated with haematuria and hypertension following a streptococcal infection which leads to an acute nephritis due to antibody cross-reactivity. A purpuric rash is not a common feature. In Goodpasture's syndrome (B), the triad of glomerulonephritis, alveolar damage and anti-glomerular basement membrane antibodies is common. Patients tend to be fluid overloaded and a systemic rash is not usually associated. In Wegener's granulomatosis (C), the lungs and kidneys are usually affected alongside small- to medium-sized blood vessels causing a necrotizing granulomatous inflammation. Symptoms tend to be of the upper respiratory system and renal failure. Meningococcal septicaemia (D) classically presents with symptoms of fever, headache, non-blanching rash and neck stiffness.

Index

Note: Italics refers to answers. In a few cases, the reader will find no mention in a question of sigificant items referenced from an answer, despite the index giving the page number for that question.

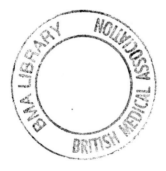